A Practical Guide to Echocardiography and Cardiac Doppler Ultrasound

Contents

Preface

Since the introduction of ultrasound imaging to the field of cardiology, echocardiography has emerged as the most effective noninvasive method for use in cardiac diagnosis. Consequently, cardiac Doppler ultrasonography has provided another complementary, noninvasive application of ultrasound that further enhances the role of echocardiography in the understanding of cardiac pathology and pathophysiology. The advances in cardiac ultrasound technology have created sophisticated ultrasound equipment and established the need for specialized technologists with a strong knowledge of cardiovascular pathology and pathophysiology, plus more refined technical skills in the use of noninvasive cardiac imaging. This knowledge and these technical skills arc called upon every time a cardiac ultrasound study is performed.

A Practical Guide to Echocardiography and Cardiac Doppler Ultrasound is designed for cardiovascular technologists and also for physicians training in cardiology who may need tutoring in the basics of ultrasonography and cardiac imaging. Whereas the discussions of cardiac pathology and pathophysiology are not intended to be exhaustive reviews of these subjects, this book uses an integrated approach, different from those employed in most standard textbooks on cardiology and more advanced textbooks on echocardiography.

This book describes the basic information needed to understand the physics of ultrasound: its applications and techniques in cardiac imaging and cardiac Doppler studies, cardiac anatomy and function, and cardiac pathology and pathophysiology. The discussions are both detailed and con-

The support of these outstanding people is greatly appreciated: Joshua Wynne, M.D., for his support in getting this book started; Priscilla Peters, B.A., for her assistance in writing Chapter 14 and supplying excellent graphics for Chapter 14; Elizabeth Juziuk, B.S., R.C.V.T., Linda Dziekan, Greg Sandidge, Darlene McBroom, R.D.M.S., and Irene Sun, R.N., R.D.M.S., for their constant encouragement and excellent graphics; and Areather Gaines and Karen Beal, for their excellent secretarial support. Most of the echocardiographic and Doppler images were obtained from the Non-Invasive Laboratories at Harper Hospital, Detroit, Michigan. Certain color flow images were supplied by Toshiba, Inc., and Advanced Technology Laboratories.

I. A. J.

I Ultrasound in Cardiology

1 Anatomy and Physiology of the Heart

The heart is located in the chest cavity (thorax), just under the anterior chest bone (sternum). It lies close to the center of the chest and protrudes toward the left side (Figure 1.1).

Anatomy

Gross Description

The heart is comprised of two atria and two ventricles. The left ventricular chamber is ellipsoid, whereas the right ventricle is triangular. Both atrial cavities are similar to a cube, with myocardial walls of approximately equal dimensions on all sides.

The right atrium and ventricle communicate through the tricuspid valve, made of three leaflets. The left atrium and ventricle communicate through the mitral valve, made of two leaflets (Figures 1.2, 1.3). The interatrial septum is a thin muscular wall that separates both atria. The interventricular septum is a thick muscular wall that separates both ventricles (Figure 1.2).

The papillary muscles are groups of cardiac muscle tissue within the ventricular chambers. Two papillary muscle groups are found in the left ventricle and are attached to the tips of the mitral valve leaflets by fibrous bands called chordae tendineae. Since the tricuspid valve is made of three leaflets, there are three groups of papillary muscles within the right ventricle, attached to the tips of the tricuspid valve leaflets.

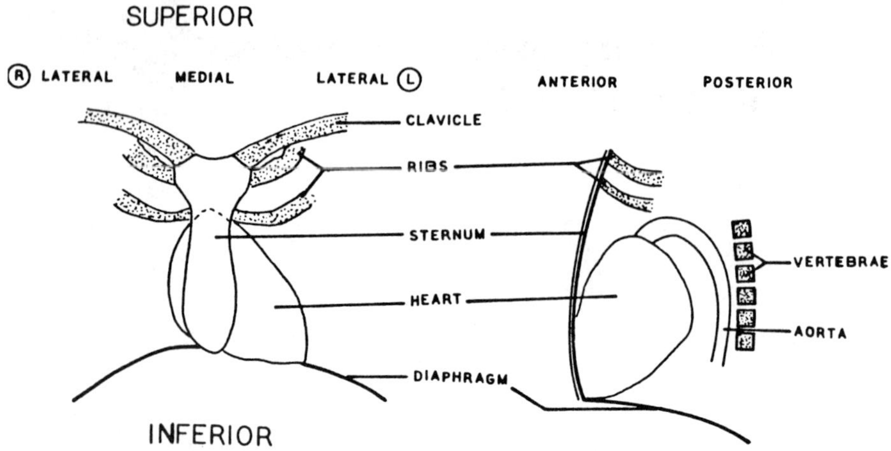

Figure 1.1
The location of the heart within the thorax.

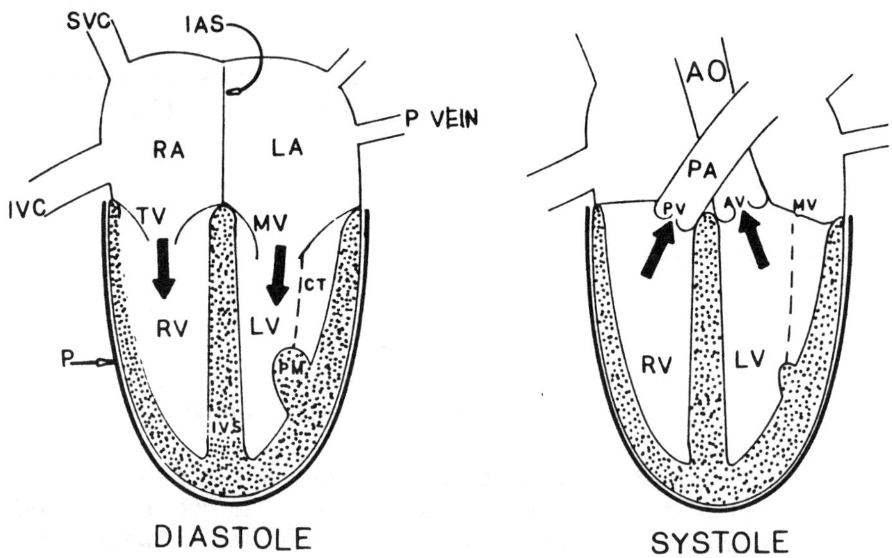

A B

Figure 1.2
A. Cross section of the heart in diastole showing its four chambers with atrioventricular valves and blood vessels entering the atria. Four pulmonic veins (P VEIN) enter the left atrium (LA). Only two are shown in this illustration. B. The plane of the cross-sectional image in systole is angulated anteriorly to show the origin of the great arteries arising from the ventricles with the semilunar valves. The pulmonary artery (PA) arises from the right ventricle (RV), anterior to the origin of the aorta (AO), which arises from the left ventricle (LV). AV = aortic valve, CT = chordae tendineae, IAS = interatrial septum, IVC = inferior vena cava, IVS = interventricular septum, MV = mitral valve, P = pericardium, PM = papillary muscle, PV = pulmonary valve, SVC = superior vena cava, RA = right atrium, TV = tricuspid valve.

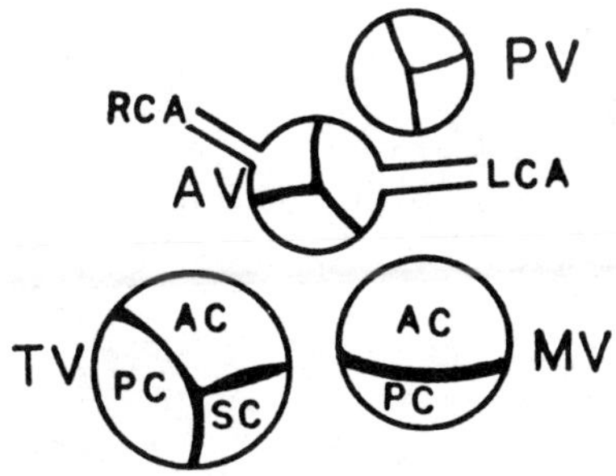

Figure 1.3
The four cardiac valves in cross section. The mitral valve (MV) is made of two leaflets, anterior (AC) and posterior cusps (PC). The tricuspid valve (TV) is made of three leaflets, anterior (AC), posterior (PC), and septal cusps (SC). The semilunar valves are made of three cusps. The aortic valve (AV) cusps are named after the coronary artery, which arises closest to the respective cusp. Hence, the left coronary cusp is closest to the left coronary artery (LCA). The right coronary cusp is closest to the origin of the right coronary artery (RCA). The third cusp is the noncoronary cusp because there is no coronary artery adjacent to it. PV = pulmonary valve.

The inner surfaces of both ventricles are made of series of muscular bridges connected together in a chaotic fashion. These are called muscular trabeculations. It is not uncommon to find one large muscular bridge connecting the right ventricular anterior wall to the right border of the interventricular septum. This is commonly referred to as the moderator band (Figure 1.4).

The superior and inferior venae cavae are large veins that open into the right atrium. The pulmonary artery is a large artery that communicates with the right ventricle through the pulmonary valve, made of three leaflets. Four pulmonary veins open into the left atrium. The aorta is a large artery that communicates with the left ventricle through the aortic valve, made of three leaflets. The pulmonary and aortic valves are called the semilunar valves because of the crescent shape of the leaflets of these two valves. The mitral and tricuspid valves are called the atrioventricular valves since they are situated between the atria and ventricles (Figures 1.2, 1.3).

The pericardium is made of two thin layers of fibrous tissue that cover the heart. The inner layer that is in direct contact with the heart muscle is called the visceral pericardium. The outer layer is called the parietal pericardium (Figure 1.2). Two coronary arteries originate from the aortic root and course along the visceral pericardium before they become buried within the cardiac muscle (Figures 1.3, 1.5). The right coronary artery supplies blood to both atria and

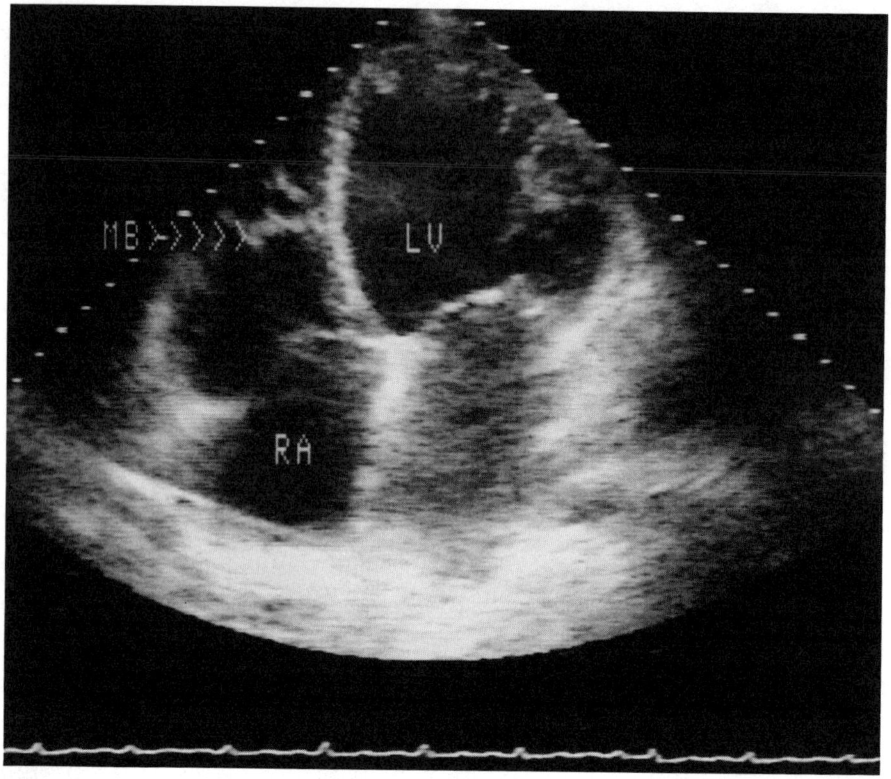

Figure 1.4
Cross-sectional two-dimensional echocardiogram of the cardiac chambers, showing the moderator band (MB) as a dense structure within the right ventricular chamber. LV = left ventricle, RA = right atrium.

the right ventricle and part of the left ventricle. The left main coronary artery divides into the left anterior descending artery and posterior circumflex artery. These arteries supply blood mainly to the left ventricle (Figure 1.5).

Venous blood coming from the cardiac muscle drains into a large, short vein called the coronary sinus, which crosses behind the heart along the junction of the left atrium and left ventricle, called the atrioventricular groove. The coronary sinus opens into the right atrium, just above the tricuspid valve (Figure 1.5).

The heart resembles a triangle in an upside-down position. The base of this triangle, i.e., the base of the heart, is situated upward, toward the head. It is comprised of both atria and all the great vessels. The tip of this triangle, i.e., the cardiac apex, is comprised of the lower portion of the left ventricle (Figure 1.2). The axis of the heart is rotated slightly to the left, so that the right ventricle lies anterior to the left ventricle. The left atrium lies posterior to the right atrium.

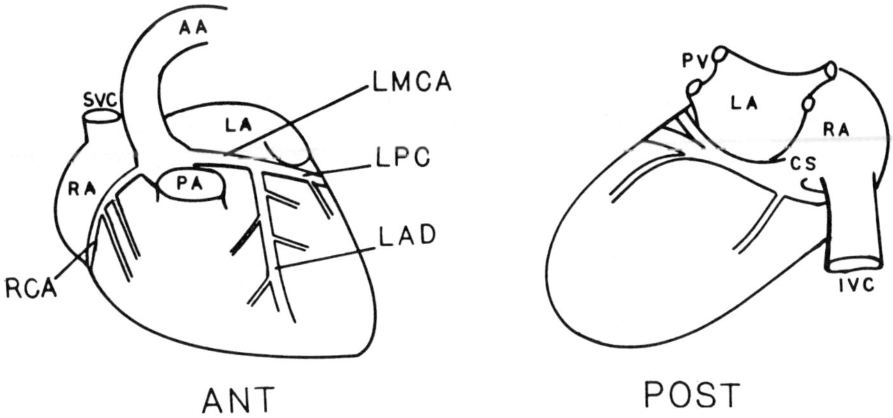

Figure 1.5
The anterior (ANT) and posterior (POST) surfaces of the heart showing the great arteries, coronary arteries, and coronary sinus. AA = aortic arch, CS = coronary sinus, IVC = inferior vena cava, LA = left atrium, LAD = left anterior descending artery, LMCA = left main coronary artery, LPC = left posterior circumflex artery, PA = pulmonary artery, PV = pulmonary veins, RA = right atrium, RCA = right coronary artery, SVC = superior vena cava.

Microscopic Description

The heart muscle is covered by two thin layers of epithelial cells that give it a smooth, glistening appearance. The epithelial cell layer that covers the inner border of the heart muscle facing the chamber cavity is called the endocardium. The epicardium is the epithelial layer that covers the outer border of the heart muscle facing the visceral pericardium. Subsequently, the portion of heart muscle adjacent to the endocardial surface is called the subendocardial muscle tissue, whereas the epicardial muscle layer lies behind the epicardial surface. The cardiac valves are made of fibrous tissue covered on both sides by endocardial layers of epithelial cells.

Cardiac Function

The heart functions as a pump that continuously circulates blood within the body. Venous blood returns to the right atrium via the superior and inferior venae cavae and also via the coronary sinus. Right atrial contraction forces blood across the tricuspid valve into the right ventricle, which in turn forces the blood into the pulmonary artery. This venous blood circulates in the lungs and accumulates oxygen; it then returns to the left atrium via the four pulmonary veins. Left atrial contraction forces blood into the left ventricle, which then forces this oxygenated blood into the aorta. This oxygenated blood circulates to the peripheral tissues, e.g., brain, kidneys, and extremities, and then returns to the right side of the heart. This cycle then repeats itself indefinitely (Figure 1.2).

The four cardiac valves are strategically situated so that blood will only flow in one direction within the cardiac chambers. For example, when the left ventricle contracts, the mitral valve closes and prevents the blood from regurgitating into the left atrium. The only route that this blood can go is across the open aortic valve into the aorta. When the left ventricle relaxes, the aortic valve closes to prevent regurgitation of blood into the left ventricle, which fills with blood coming from the opened mitral valve.

The Cardiac Cycle

In order to be effective, atrial and ventricular contractions are not simultaneous. When both atria contract, the ventricles are relaxing in order to fill with blood coming through the mitral and tricuspid valves. During ventricular contraction, the atria are relaxing in order to fill with blood returning from the venous circulation. This sequence of contraction and relaxation is governed by electrical stimulation of cardiac muscle. Electrical activity is generated in the sinoatrial node (SA node) (Figure 1.6), a specialized group of cardiac muscle tissues located in the right atrium, which spontaneously discharge electrical currents in a rhythmic fashion.

This electrical activity propagates to the closely surrounding cardiac muscle which, when electrically stimulated, will contract. Since the SA node is situated in the right atrium, activation of both atria will occur first, when the ventricles are relaxing. The electrical activity will then propagate to the atrioventricular node (AV node), which is a group of specialized cardiac muscle tissue located between the atria and ventricles at the junction of the interatrial septum and the interventricular septum. At this point in time, atrial muscle will start to relax, whereas the ventricular chamber is still inactive. Later on, the electrical current arrives to the His bundle and then propagates to the ventricular muscle via the Purkinje fibers, and mechanical contraction occurs (Figure 1.6). Finally, there is a period of complete electrical inactivity when none of the cardiac chambers are contracting. This

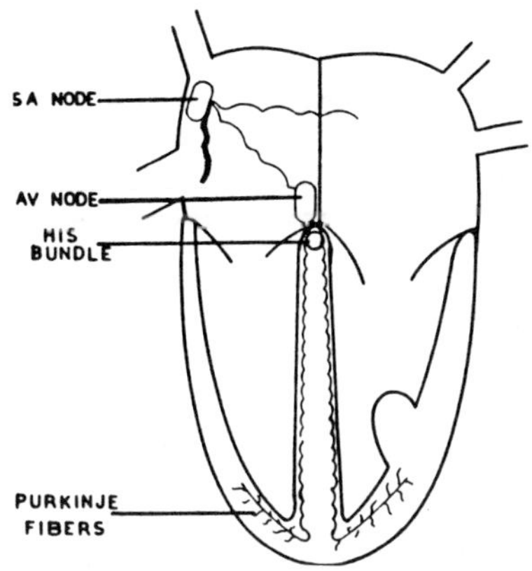

Figure 1.6
The normal propagation of electrical activity in the heart. Electrical impulses generated in the sinoatrial node (SA NODE) propagate through specialized channels to the atria and the atrioventricular node (AV NODE), and then to the ventricles via the His bundle and Purkinje fibers.

period lasts until the next spontaneous depolarization of the SA node, which starts another cardiac cycle.

The Electrocardiogram

The sequence of electrical depolarization and repolarization of the cardiac muscle generates electrical currents that are strong enough to be recorded by electrodes placed on the skin surface. Usually ten electrodes are utilized; one on each extremity and six on the chest wall along the outer borders of the heart. For echocardiographic and Doppler recordings, only three or four electrodes may be enough to record the cardiac electrical activity.

The electrocardiogram (ECG) will typically reflect the electrical activity of the heart (Figure 1.7). The P wave represents atrial depolarization. This is followed by a short pause that is terminated by ventricular depolarization, which produces a series of electrical currents commonly referred to as the QRS complex. After a short pause the T wave occurs. This represents the electrical recuperation of ventricular muscle after contraction. There is no electrical activity between the end of the T wave until the beginning of a new cardiac cycle with another P wave (Figure 1.7).

From the preceding discussion, it becomes evident that electrical activation is immediately followed by mechanical contraction of the activated cardiac muscle. Hence, the P wave on the ECG represents atrial contraction and the QRS complex represents ventricular contraction. The time inter-

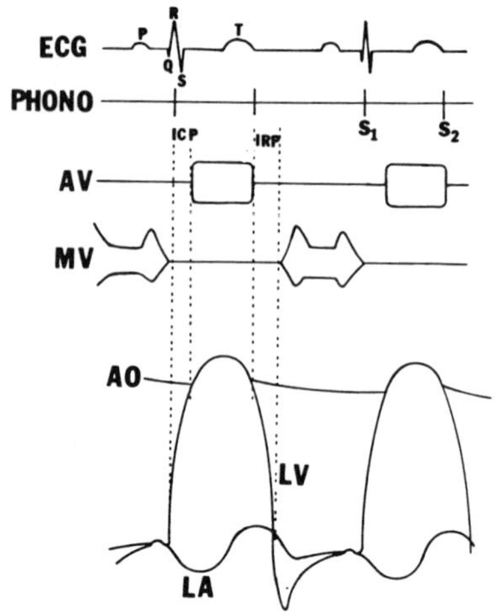

Figure 1.7
The simultaneous motion of the mitral and aortic valves together with the pressure recordings in the aorta (AO), left ventricle (LV), and left atrium (LA). A simultaneous ECG and phonocardiographic recording (PHONO) of mitral and aortic valve closure sounds are also shown. The first heart sound (S_1) occurs with mitral valve closure at the crossover of left ventricular and left atrial pressures in early systole. The second heart sound (S_2) occurs with aortic valve closure at the crossover of left ventricular and aortic pressure in late systole. The time interval between mitral valve closure and aortic valve opening is the isovolumic contraction period (ICP). The time interval between aortic valve closure and mitral valve opening is the isovolumic relaxation period (IRP). AV = aortic valve, MV = mitral valve.

val during which the cardiac muscle contracts is called systole. Ventricular systole starts with the beginning of the QRS complex on the ECG and usually ends close to the termination of the T wave. Ventricular diastole refers to the remaining period of the cardiac cycle when the ventricular muscle is relaxing. Ventricular diastole starts with the termination of the ventricular systole and ends with the beginning of the new QRS complex on the ECG. Since atrial contraction always precedes ventricular contraction in the normal situation, it becomes evident that atrial systole occurs during ventricular diastole. All cardiac chambers are in diastole during the time interval between the termination of the T wave and onset of the new P wave.

Heart Sounds

During atrial contraction, the mitral and tricuspid valves are open. Once ventricular contraction starts, there is a rapid buildup of intraventricular pressure. When this pressure exceeds the left atrial pressure, the mitral valve leaflets drift toward each other early in systole and cause a snapping sound as the mitral valve closes. A similar sound of less intensity occurs shortly afterward and represents closure of the tricuspid valve. These two events occur almost simultaneously and produce one single heart sound. Since this sound occurs shortly after the QRS complex in the beginning of ventricular systole, it is called the first heart sound (S_1) (Figure 1.7).

As ventricular contraction progresses, there is an adequate buildup of intraventricular pressure, which forces the pulmonary and aortic valves to open, and blood is ejected into the pulmonary artery and aorta, respectively. At the completion of ejection at the end of systole, the aortic valve leaflets drift toward each other and cause a snapping sound as the aortic valve closes. This is followed by another sound representing the closure of the pulmonary valve. The closure sounds of these two valves can be heard as two discrete clicks close to each other. These sounds are referred to as the second heart sound (S_2). A_2 and P_2 denote the aortic and pulmonary components of the second heart sound, respectively (Figure 1.7); only the aortic component of S_2 is depicted in Figure 1.7.

Ventricular Systole

Electromechanical Delay

Electromechanical delay is a very brief period when electrical activation of the ventricle occurs, but mechanical contraction has not yet started. This time interval is approximately 35 milliseconds long.

Isovolumic Contraction Period

Once ventricular contraction starts, there is a buildup of intraventricular pressure, which induces closure of the atrioventricular valves. This causes cessation of blood flow into the ventricles; however, the semilunar valves are still closed in early systole. Hence, ventricular contraction occurs without any change of chamber volume, since all the cardiac valves are closed. This interval is referred to as the isovolumic contraction period (ICP) (Figure 1.7).

Ejection Phase

Once intraventricular pressure exceeds the pressure in the aorta and the pulmonary artery, the aortic and pulmonary valves are forced to open and ventricular ejection begins.

This phase is terminated at the end of systole, close to the end of the T wave on ECG. Once ejection is completed, the aortic and pulmonary valves close; thus, ejection ends with the onset of S_2 (Figure 1.7).

Ventricular Diastole

Protodiastole

Protodiastole is a very brief interval when ventricular ejection stops but aortic or pulmonary valves are still in the process of closing.

Isovolumic Relaxation Period (IRP)

As ventricular relaxation proceeds, the semilunar valves are closed, whereas the atrioventricular valves have not yet opened. Therefore, ventricular relaxation occurs without any change in chamber volume, since all cardiac valves are closed during this period in early diastole (Figure 1.7).

Rapid Filling Period

Following IRP, ventricular pressure drops below atrial pressure. This causes the mitral and tricuspid valves to open, and accumulated blood in the atria rushes into the ventricles (Figure 1.7).

Diastasis

By the end of the rapid filling period, both atria have emptied most of the blood contents into the respective ventricles. Thus, this phase in diastole marks the beginning of slow ventricular filling.

Atrial Contraction

The onset of a new atrial electrical activation (P wave) causes mechanical atrial contraction. This generates enough intra-atrial pressure to force more blood into the respective ventricles. This is the last phase in ventricular diastole and is terminated by the onset of electrical ventricular activation with a new QRS complex. However, it is to be noted that ventricular filling persists in early systole until the closure of the mitral and tricuspid valves with the onset of S_1 (Figure 1.7). The diastolic filling period is comprised of the last three phases of diastole.

2 Principles of Sound and Ultrasound

When two persons are talking together, sound is generated from the vocal cords of one and is transmitted through air to the ears of the other person. Sound is generated by the subject's vocal cords as they vibrate and cause to-and-fro displacement of air particles in the immediate proximity. This back-and-forth motion is then transmitted to the next layer of air particles in succession throughout the distance to the ear drums of the other person, which then vibrate in a similar manner. This to-and-fro motion of the air particles creates multiple layers of densely compressed air particles (dense air, compression) alternating with layers of air particles spread apart (thin air, rarefaction). These series of compression and rarefaction constitute a sound wave (Figure 2.1).

Definitions (Figure 2.1)

Cycle: One cycle is composed of one compression and one rarefaction layer adjacent to each other.

Wavelength: This is the distance in space between any two consecutive rarefaction layers.

Amplitude: This denotes the degree of compression or rarefaction. It reflects how densely the air particles are compressed together, or how thinly they are spread apart.

Frequency: The number of cycles in a unit of time, usually 1 second, is the frequency. The unit of frequency is hertz (Hz), where 1 Hz is equal to 1 cycle/sec. The human ear can perceive sound frequencies ranging from 2000 to 20,000 Hz.

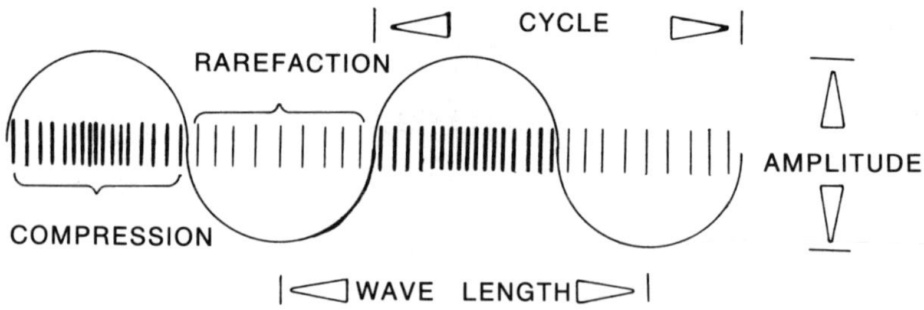

Figure 2.1
Compression and rarefaction phases of a sound wave.

Sound frequency greater than 20,000 Hz is referred to as ultrasound. For the purpose of ultrasound imaging, frequencies of 1.5 to 10.0 million Hz are used. One thousand Hz equals 1 kilohertz (kHz); 1 million Hz equals 1 megahertz (MHz).

Velocity: Velocity of the sound wave reflects the speed of transmission of the wave in a particular medium. It is equal to the product of frequency and wavelength.

Principles of Ultrasound Imaging

The basic principle of ultrasonic imaging is to generate an ultrasound pulse by a transducer and direct the beam through a certain medium, and then analyze the echoes reflected to the same transducer from various objects along the path of the ultrasound beam. In order to achieve this goal, one has to understand the interplay of various independent parameters pertaining to the physical properties of the ultrasound wave being employed and the object being imaged.

Acoustic Impedance

Sound waves travel in a straight line in a homogeneous medium. When the sound beam reaches an interface between two media of different densities, it undergoes certain physical changes. Acoustic impedance is defined as the product of the velocity of sound and the density of the medium that the sound wave is traveling through. The degree of distortion of the sound waves traveling across an interface between two different media is dependent on the relative difference of their acoustic impedances.

Angle of Incidence

The interface between two media of different acoustic impedances acts as a barrier to the propagation of ultrasound

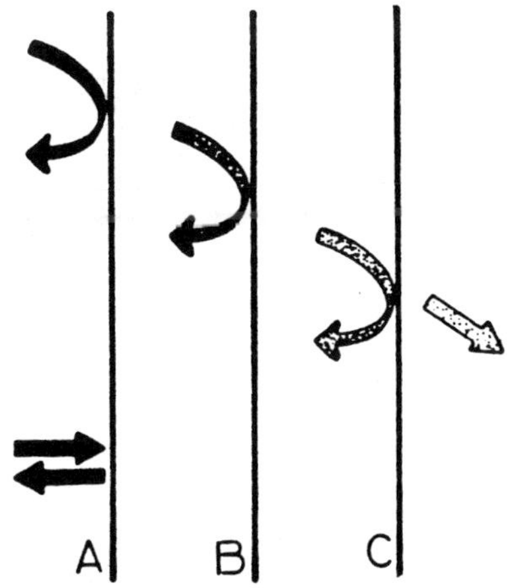

Figure 2.2
Reflection and refraction of sound. The black straight arrow represents a sound wave arriving at an interface A at a 90-degree angle of incidence. This sound wave will be largely reflected with minimal loss of intensity. On the other hand, when the sound wave arrives to interface A at an angle of incidence less than 90 degrees, a portion will be reflected, while the remaining portion will be refracted into the other medium. As this sound wave is refracted at multiple interfaces, its intensity will be greatly diminished.

from one medium to the other. As the ultrasound wave reaches this interface, a portion of this wave is reflected back (reflected wave, echoes). The remaining portion penetrates through into the second medium; however, the path of the ultrasound beam is altered in a new direction (refracted wave) (Figure 2.2). The proportions of the reflected and refracted waves depend on the angle of incidence θ between the path of the original ultrasound beam relative to the interface between the two media. Hence, an angle of incidence θ of 90 degrees implies that most of the incident ultrasound beam is reflected as echoes with minimal refraction into the second medium. More and more of the ultrasound beam will be refracted and thus, less and less will be reflected as the angle of incidence θ decreases.

Size of Object

Since the primary focus of ultrasonic imaging is on the analysis of reflected ultrasound waves, the interplay between the size of the object being imaged and the relative characteristics of the ultrasound wave employed for imaging needs to be emphasized. In general, the wavelength of the ultrasound waves should be a maximum of 4 times the thickness of the object being imaged. In other words, smaller objects need

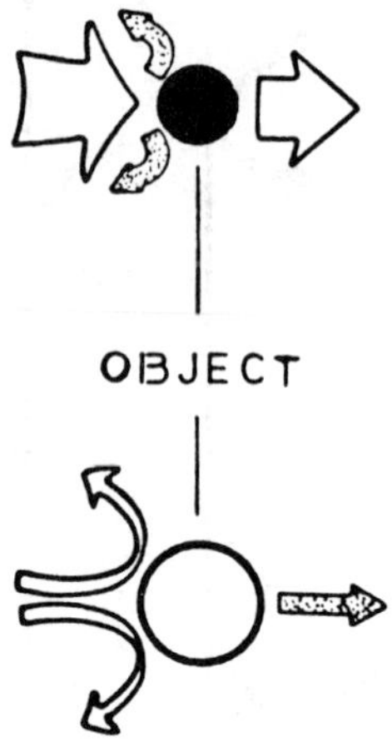

Figure 2.3
Relation of object size to the frequency of ultrasound. A small object insonated by ultrasound of long wavelength and low frequency will reflect echoes of low intensity (small curved arrows). On the other hand, a large object insonated with short-wavelength and high-frequency ultrasound will reflect echoes of high intensity (large curved arrows).

shorter wavelengths (higher frequency) of ultrasound for adequate imaging (Figure 2.3).

Effect of Multiple Interfaces

The clinical application of ultrasound for cardiac imaging involves transmission of ultrasound waves through multiple layers of tissues within the chest. Most of these tissue layers are not strictly homogeneous; ultrasound waves passing through are scattered and absorbed so that the intensity of the wave is attenuated and diminishes across the thickness of the tissue layer. Half-power distance is a term used to ascribe a numerical value to compare different tissues and media to each other. It denotes the distance an ultrasound wave travels within the tissue before its intensity is reduced by one-half. Because of the interplay of frequency versus size of object, the half-power distance of any particular tissue varies according to the frequency of the ultrasound employed for imaging. In general, the half-power distance of a particular tissue or medium is higher when using low-frequency ultrasound than the half-power distance of the same tissue when using a higher frequency ultrasound. In other words, deeper penetration is obtained when using lower frequency ultrasound. Tissues with very low half-power distance may cause significant attenuation of the ultrasound wave so that very little ultrasound energy penetrates to the distal layers. This creates an acoustic shadow whereby objects distal to this particular tissue cannot be imaged by ultrasound (Figure 2.4A). On the other hand, a particularly dense structure with high acoustic impedance may create a strong interface that reflects most of the ultrasound beam. Hence, minimal ultrasound energy is refracted through this medium, thereby producing acoustic shadows and impeding adequate imaging of distal objects (Figure 2.4B).

The heart is situated within the thoracic cavity and is separated from the chest wall by multiple layers of tissues of different densities and acoustical impedances. Moreover, a thin layer of air may separate the ultrasound transducer from the chest wall, thus creating two more interfaces (transducer versus air, air versus skin of the chest wall). Hence, the ultrasound wave generated by the transducer undergoes attenuation, scattering, reflection, and refraction at multiple interfaces before it arrives to the cardiac structures to be imaged. In general, air, lung tissue (filled with air), and bone create the biggest obstacles to adequate cardiac imaging. These tissues possess very low half-power distances. Blood and fat tissue have much higher half-power distance. The half-power distance of muscle tissue is intermediate. With these differences in mind, technical difficulties are unavoidable during cardiac imaging with ultrasound. One can apply special gels to eliminate the air interface between the ultrasound transducer and chest wall. As will be discussed in the next chapter, special positions for the transducer along the chest wall may allow the ultrasound beam to bypass bone and lung tissue along its path to the heart, thereby avoiding these potential obstacles for cardiac imaging.

Methods of Ultrasonic Imaging

The ultrasound transducer intermittently generates an ultrasound wave at a predetermined rate referred to as pulse repetition frequency (PRF). In between each pulse of ultrasound emitted, the transducer acts as a receiver for reflected waves. When an ultrasound wave is emitted from the transducer, the ultrasound unit measures the time interval elapsed between emission of the ultrasound pulse and reception of the reflected echoes. Knowing the speed of propagation of ultrasound in human tissue, approximately 1540 m/sec or 154 cm/msec, the ultrasound unit estimates the depth location of the object from the transducer:

$$d = ct/2 \qquad \text{(Equation 2.1)}$$

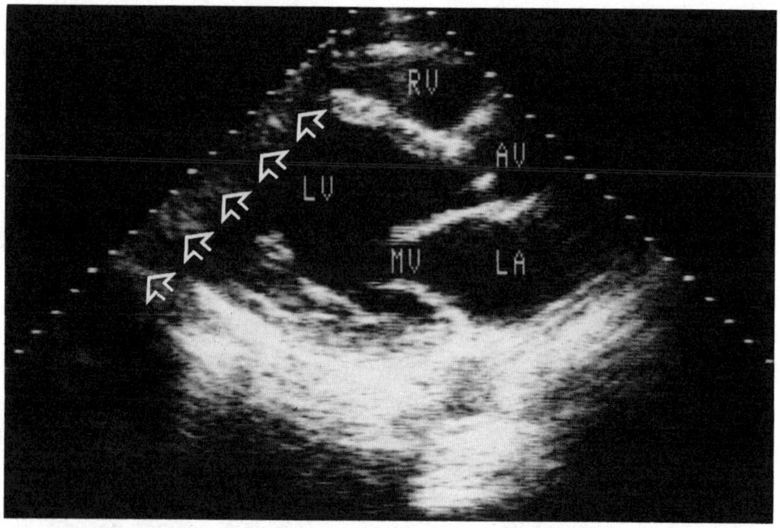

A

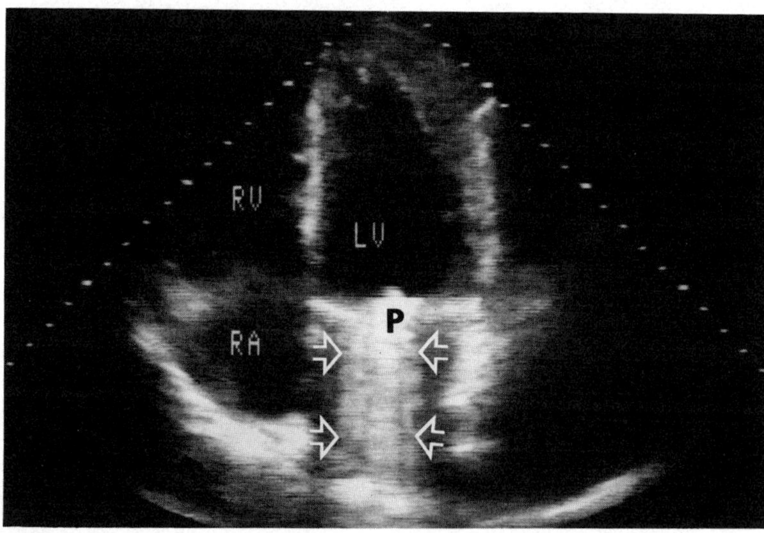

B

Figure 2.4
A. The ultrasound transducer was positioned on a rib at the chest wall. A portion of the ultrasound beam was significantly attenuated by the rib, thus creating an acoustic shadow (arrowheads). Cardiac structures are not visualized within this acoustic shadow. B. A metallic valve prosthesis (P) in the mitral valve position creates a strong interface that ultrasound cannot penetrate. The left atrium is completely obliterated by the acoustic shadows (arrowheads) from this valve prosthesis.

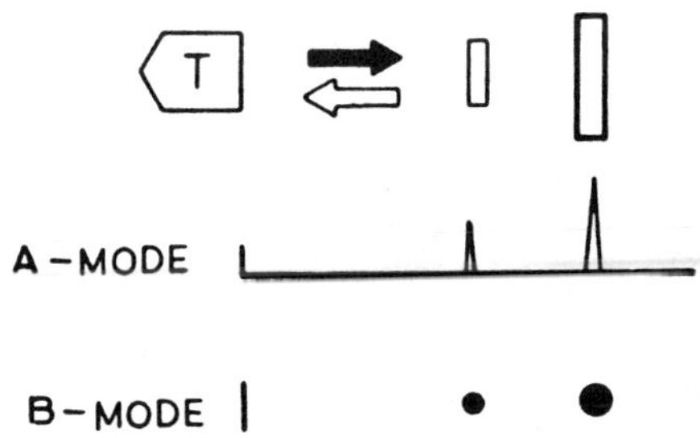

Figure 2.5
Modes of ultrasound imaging. A transducer (T) emits ultrasound that is reflected from two objects of different acoustic impedances. A-mode imaging depicts two spikes on the oscilloscope, with the distal object of higher acoustic impedance represented by the bigger spike. B-mode imaging depicts two dots, the larger one representing the distal object.

where d is the distance between the transducer and the reflecting object, c is the speed of propagation of ultrasound in tissue, and t is the time interval elapsed between emission of the ultrasound pulse and reception of reflected echoes. The right-hand side of this equation is divided by 2 since the ultrasound wave travels twice the distance between the transducer and the reflecting object. For example, if the elapsed time from emission to reception of the sound wave is 0.13 milliseconds, then by applying Equation 2.1, the object is situated 10 cm away from the transducer:

$$d = 154 \text{ cm/msec} \times 0.13 \text{ msec} \times \tfrac{1}{2} = 10 \text{ cm}$$

Signals reflected from multiple objects along the path of the ultrasound beam will reach the transducer at different time intervals; hence, their respective depth location can be determined. Moreover, the ultrasound unit analyzes the intensity of the signals reflected from each object. A highly refractile (echogenic) object will reflect a greater proportion of the ultrasound beam than a less refractile object.

A-mode Imaging

In A-mode imaging, the ultrasound unit displays each imaged object as a spike on the monitor. The distance of this spike from the reference point on the monitor corresponds to the elapsed time for the reception of signals reflected from that particular object. The intensity of the reflected signal is depicted as the amplitude of the spike. A strong signal causes a higher amplitude spike than a weaker signal (Figure 2.5).

As the object moves back and forth, the location of the

spike on the monitor shifts accordingly. Cardiac imaging with A-mode is not practical because the multiple moving echoes reflected from various cardiac walls and valves along the path of the ultrasound beam generate a confusing array of constantly moving and overlapping spikes of various amplitudes.

B-mode Imaging

Each imaged object in the B-mode is displayed as a dot on the monitor instead of a spike (Figure 2.5). The intensity of the signal is depicted by varying the brightness of the dot. Thus, a strong echo signal exhibits a bright dot, whereas a weak echo signal exhibits a faint dot on the monitor. As the object moves back and forth, so does the dot. The B-mode is the preferred method for cardiac imaging as will be discussed in the next section.

M-mode Echocardiography

Using the B-mode, a continuously moving object generates multiple dots with variable depth locations relative to the transducer. Hence, as time elapses, echoes reflected from this object will overlap on each other as the object moves back and forth. One can trace the motion of this dot with respect to time by examining serial still-frame images taken at variable time intervals. Each frame displays the dot at a different depth location corresponding to its actual depth during that particular point in time when the still-frame image was taken. If all the frames are viewed side by side, the actual motion of the dot can be traced with respect to time (Figure 2.6).

M-mode echocardiography employs the same principle just described. The series of dots generated by a moving object is recorded on a strip of paper rolling at a steady speed. Because the speed of the rolling paper is very slow relative to the rate of the B-mode imaging, the dots will be displayed very close to each other and simulate a continous wavy line on the M-mode recording (Figure 2.6). A high intensity of reflected echoes causes a bright dot on the B-mode and a dark line on the M-mode tracing.

When the heart is imaged with M-mode echocardiography, multiple lines will be generated at various depth locations corresponding to the various cardiac structures that are imaged simultaneously. The heart is a three-dimensional object. One cannot image all the cardiac chambers and valves simultaneously with the unidimensional ultrasound beam of M-mode echocardiography. Only small segments of the

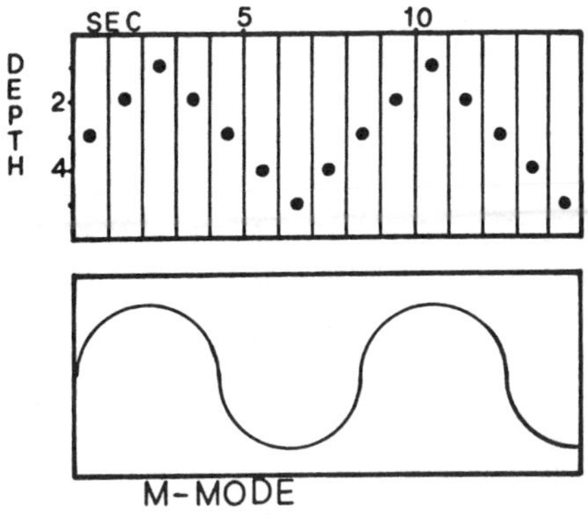

Figure 2.6
M-mode imaging. B-mode images of an oscillatory object are taken at the sampling rate of 1-second intervals. Each image depicts the object at a certain depth relative to the ultrasound transducer. M-mode imaging utilizes a very high sampling rate so that the dots are very close to each other and simulate a continuous line.

heart are imaged at any one time. The operator must manually alter the direction of the ultrasound beam across the heart for adequate imaging (Figure 2.7).

Real-Time Two-Dimensional Echocardiography

With a single ultrasound beam, only a very small portion of a relatively large object can be imaged at any one time with the B-mode. In order to visualize a large object, the ultrasound beam can be moved along the length of the object, thus creating multiple still-frame images of various segments of this object. By superimposing these multiple images, a final cross-sectional image is obtained (Figure 2.8). Such cross-sectional images also can be obtained by generating multiple ultrasound beams, side by side, so that the whole object can be imaged throughout its length. This technique of cardiac imaging is commonly referred to as cross-sectional or two-dimensional echocardiography. Since the various cardiac structures are constantly moving with respect to time, real-time imaging is achieved by recording the instantaneous images on videotape.

The Ultrasound Equipment

Cardiac imaging (echocardiography) is achieved by applying the principles and methods of ultrasound imaging discussed previously. The basic ultrasound unit consists of:

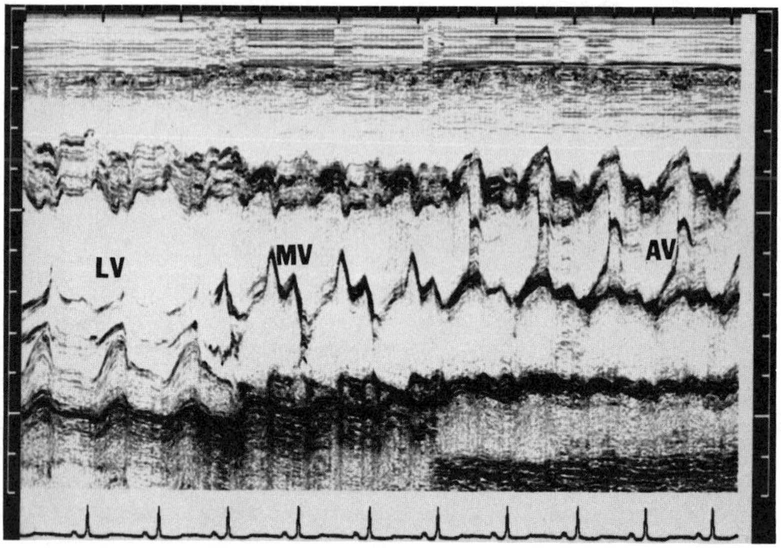

Figure 2.7
M-mode sweep. The path of the ultrasound beam is manually rotated during a continuous M-mode recording of the heart. In this example, the ultrasound beam travels through the left ventricle (LV), mitral valve (MV), and aortic valve (AV).

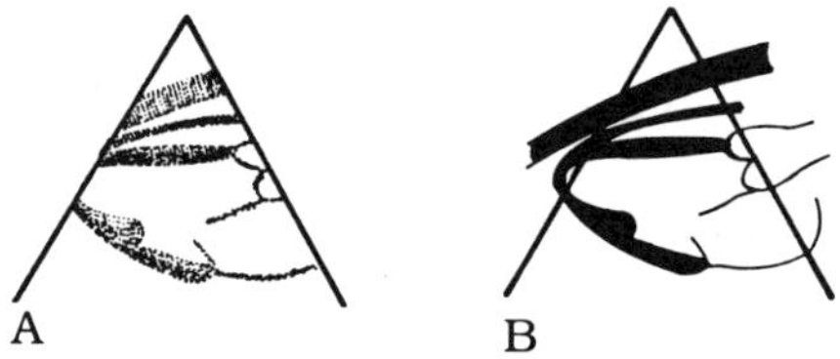

Figure 2.8
The path of the ultrasound beam is rapidly rotated through an arc that transects various cardiac chambers and valves. The resulting B-mode images are displayed side by side on the monitor and form one cross-sectional image of the heart. A. Only cardiac structures that lie within the path of the ultrasound beam are imaged. B. Cardiac structures outside this path are not visualized.

1. An ultrasound transducer used to generate ultrasound waves and receive reflected echoes;
2. A computer system to analyze reflected signals; and
3. An oscilloscope or TV monitor with or without a paper recorder to display the final echocardiographic images.

The Ultrasound Transducer

The ultrasound transducer is analogous to a loudspeaker. When subjected to an electrical current, the magnetic ele-

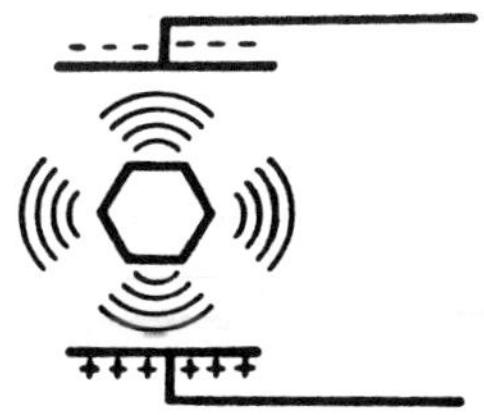

Figure 2.9
The shape of the piezoelectric crystal changes rapidly, at the same rate of alternation of the electrical current. This creates a series of compression and rarefaction of sound.

ments in a loudspeaker cause a special diaphragm to vibrate. The to-and-fro motion of this diaphragm causes displacement of the adjacent layer of air particles, thereby creating a series of compression and rarefaction of sound waves.

In a similar fashion, special piezoelectric crystals housed in the ultrasound transducer change their shape when subjected to an electrical field. If the polarity of the electrical field is rapidly alternated, the associated rapid alteration of the shape of the piezoelectric crystals causes to-and-fro displacement of the adjacent elements in the transducer and thus generates the series of compression and rarefaction of sound waves (Figure 2.9). The frequency of these sound waves is related to the rapidity of alternation of polarity of the electrical field and on the physical characteristics of the crystals; hence, a very rapid rate generates ultrasound waves. On the other hand, ultrasound waves returning to the transducer cause the piezoelectric crystals to change in shape accordingly, thereby generating an electrical current that is then transmitted to the computer in the ultrasound unit for analysis.

The ultrasound waves generated by a single piezoelectric crystal travel in all directions in space. However, by prearranging multiple small crystals side by side or by using a larger single crystal with a specific geometric configuration, the resulting multiple ultrasound waves will travel predominantly in one direction only. This is also achieved by employing special material within the transducer housing to limit the direction of the ultrasound waves. As these multiple waves exit the transducer, they travel in a straight line parallel to each other for a limited distance only (near field), beyond which they begin to diverge (far field) (Figure 2.10). The higher intensity of more parallel ultrasound waves in the near field allows better imaging of the objects located in this field than of objects situated farther away in the far field where the waves are divergent and of less intensity.

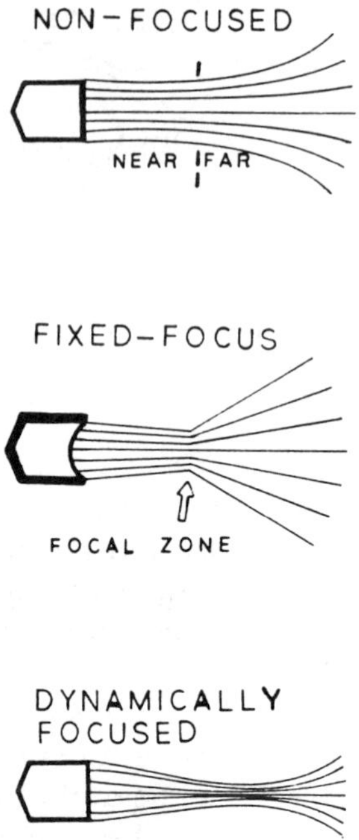

Figure 2.10
Ultrasound waves generated by a nonfocused transducer remain parallel for a short distance (near field), beyond which they diverge (far field). Fixed focusing creates a high-intensity ultrasound beam at a narrow focal zone, beyond which they diverge. Dynamic focusing creates a longer focal zone than fixed focusing.

The characteristics of the near field are dependent on the size of the transducer and the wavelengths of ultrasound. A longer near field is produced by a larger transducer that emits ultrasound of a smaller wavelength (higher frequency). For a circular transducer, the depth (d) of the near field is measured as:

$$d = \lambda r^2 \qquad \text{(Equation 2.2)}$$

where r is the radius of the transducer and λ is the wavelength.

The heart's location within the chest cavity necessitates the use of transducers with a relatively long near field. Thus, a large transducer that employs high-frequency ultrasound waves seems to be ideal. However, the boney rib cage limits transducer size, which should not be significantly wider than the widths of the intercostal spaces. On the other hand, as discussed in the previous sections, adequate penetration of ultrasound through tissues necessitates the use of a relatively low-frequency ultrasound. These physical limitations restrict the use of a large transducer with high-frequency ultrasound. In order to circumvent this problem, one can use artificial means to improve the near field.

Using the same principles of concave or convex lenses that distort the path of a light beam, one can use specially curved transducer surfaces or attach special acoustic lenses that cause the ultrasound waves to focus at particular depth locations. The focal zone represents the particular depth at which the ultrasound waves are most parallel to each other and the beam is at its highest intensity (Figure 2.10).

The focal zone of such fixed-focus transducers may still be limited in length. This issue was resolved by introducing phased array transducers. Such a transducer utilizes multiple small piezoelectric crystals that are electronically triggered at different time intervals in succession. The resulting ultrasound beam is dynamically focused at a longer focal zone (Figure 2.10). The shapes and sizes of these complex ultrasound beams are dependent on the number of piezoelectric crystals and their geometric arrangement (circular, rectangular, or squarelike) within the transducer housing.

Adequate focusing serves multiple purposes. A focused ultrasound beam has a relatively homogeneous intensity at the focal zone. In general, the intensity of the ultrasound beam is highest at its center, with progressive diminution of the intensity toward the periphery. When two objects, situated side by side, are hit by a wide beam of ultrasound, both objects will be imaged simultaneously and their echoes will be superimposed or displayed one behind the other. This occurs because of lack of lateral resolution. Focusing generates a narrower beam width so that the two objects will not be imaged simultaneously, thus eliminating this potential artifact (Figure 2.11).

The multiple ultrasound beams needed for two-dimensional imaging can be generated by mechanically altering the direction of the ultrasound beam. There are different ways to achieve this purpose, although the basic principle relies on an electrical motor, within the transducer housing, that continuously rotates the piezoelectric elements or causes these elements to oscillate. Hence, each ultrasound pulse travels in a different direction. One complete rotation or oscillation (sweep) of the piezoelectric elements creates one cross-sectional image (Figure 2.12).

The second method to create two-dimensional images employs the use of a phased array transducer, whereby triggering of the piezoelectric elements is electronically controlled to steer the direction of the ultrasound beam. This eliminates the need for the electrical motor (Figure 2.13).

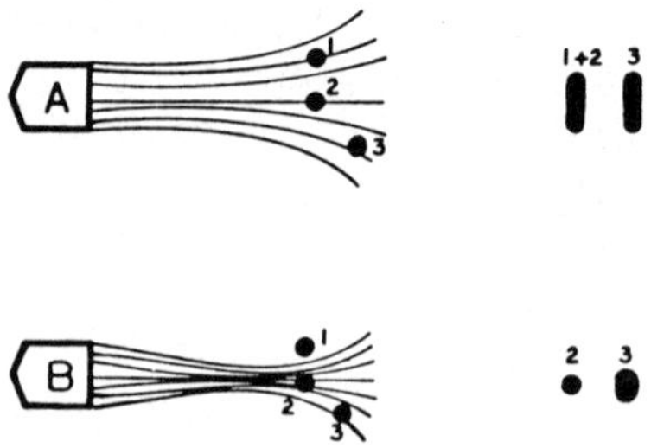

Figure 2.11
Objects 1 and 2 are at the same distance from the transducer, while object 3 is more distal and lies within the far field. Using a nonfocused transducer (A), the images of objects 1 and 2 will be superimposed. The image of object 3 is significantly distorted. However, the ultrasound beam generated by a dynamically focused transducer (B) is narrow, with a long focal zone. Objects 1 and 2 are better defined because each object is imaged separately. There is less distortion of object 3 because the ultrasound waves are less divergent. Thus, a dynamically focused transducer provides better lateral resolution.

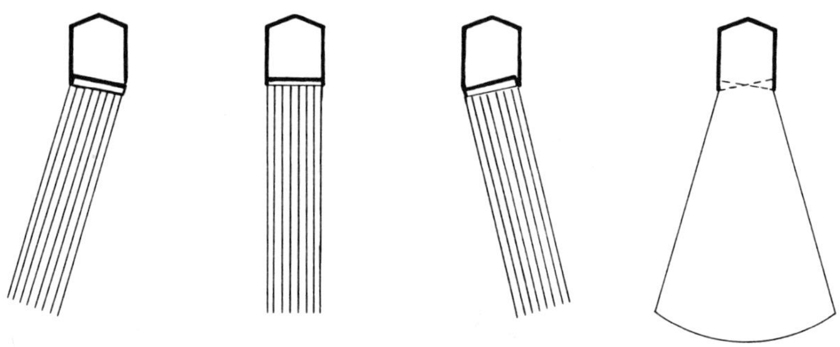

Figure 2.12
The direction of the ultrasound beam is mechanically rotated so that one full rotation defines the arc of the imaging field.

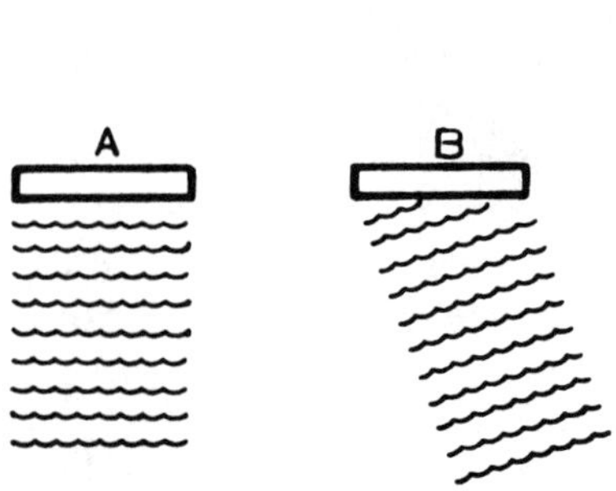

Figure 2.13
Sequential electronic triggering of multiple piezoelectric crystals (A) creates an ultrasound wave that travels in predominantly one direction (B).

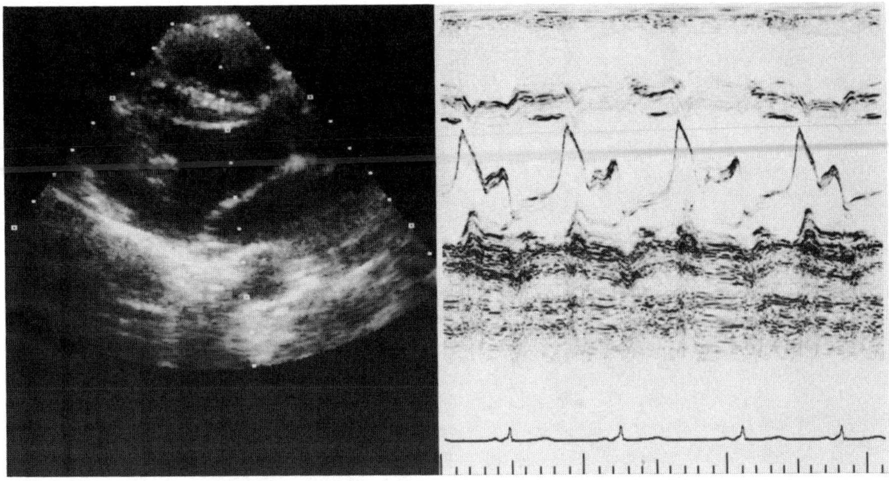

Figure 2.14
Simultaneous M-mode and two-dimensional echocardiogram. The cursor (the vertical dotted line superimposed on the two-dimensional image) depicts the path of the ultrasound beam employed for M-mode imaging.

In general, mechanical transducers are larger than phased array transducers because of the need to incorporate the electrical motor within the transducer housing, as well as to allow space for the rotatory or oscillatory motion of the piezoelectric elements. Because of technical considerations, dynamically focused phased array transducers are usually larger than nonfocused or fixed-focus transducers. Moreover, the lower the ultrasound frequency of the transducers, the larger its size is. Finally, unlike mechanical transducers, phased array transducers allow simultaneous M-mode and two-dimensional imaging. This is achieved by electronic control of the triggering of the piezoelectric element through a time-sharing process. A portion of the time is used for the M-mode imaging, whereas the rest of the time is used for two-dimensional imaging. In this context the TV monitor is split with the two-dimensional image on one side and the M-mode image on the other side. A cursor line, superimposed on the two-dimensional image, depicts the direction of the ultrasound beam employed for M-mode imaging (Figure 2.14). Such transducers may also be capable of generating two M-mode scans simultaneously with the two-dimensional image.

Analysis of Reflected Echoes

Multiple objects encountered along the path of the ultrasound beam reflect echoes of various intensities that return

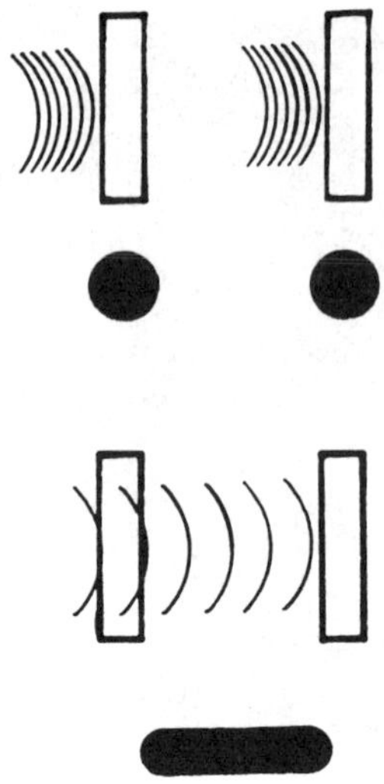

Figure 2.15
Echoes reflected from two close objects may be superimposed when imaged with a low-frequency, long-wavelength, ultrasound pulse that hits both objects simultaneously. On the other hand, an ultrasound pulse of high frequency and short wavelength generates two separate echoes, hence providing better axial resolution.

to the transducer during different time intervals. The electronic signals generated by these reflected echoes are transmitted to the computer system within the ultrasound unit for analysis. The most important element of such analysis is the timing of reception of these signals in order to estimate the depth location of each individual object encountered by the ultrasound beam. Moreover, analysis of the intensities of these signals provides valuable information pertaining to the characteristics of the objects being imaged, i.e., valve structure versus muscle tissue, etc. The computer analysis system plays an important role in the final display of these signals on the oscilloscope, TV monitor, or paper recorder.

When two objects are situated far from each other, the computer analysis system can easily distinguish them. However, if two objects are very close to each other, such distinction becomes very dependent on the frequency of ultrasound employed (higher frequency allows better resolution) and the capabilities of the analysis system (Figure 2.15). In general, the dot on the B-mode becomes larger and brighter as the intensity of the signal increases (Figure 2.5). Hence, the dots depicting two closely situated objects may partially overlap if the intensities of the reflected echoes are sufficiently high. If this occurs, then these two objects cannot be distinguished

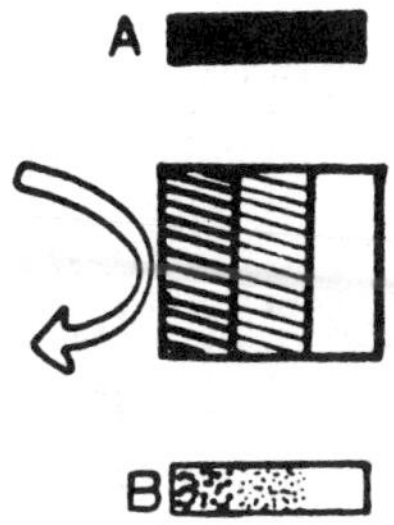

Figure 2.16
Closely adjacent objects create a single distorted echo (A), unless gray scale analysis is utilized (B). This separates the images according to the intensity of reflected echoes from each object.

from each other. Most commercial ultrasound units employ the process of "differentiation," whereby a signal of high intensity is primarily depicted as a bright dot without significantly affecting its size. In this context, the two objects are displayed as two distinct bright dots that do not overlap.

Because of the variable acoustic impedances of various cardiac structures, echoes reflected from these structures are of different intensities. Gray scale analysis has been developed to grade the intensities of such reflected echoes. By doing that, gray scale analysis provides the added benefit of distinguishing closely adjacent objects from each other, based on the relative intensities of individual echoes reflected from these objects (Figure 2.16). By this technique, the intensities of multiple signals are represented by various shades of gray. The higher the intensity of a particular signal, the lighter the shade of gray displayed on the monitor. Gray scale analysis has greatly enhanced the role of echocardiography in imaging cardiac muscle tissue or pathologic masses such as tumors or clots, which predominantly produce scattered echoes of low intensity.

All electronic signals returning to the computer for analysis are contaminated by electronic noise as well as low-intensity signals reflected from minor interfaces within the cardiac structures. Such low-intensity signals are routinely eliminated during the analysis. On the other hand, very high-intensity signals may exceed the limits of the system for analysis. The term dynamic range denotes the range between the minimal low-intensity and maximal high-intensity signals that a particular system is capable of analyzing (Figure 2.17). The gradations of gray scale in the ultrasound equipment represent its dynamic range. A higher dynamic range provides a wider gray scale and better distinction of echoes of slightly different intensities. The dynamic range of any particular system can be increased through

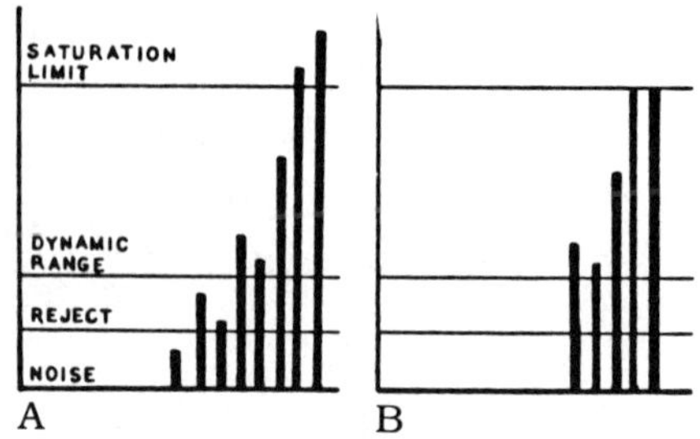

Figure 2.17
Dynamic range. A. The bars represent the raw intensities of different signals perceived by the ultrasound unit. B. Very low-intensity signals (noise) and other signals of low intensity are rejected from analysis. Very high-intensity signals are cut off. The spectrum between the lowest and the highest signals processed by the ultrasound equipment represents its dynamic range.

computer processing. Echoes of very high intensity that exceed the upper limit of the dynamic range are partially suppressed to fall within the dynamic range. Weak echoes are also suppressed, but to a lesser degree. This decremental suppression follows a logarithmic scale, and hence the term logarithmic compression.

Image Display Methods

The process of transformation of processed electronic signals into image format represents the final step in echocardiographic imaging. It is this final product, i.e., the echocardiographic image, that we rely on for the evaluation of cardiac anatomy and function.

For the purpose of the M-mode examination, the rate of motion of the various cardiac structures is relatively slow compared to the rate of M-mode imaging where the PRF is approximately 1000 times per second. Hence, there is excellent identification of the sequence of cardiac events as depicted by the M-mode echocardiogram. Such echocardiographic images are often displayed on an oscilloscope or TV monitor. Permanent record can be stored on a videotape, Polaroid pictures, or a strip chart recorder. The availability of gray scale on strip chart recorders has greatly enhanced the quality of the M-mode images (Figures 2.7, 2.14).

With respect to two-dimensional imaging, several important issues must be considered. Recall that in order to obtain a single two-dimensional image, the ultrasound beam must be moved across a certain path, with a full sweep representing one complete cycle from one end to the other. The

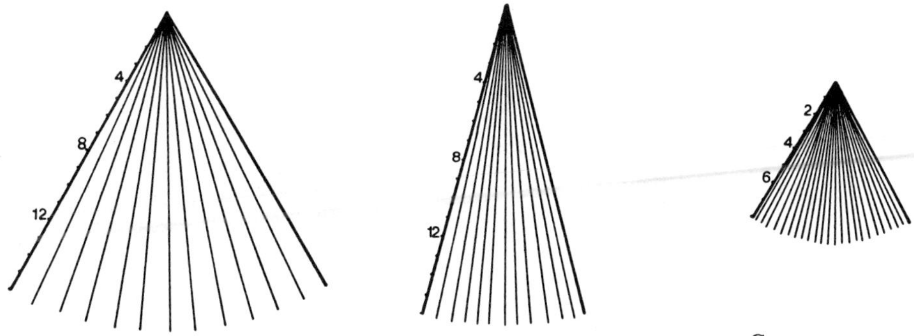

A B C

Figure 2.18
For a given sweep rate (fixed number of sweeps per second), a greater number of lines per sweep with better resolution can be achieved by using a smaller arc (B versus A). This can also be achieved by using a closer depth field of examination (C versus A) whereby the ultrasound pulse travels a shorter distance.

transducer emits multiple ultrasound pulses, each going in a different direction to complete the sweep. Each ultrasound pulse generates one line of information. Given a fixed sweep rate, the ultrasound unit varies the number of lines per sweep, the PRF, according to the size of the sweep. All other parameters being constant, the wider the sweep (i.e., 30-degree arc versus 90-degree arc), the less the number of lines per sweep. Moreover, enough time should be given to allow each burst of ultrasound wave to travel back and forth to the transducer. The greater the depth field being examined (i.e., 10 cm versus 20 cm away from the transducer), the longer the time interval needed for the reflected echoes to arrive to the transducer (Figure 2.18).

Two-dimensional images are usually displayed on a TV monitor. Such monitors display 30 frames/sec with each frame made of two fields, 1⁄60 second each. The usual sweep rate is 60 sweeps/sec to correspond to one field on the TV monitor. Since each ultrasound pulse represents one line of information for a given sweep rate, the number of lines (PRF) varies depending on the width of the sweep and the depth of the field of examination. Image quality depends on the number of lines per sweep. The higher the line density per sweep, the clearer the two-dimensional image is. This can be achieved by decreasing the sweep rate, decreasing the arc of the sweep, or decreasing the depth range of the examination field. However, it may not be feasible to alter these parameters during every routine echocardiographic examination.

There are different ways to improve image quality without changing the line density per sweep. One such approach is

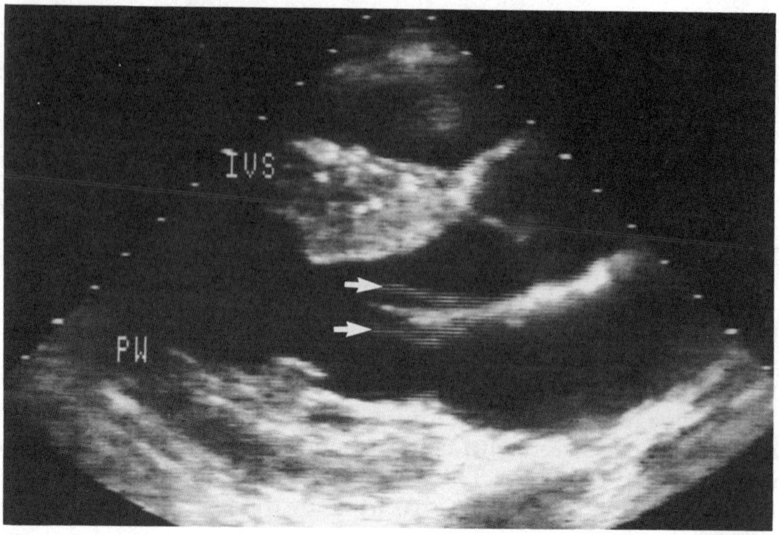

Figure 2.19
Persistence. A relatively fast moving anterior mitral leaflet creates persistence with two faintly visualized ghost images of this leaflet (arrowheads). During normal playback speed of the videotaped images, persistence allows smooth transition between successive frames. IVS = interventricular septum, PW = posterior wall.

by means of "persistence." This is achieved by adjusting the TV monitor screen so that a relatively longer time elapses before each projected image fades off the screen (Figure 2.19). In this way, the gaps in between lines are less conspicuous and the image appears more homogeneous. Current computerized image enhancement systems generate images that greatly eliminate the gaps in between the lines.

Imaging Controls

Overall image quality can be adjusted by several features controlled by the operator. Electronic noise and other low-intensity echoes can be deleted from the final image by using the reject control. This feature rejects all echoes with intensity below a certain value without affecting other echoes of higher intensity (Figure 2.20).

In situations where most of the returning echoes are of relatively low intensity, one can enhance these echoes by adjusting the gain control. This feature amplifies the intensity of all reflected echoes including those related to noise (Figure 2.21). Proper gain and reject settings are crucial for adequate imaging. Too much reject may eliminate important low-intensity echoes in certain cardiac pathologic states. On the other hand, too much gain may falsely enhance artifacts and lead to misinterpretation of the echocardiogram.

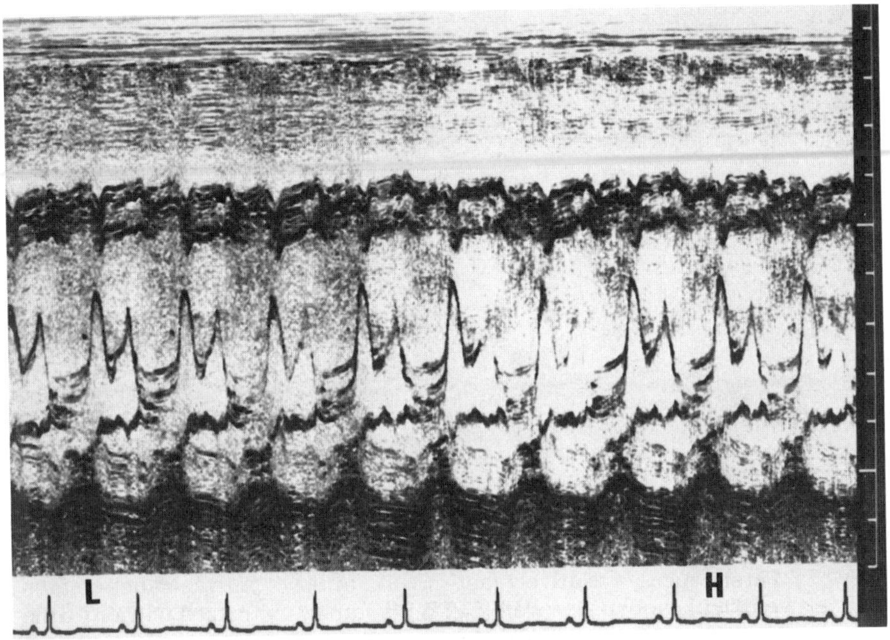

Figure 2.20
The reject control eliminates low-intensity echoes as selected by the operator without affecting other echoes of higher intensity. H = high reject control, L = low reject control.

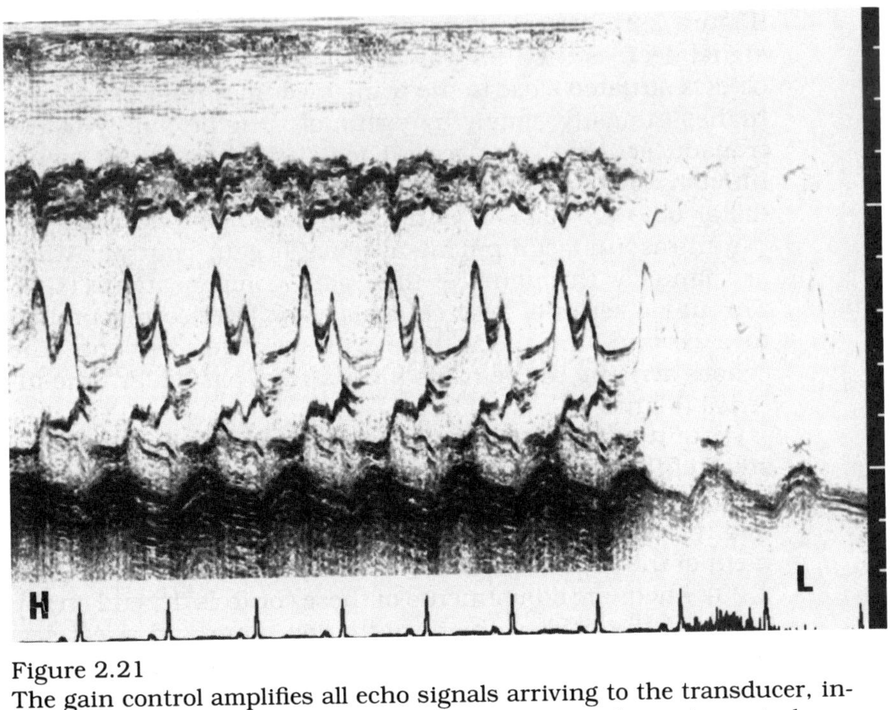

Figure 2.21
The gain control amplifies all echo signals arriving to the transducer, including noise artifacts. H = high gain control, L = low gain control.

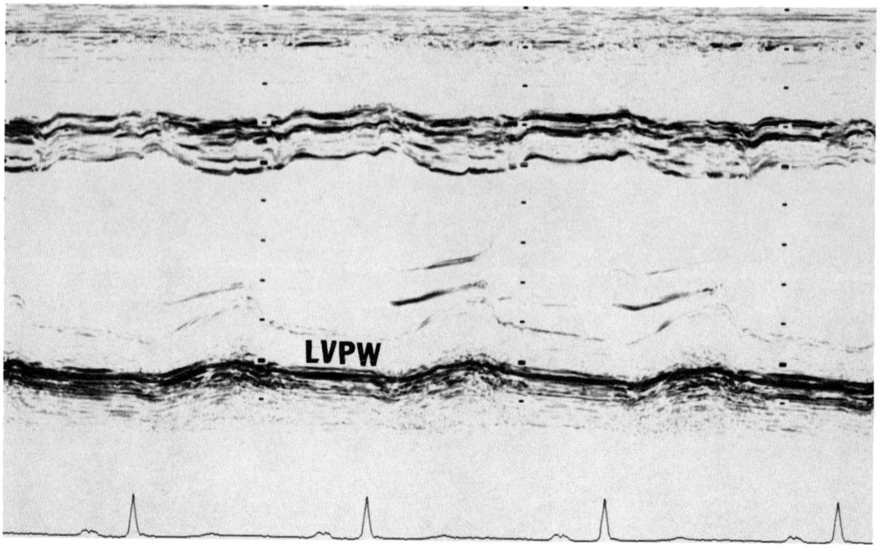

Figure 2.22
The left ventricular posterior wall (LVPW) is faintly visualized without time gain compensation (compare with Figure 2.7).

As the ultrasound beam travels through the chest wall, it undergoes reflection, refraction, attenuation, and scattering (Figure 2.2). In a similar way, the intensity of the reflected signal decreases on its way back to the transducer. Hence, objects situated close to the transducer may reflect echoes of higher intensity simply by virtue of their proximity to the transducer. One can account for such variation of signal intensity by preferentially enhancing echoes reflected from distal objects. This is either performed automatically by the ultrasound equipment automatic gain control (AGC), or manually through the time gain compensation (TGC). Through a series of lever controls, each lever corresponding to a certain time delay, one can selectively enhance the echoes arriving to the transducer after a particular time interval (Figure 2.22).

Certain ultrasound equipment provides knob controls instead of the TGC. One control identifies the depth zone closest to the transducer where gain adjustment is not needed, and the other control is used to adjust the rate of enhancement of the gain setting in the far depth zone (ramp) (Figure 2.23). Adequate adjustments of these controls depend on the depth of the field of the examination, gain and reject settings, as well as the intrinsic cardiac structures being evaluated.

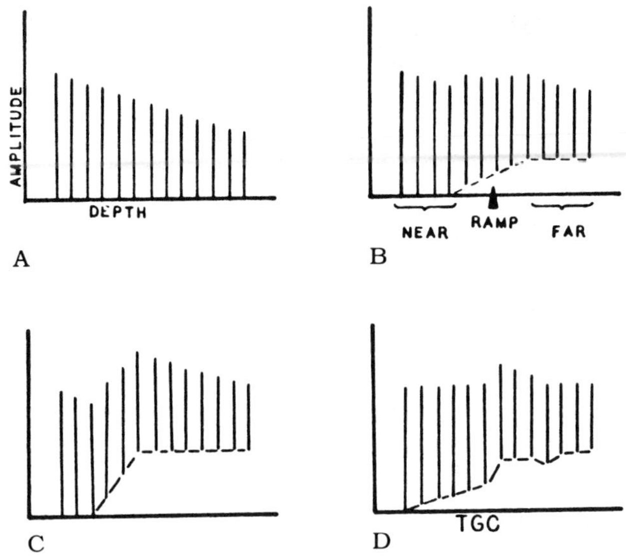

Figure 2.23
A. More distal objects produce images of lower intensity. B and C. Time gain compensation is achieved by near and far zone controls. D. Time gain compensation (TGC) is achieved by series of levers with selective enhancement of signals reflected from the midfield of examination.

Pitfalls in Echocardiography

Despite the major advances in ultrasound technology in improving overall image quality, particular circumstances may produce image artifacts leading to misinterpretation of the echocardiogram. The issue of beam width has already been addressed (Figure 2.11).

Reverberation of ultrasound represents another common imaging artifact. In simple terms, reverberations signify the presence of multiple echoes reflected from the same object. This is analogous to the situation where a subject screams while in a valley between two mountains. The sound waves generated by this subject keep bouncing between these two mountains so that one hears multiple echoes. During the ultrasonic examination, when an echo of relatively strong intensity returns to the transducer surface, a portion of this echo signal is reflected back into the chest cavity, and hits the same object again before it returns once more to the transducer. Hence, two echoes of the same object are generated from a single ultrasound pulse. The time delay inherent to the second echo signal causes the ultrasound unit to dis-

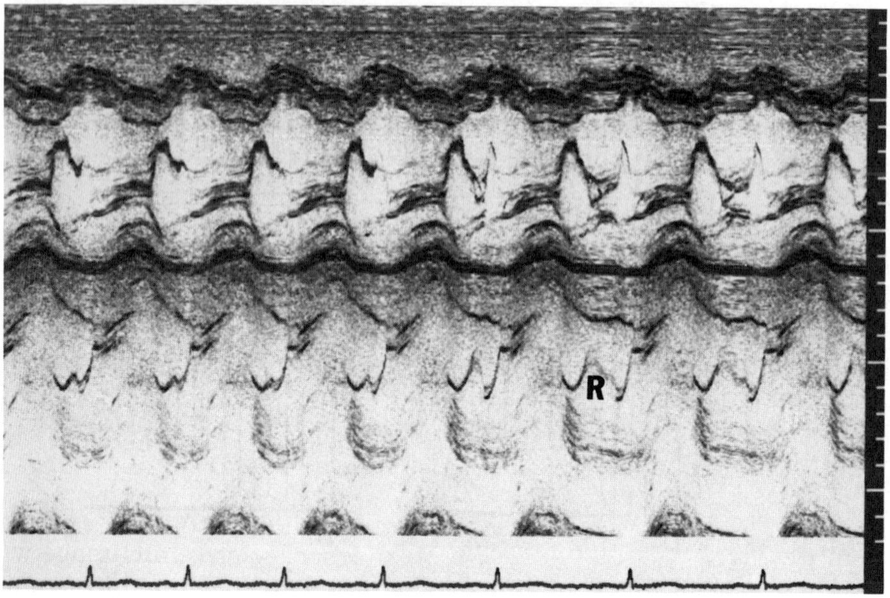

Figure 2.24
Reverberation (R) of the mitral valve echoes are noted at twice the true depth location and exhibit exaggerated leaflet motion.

play a second image of the object at twice the original depth location. In the same manner, the motion of a moving object appears to be exaggerated in the reverberating echoes (Figure 2.24).

Reverberations can occur at strong tissue interfaces other than the transducer surface. The depth location where such reverberating echoes are displayed depends on the time delay for these echoes to return to the transducer. In general, reverberating echoes are displayed outside the borders of the heart on the echocardiogram. Occasionally, such reverberations may appear within the cardiac structure and may cause confusion. Such artifacts may be eliminated by repositioning of the transducer at the chest wall so that the direction of the ultrasound beam is slightly altered.

Another potential artifact is that of side lobes, most commonly noted with phased array transducers. Recall that the ultrasound waves generated by piezoelectric crystals travel in all directions. Special transducer design, coupled with computer-controlled triggering of these crystals, generates a single beam of ultrasound that travels predominantly in one direction. However, this process is not perfect. Multiple ultrasound beams of weaker intensity may still originate and will travel in a slightly different direction than the original beam. Because of the weaker intensity, echoes reflected from

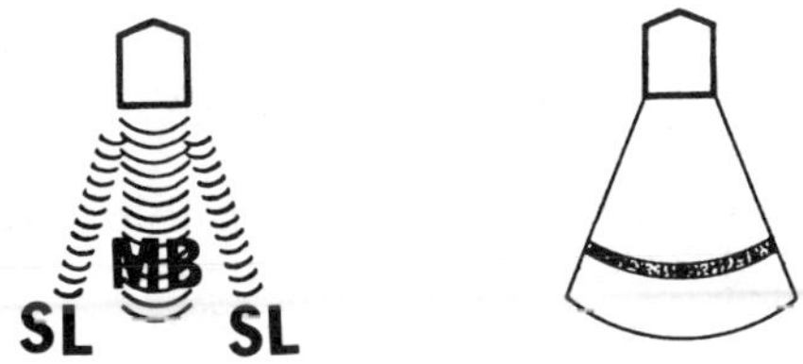

Figure 2.25
Echoes reflected from the secondary ultrasound beams (side lobes) may be of sufficient intensity to be processed by the ultrasound equipment and displayed on the monitor, thereby creating an artifact. MB = main ultrasound beam, SL = side lobes.

these secondary ultrasound beams are also weak and commonly rejected in the final image processing. However, when such weak ultrasound beams are reflected from a strong interface, the resulting echoes may be of sufficient intensity to be recorded. Hence, the final echocardiographic image will display a strong echo originating from the main ultrasound beam, together with weaker, ill-defined echoes on either side, extending throughout the edges of the sweep (Figures 2.4B, 2.25). This imaging artifact may be avoided by adjusting the reject and gain controls to eliminate these weaker echoes. Repositioning of the transducer at the chest wall does not necessarily eliminate this artifact.

Energy of Ultrasound

Sound, light, x-ray, and heat all represent different forms of energy. The energy of ultrasound waves has long been used to generate heat commonly used in physical therapy. This has raised certain issues regarding the safety of ultrasound in echocardiography. However, when one estimates the amount of energy delivered to the body during a routine echocardiographic examination and the amount of heat generated, it becomes evident that this amount is negligible and is of no concern.

Earlier studies suggested that ultrasound may cause certain chromosomal changes that could affect a developing fetus during obstetric applications of ultrasonography. However, such observations have not been confirmed.

Gaseous microcavitations have also been attributed to the rarefaction portion of an ultrasound wave. This physical phenomenon has not been substantiated and appears to have no ill effects.

Hence, to date, there is no evidence to suggest any significantly harmful effect of routine echocardiography to the heart or surrounding structures. Echocardiography is a safe means of noninvasively evaluating the heart, thus avoiding invasive procedures such as cardiac catheterization in many patients.

Echocardiography is preferable to radiologic techniques in the evaluation of cardiac size and function. Moreover, the potentially harmful effects of the x-ray may become an issue in serial radiographic examinations. There are no known ill effects, however, of serial echocardiographic studies.

3 Principles of Doppler Ultrasonography

The Doppler Principle

The term Doppler refers to the physicist, Christian Doppler, who first noticed the physical phenomenon that is currently called the Doppler shift, the Doppler effect, or the Doppler principle. The basic principle of the Doppler shift refers to a situation whereby the frequency of sound waves perceived by a sound receiver may be slightly different from the original frequency emitted from the sound source. This occurs when either the sound source or the receiver, or both, are moving in relation to each other. If the sound source and sound receiver are both stationary, there will be no significant difference between the frequency of the emitted sound signal (f_o) and the frequency of the received signal (f_l). However, if either the sound source or sound receiver is moving toward the other, then f_l will be higher than f_o. If either the sound source or sound receiver is moving away from the other, then f_l will be smaller than f_o. The difference between f_o and f_l is called the frequency shift (f_d) (Figure 3.1).

$$f_d = f_l - f_o \qquad \text{(Equation 3.1)}$$

As anticipated from Equation 3.1, f_d may be positive or negative depending on the relative motion of the sound source and receiver. The magnitude of the frequency shift can be determined from the Doppler equation:

$$f_d = \frac{2f_o(V)(\cos\theta)}{c} \qquad \text{(Equation 3.2)}$$

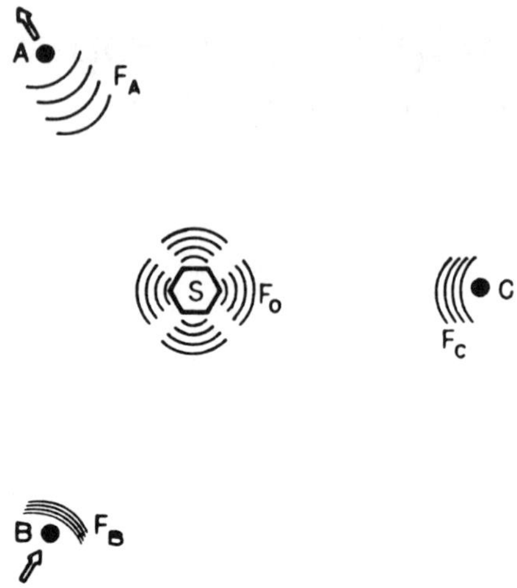

Figure 3.1
The sound source (S) emits ultrasound at frequency f_o. There is no frequency shift of ultrasound reflected from the stationary object C; $f_c = f_o$. Object A is moving away from the transducer. The reflected ultrasound has frequency f_a, which is less than f_o. Object B is moving toward the transducer with a resulting reflected ultrasound frequency, f_b, which is larger than f_o.

Where f_d is the frequency shift, f_o is the frequency of emitted sound wave, V is the velocity of the sound reflector relative to the sound source, c is the velocity of sound in the medium, and θ is the angle of incidence between the direction of motion in space of the sound reflector relative to the path of the sound wave (Figure 3.2).

The Doppler effect is applied in cardiovascular medicine to measure the velocity of moving particles in the blood, mainly red blood cells. An ultrasound transducer is used as a sound source. The ultrasound waves are directed toward the blood vessels or cardiac chambers; the reflected ultrasound signal from red blood cells and other blood elements is received by the transducer and the frequency shift is measured. Knowing the original frequency f_o, the velocity of sound in biologic tissue (approximately 1540 m/sec), and the angle θ, the velocity and direction of motion of the red blood cells relative to the transducer can be estimated.

$$V = \frac{cf_d}{2f_o(\cos \theta)} \qquad \text{(Equation 3.3)}$$

Knowledge of the velocity of blood and direction of motion within the blood vessels and cardiac chambers is of great practical significance in the understanding and diagnosis of

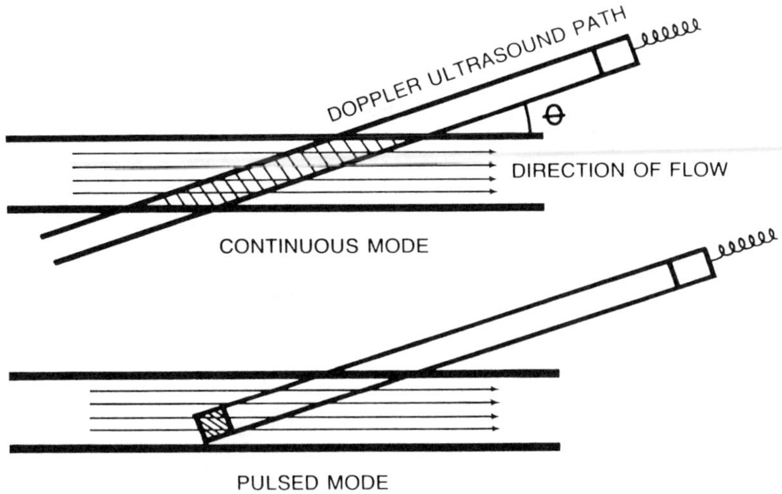

Figure 3.2
The angle of incidence θ defines the path of the ultrasound beam relative to the direction of flow. This applies to both continuous and pulsed mode Doppler ultrasound. See text for details.

various disease states. Originally, the Doppler effect was applied to examine blood flow characteristics in peripheral arteries and veins. This provided useful information in the diagnosis of arterial stenosis and venous thrombosis. Blood flow is variable within the different cardiac chambers and great vessels, as well as with respect to the cardiac cycle. Recently, advances in technology have made it possible to apply the Doppler effect to examine blood flow in a complex structure such as the heart. The frequency shifts recorded during cardiac Doppler examinations happen to be within the frequency range that can be heard by the human ear. These acoustic signals have significant value during the cardiac Doppler recording and data interpretation, as will be discussed later.

As is evident from the Doppler equation, for any given incident frequency, f_o, the frequency shift, f_d, is directly proportional to the velocity of the moving particles, provided the angle of incidence, θ, is the same. Moreover, since f_d is also directly proportional to f_o, then using a transducer with a higher f_o, one may record a higher f_d if the velocity and angle θ are constant (Figure 3.3). It is important to know the angle of incidence θ, since the numerical value of cosine θ may vary widely. An angle θ of zero or 180 degrees (i.e., the direction of blood flow is parallel to the direction of the ultrasound beam) will have a cosine value of one, while an angle θ of 90 degrees or 270 degrees (i.e., the direction of blood flow is perpendicular to the direction of the ultrasound beam) will have a cosine

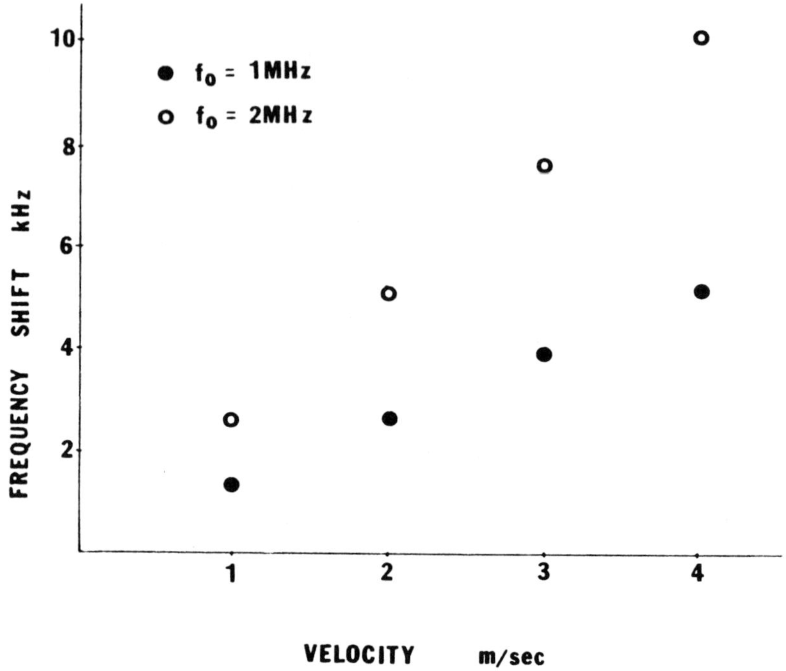

Figure 3.3
A greater frequency shift is achieved by increasing the velocity of flow or increasing the frequency of emitted ultrasound. f_o = frequency of emitted sound signal.

value of zero. Hence, if one attempts to estimate velocity using the Doppler equation without correction for the angle θ, the recorded velocity may seriously underestimate the true velocity (Figure 3.4). For all practical purposes, correction for angles less than 20 degrees is not necessary since the true velocity will not be significantly underestimated.

Physics of Blood Flow

The information provided by using the Doppler principle is obtained from a relatively small number of red blood cells. This underscores the importance of properly understanding certain physical properties of blood flow, because the information provided by the Doppler equation may be misleading and may not be an adequate representation of the actual events in the heart.

Blood as a Fluid

Whole blood is made of two main components: (1) plasma, with various macromolecules and proteins; and (2) blood

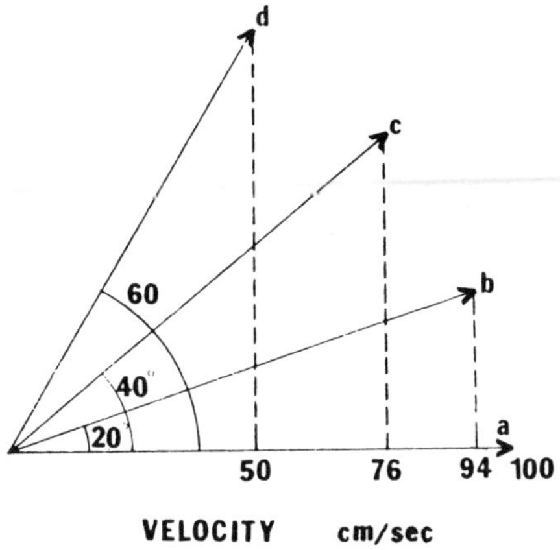

Figure 3.4
Effect of angle θ on velocity measurements. Velocity of 100 cm/sec parallel to the ultrasound beam (a) will be underestimated as the angle of incidence increases (b, c, and d). The estimated velocities at angles 20, 40, and 60 degrees will be 94, 76, and 50 cm/sec, respectively. An angle θ of less than 20 degrees is acceptable during clinical applications of the Doppler principle.

cell elements, mainly red blood cells, white blood cells, and platelets. The blood cell elements are uniformly suspended in the plasma within the cardiac chambers and great vessels. For all practical purposes, whole blood demonstrates physical properties more similar to fluids than solids.

Fluid Dynamics

The important properties of fluid dynamics to be recognized are:

1. Inertia, which is defined as the resistance to motion, acceleration, deceleration, or change of direction. This property is inherent in most fluids as well as solids.
2. Viscosity, which is defined as the degree to which a fluid resists flow when a force is applied to it, e.g., syrup is a very viscous fluid compared to water, which flows easily. Blood is slightly more viscous than water. The endothelial lining of blood vessels and cardiac chambers tends to minimize the effect of blood viscosity on flow.
3. Patterns of flow. In general, two common patterns of blood flow are usually encountered (Figure 3.5).
    a. Laminar flow, where fluid particles move in the same direction.
    b. Turbulent flow, where fluid particles move in different directions. This is most commonly seen in poststenotic flow jets.

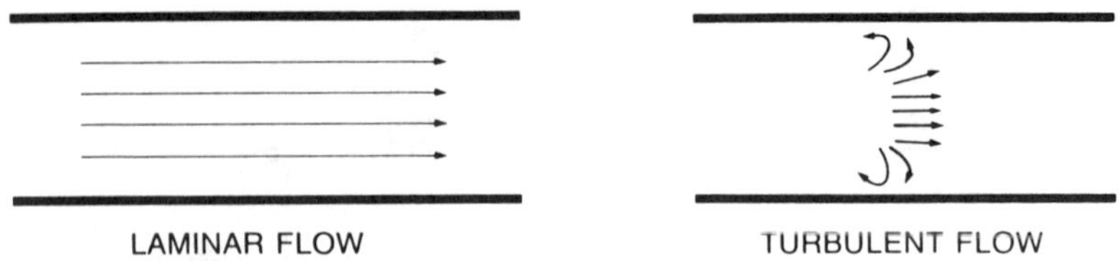

Figure 3.5
Patterns of flow. A flow in which all the fluid particles are moving in the same direction is said to be laminar. Turbulent flow occurs when the fluid particles are moving in different directions relative to each other.

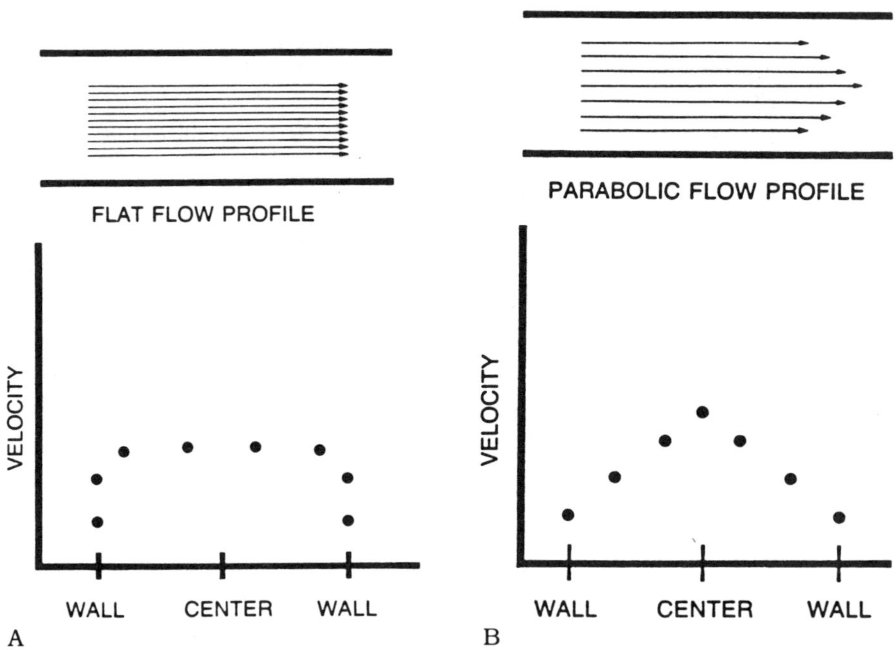

Figure 3.6
Flow profile. A flat flow profile occurs when most of the fluid particles are moving at the same velocity. Only fluid particles in close proximity to the wall of the vessel may be moving at a slower velocity. A parabolic flow profile occurs when the fluid particles at the center of the vessel are moving at the highest velocity with gradual decrement of the velocity of neighboring particles closer to the vessel wall.

4. Flow profile. In general, two types of blood flow profiles are encountered (Figure 3.6).

a. Flat flow profile, where most fluid particles are moving at relatively the same velocity.

b. Variable flow profile, where the fluid particles are moving at different velocities, although in the same direction.

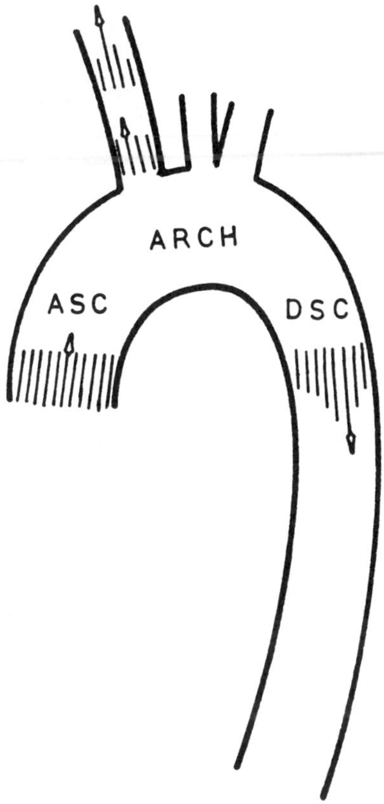

Figure 3.7
The flow profiles change according to the geometric area of flow. A flat profile is observed in the ascending aorta (ASC) and at the origin of the major branches. The profile becomes parabolic distally in the artery. The curvature in the aortic arch distorts the flow profile in the descending aorta (DSC).

Normal blood flow in the cardiac chambers and great vessels usually has a laminar pattern with a flat profile. However, blood flow is pulsatile and variable throughout the cardiac cycle. Also, blood flows through channels of different sizes and geometric configurations within the cardiac chambers and great vessels. The blood flow profiles will differ accordingly (Figure 3.7).

Modes of Doppler Ultrasound

There are two modes available for the cardiac Doppler ultrasound examination. These two modes are considered to be complementary.

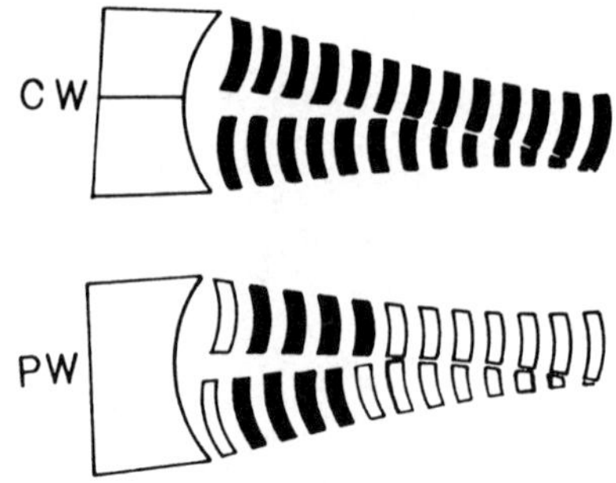

Figure 3.8
Modes of Doppler ultrasound. Continuous wave (CW) mode utilizes two transducer elements, one for emission and the other for reception of ultrasound waves. Pulsed wave (PW) mode utilizes only one transducer element to emit short bursts of ultrasound and receive reflected signals after a certain time delay.

Continuous Wave

In the continuous wave (CW) mode, two adjacently positioned transducer elements are utilized. One element constantly emits waves and the other continuously receives reflected signals (Figures 3.8, 3.9). The signals received by the transducer could have been reflected from anywhere along the path of the ultrasound beam; thus, in this mode it is not possible to determine the exact location within the cardiac chambers or great vessels from which the ultra-

---

Figure 3.9
A. Apical two-dimensional view showing the left ventricle (LV) and left atrium (LA) with the white cursor line depicting the path of the Doppler ultrasound beam. The simultaneous CW Doppler recording detects blood flow along the path of the ultrasound beam in this patient who has mitral regurgitation and abnormal flow pattern in systole. B. PW recording along the same path of the Doppler ultrasound beam. The square on the two-dimensional image depicts the location from which the simultaneous Doppler recording is obtained. At this location, only normal transmitral flow in diastole is recorded. C. PW Doppler recordings are obtained from a location within the left atrium close to the mitral annulus. At this location, PW recording depicts the normal diastolic flow, as well as the abnormal systolic regurgitant flow. Hence, CW Doppler was utilized to detect the abnormal flow pattern, whereas PW Doppler localized the abnormal flow pattern within the left atrium only. PRF = pulse repetition frequency, CAL = calibration.

Note the difference in recording of the systolic regurgitant transmitral flow between A and C. The CW recording in A shows flow predominantly in one direction in systole, whereas the PW recording in C shows flow above and below the baseline, consistent with frequency aliasing. See text for details.

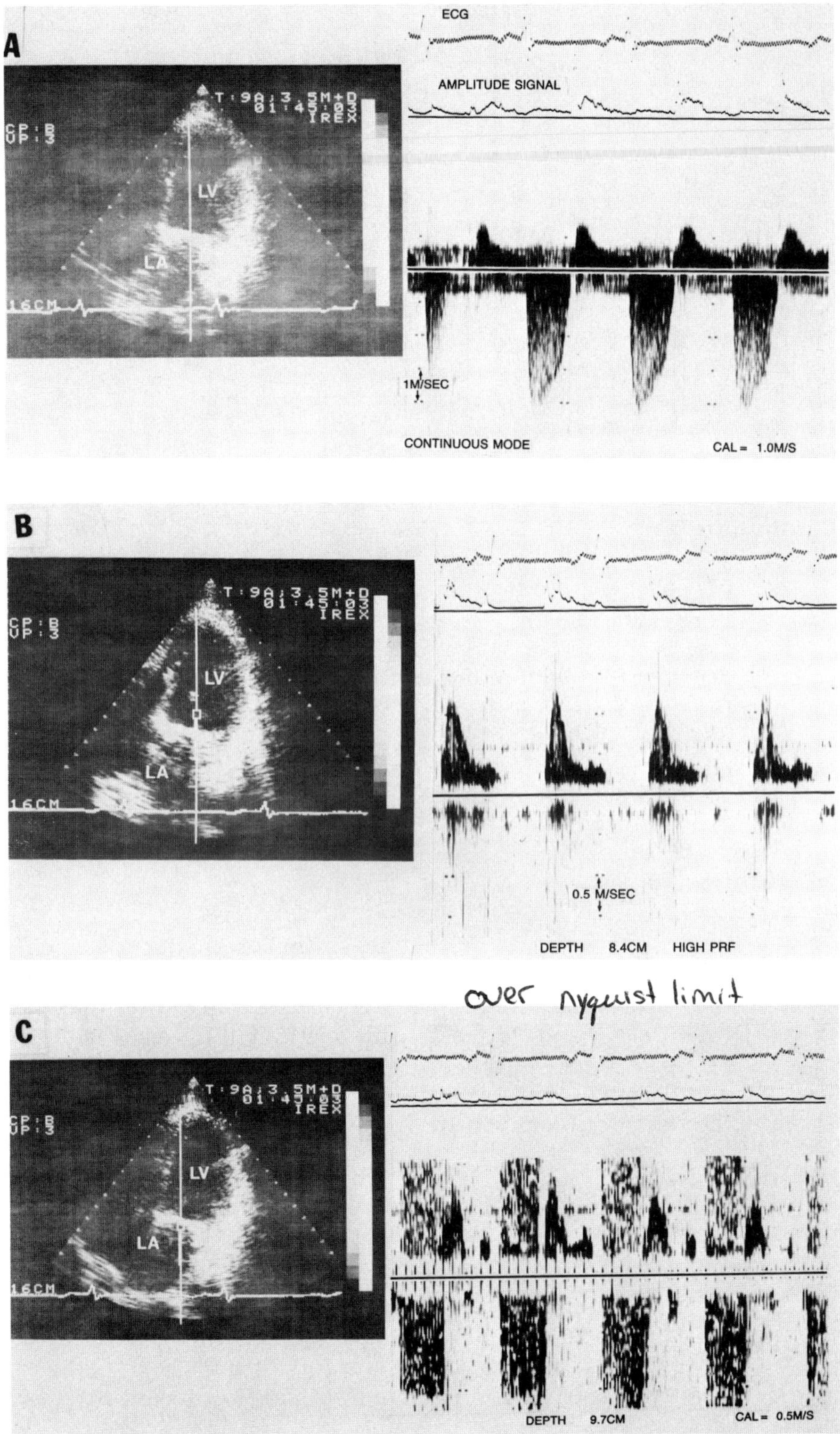
A
T:9A;3.5M+D
01:45:03
IREX
CP:B
VP:3
LV
LA
16CM
ECG
AMPLITUDE SIGNAL
1M/SEC
CONTINUOUS MODE
CAL = 1.0M/S
B
LV
LA
16CM
0.5 M/SEC
DEPTH 8.4CM HIGH PRF
C
LV
LA
16CM
DEPTH 9.7CM
CAL = 0.5M/S

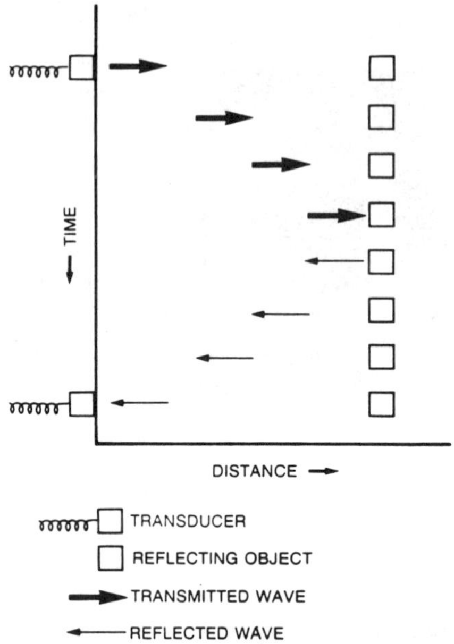

Figure 3.10
In the PW mode, the transducer is controlled to receive reflected signals after a specific time delay that corresponds to a desired depth location within the heart. The ultrasound pulse travels twice the distance as it goes back and forth to the transducer (see Figure 3.11).

sound waves are being reflected. This is particularly important in disease states with abnormal flow patterns.

Pulsed Wave

In the pulsed wave (PW) mode, a single transducer element intermittently emits ultrasound waves at predetermined time intervals and receives reflected signals after specific time delays as selected by the operator (Figures 3.8, 3.9). The transducer rejects any signals that are received during a time period other than the specific period selected by the operator (gate width).

$$d = ct/2 \qquad \text{(Equation 3.4)}$$

Knowing the velocity of sound in tissue, c, and the time delay, t, the distance of the reflecting surface from the transducer, d, can be estimated. The right-hand term in Equation 3.4 is divided by 2 since the ultrasound wave has to travel twice the distance, d, going back and forth to the transducer (Figure 3.10). This is similar to M-mode echocardiography where the time delay for the signals to return to the transducer is used to estimate the distance of cardiac structures from the transducer. However, major differences occur. In M-mode echocardiography, all reflected signals are analyzed, while in PW Doppler ultrasound, only the reflected signals arriving at particular time intervals (gate width) will be analyzed. The other difference involves the pulse repetition frequency (PRF), which is the number of ultrasound pulses emitted by the transducer per second. M-mode echocardiography employs a relatively low PRF, approximately 1000 Hz. Such low PRF is inadequate for PW Doppler ultrasound to examine constantly changing blood velocities with pulsatile flows. Higher PRFs, generally greater than 5000 Hz, are needed. However, there is a relative limit as to how high the PRF can be in the PW mode. Time should be allowed for any single burst of ultrasound to travel back and forth to the transducer before another ultrasound pulse is emitted. If more than one ultrasound pulse is traveling within the heart at any single point in time, the Doppler unit cannot determine which reflected signal has originated from which emitted pulse and, hence, confusion may arise as to the true depth location of the reflecting object within the heart. In general, a farther depth selection imposes a lower PRF to avoid this confusion.

Range Ambiguity

A potential source of confusion develops when the PRF, which is appropriate for a normal-sized heart, is inappropriate for a markedly dilated heart with abnormal flow patterns. This occurs when a transmitted ultrasound pulse travels a longer distance within the dilated heart before it is reflected back to the transducer. If this reflected signal happens to reach the transducer when it is receiving signals from a second burst of ultrasound, the Doppler unit will interpret this delayed signal as a reflection of the second ultrasound pulse and will display the estimated depth location as that depth corresponding to the time delay from the second pulse wave, which is different from the depth of the true sample location (Figure 3.11). This is known as range ambiguity. Therefore, in order to determine the true depth location of these ambiguous signals, it is important to know the PRF when these signals are recorded. The pulse interval is the time interval between each two bursts of ultrasound:

$$T = \frac{1}{PRF} \quad \text{(Equation 3.5)}$$

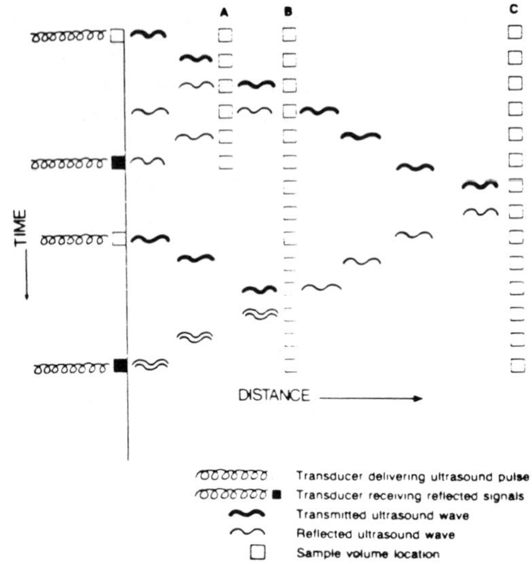

Figure 3.11
Range ambiguity. The transducer is set to receive reflected signals after a time delay corresponding to the depth location B. Signals reflected from depth location A arrive too early and are not processed. Signals reflected from depth location C travel a longer distance and are delayed. In the mean time, the transducer has already emitted another pulse of ultrasound. The delayed signals reflected from location C arrive at the transducer simultaneously with the signals reflected from location B from the second pulse wave. The Doppler unit will interpret both signals as if they originated from depth location B, thus causing range ambiguity.

The total time delay for this ambiguous signal, T_a, is

$$T_a = T + t \qquad \text{(Equation 3.6)}$$

where T is the pulse interval and t is the original time setting as selected by the operator.

Therefore, the true depth location, d_a, can be estimated by modification of Equation 3.4:

$$d_a = c(T + t)/2 \qquad \text{(Equation 3.7)}$$

$$d_a = cT/2 + ct/2 \qquad \text{(Equation 3.8)}$$

where cT/2 is the distance corresponding to the time delay, T.

If this is added to the depth location as displayed by the Doppler unit, the true depth location can be estimated (Figure 3.12).

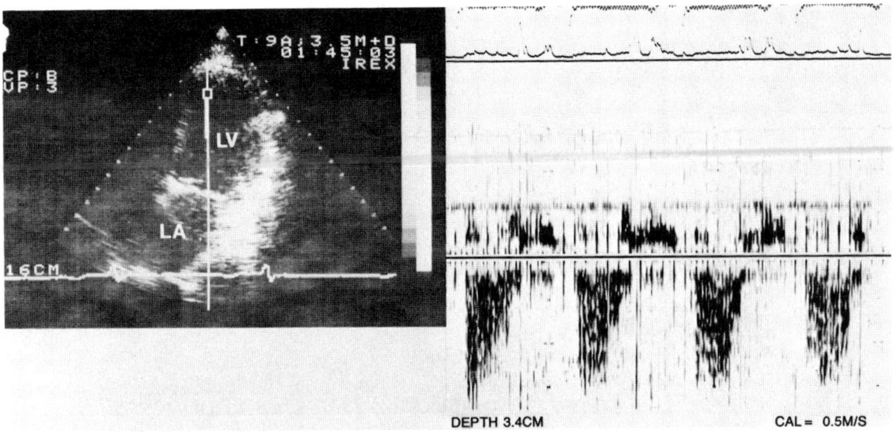

Figure 3.12
Range ambiguity. Doppler recordings obtained from the same patient shown in Figure 3.9. The transducer is set to receive signals reflected from within the left ventricular apex (square on the two-dimensional image). At this location, PW Doppler recordings exhibit an abnormal flow pattern in systole, which actually occurs within the left atrium (LA) and not the left ventricular apex. LV = left ventricle, CAL = calibration.

Sample Volume

In the CW mode, sampling of flow occurs at all depths along the ultrasound path. In the PW mode, sampling of flow occurs at specified depths referred to as the sample volume location (Figures 3.9, 3.10). The sample volume represents the actual dimensions of the biologic medium from which reflected signals are being interrogated. The dimensions are dependent on the nature of the transducer, whether it is focused or nonfocused, and the length in time of the ultrasound pulse, known as the pulse width. The sample volume can be changed in its longitudinal dimension by altering the time interval during which the transducer is emitting sound waves (pulse width). The time interval during which the transducer is receptive to reflected signals is referred to as the gate width (Figure 3.13).

Frequency Aliasing

If the reflected ultrasound wave is superimposed on the original ultrasound wave, one can realize that they are not identical due to the frequency shift, f_d (Figure 3.14). The phase lag, ΔQ, between these two sound waves can be measured. Knowing the pulse interval, T, the frequency shift can be determined:

$$\Delta Q = 360 \text{ degrees} \times f_d \times T \qquad \text{(Equation 3.9)}$$

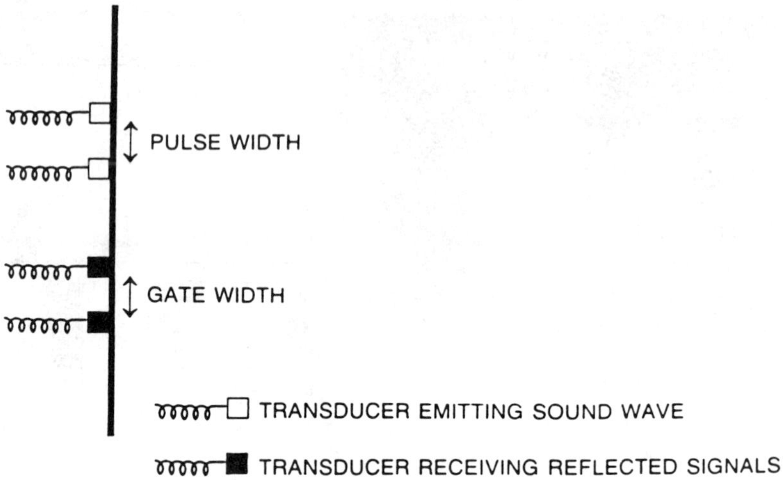

Figure 3.13
In the PW mode, pulse width represents the time interval during which the transducer emits ultrasound waves. Gate width represents the time interval during which the transducer receives reflected signals.

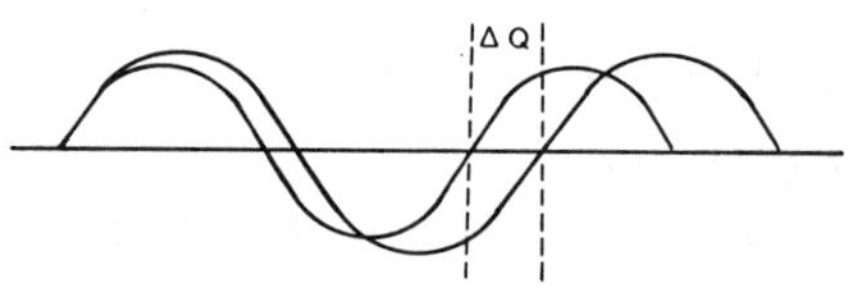

Figure 3.14
When two sinusoidal waves representing the emitted and reflected ultrasound waves are superimposed, the frequency shift is represented by the phase lag ΔQ.

Since T = 1/PRF (Equation 3.5), then Equation 3.9 can be rewritten as follows:

$$\Delta Q = \frac{360 \text{ degrees} \times f_d}{\text{PRF}} \qquad \text{(Equation 3.10)}$$

If the phase lag is equal to 180 degrees, then f_d would be equal to one-half the PRF. If the phase lag is greater than 180 degrees in one direction, confusion may arise as to whether this phase lag is truly greater than 180 degrees in one direction, or less than 180 degrees but in the opposite direction (Figure 3.15). In this situation, the Doppler recording will display flow pattern in both directions. This physical phenomenon is referred to as frequency aliasing.

The Nyquist limit is the numerical value of one-half the PRF. If f_d exceeds this Nyquist limit, then frequency aliasing

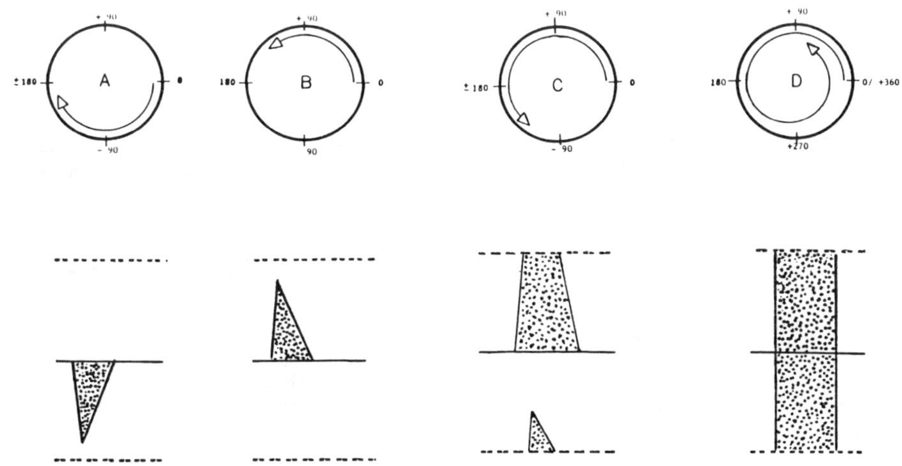

Figure 3.15
The phase lag (arrows) in A and B are −150 degrees and +120 degrees, respectively. There is no confusion in regards to the direction and magnitude of the frequency shifts when the phase lag is less than 180 degrees in either direction. The phase lag in C is +220 degrees. The Doppler instrument will interpret this as +180 degrees in one direction, and −40 degrees in the other direction. A phase lag greater than 360 degrees in either direction will create total confusion in regards to the direction and magnitude of flow (D).

will occur and the resultant signal will be distorted with respect to the magnitude and direction of the flow being examined (Figure 3.9). The maximum limit of frequency shift or velocity that can be measured without the distortion of frequency aliasing with PW mode Doppler ultrasound is a function of the range of the sample volume and frequency of the emitted signal (f_o). It becomes obvious that a higher PRF will give a higher Nyquist limit and, hence, allow adequate recordings of a higher f_d and velocity. However, if a relatively high PRF is used, more than one ultrasound pulse may be traveling in the heart at one time, thus causing another problem, namely that of range ambiguity. If the frequency aliasing is not severe, then shifting the zero baseline on the Doppler tracing allows adequate recording of the original velocity and eliminates the aliasing (Figure 3.16). One may consider CW mode to be similar to PW mode with an infinite PRF; hence, f_d cannot exceed the Nyquist limit. The trade-off in this situation is the loss of range resolution (Table 3.1).

High Pulse Repetition Frequency

PW mode Doppler ultrasound is used to locate the origin of frequency shifts within the cardiac chambers and great ves-

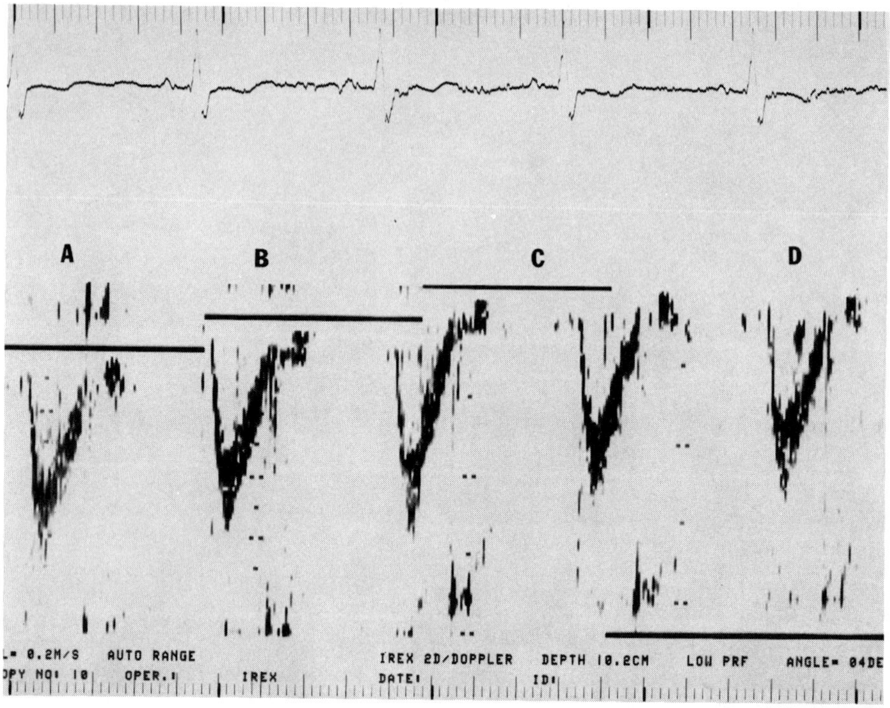

Figure 3.16
PW recording of transaortic flow. The dark horizontal line depicts the zero baseline, which was moved up along the tracing (A, B, and C). In D, the zero baseline is at the bottom of the Doppler tracing. Hence, transaortic flow in D is depicted at the top of the tracing. CAL = calibration, PRF = pulse repetition frequency.

Table 3.1
Comparison of continuous and pulsed mode Doppler ultrasound

	Continuous wave	Pulsed wave
Recording of high velocities	Possible	Frequency aliasing may occur
Depth resolution	Impossible	Possible if no range ambiguity occurs
Reflected signal intensity	Higher	Lower
Sensitivity to small frequency shifts	Lower	Higher
Combination with M-mode echocardiography	Not practical	Limited value
Combination with two-dimensional echocardiography	Very useful	Very useful

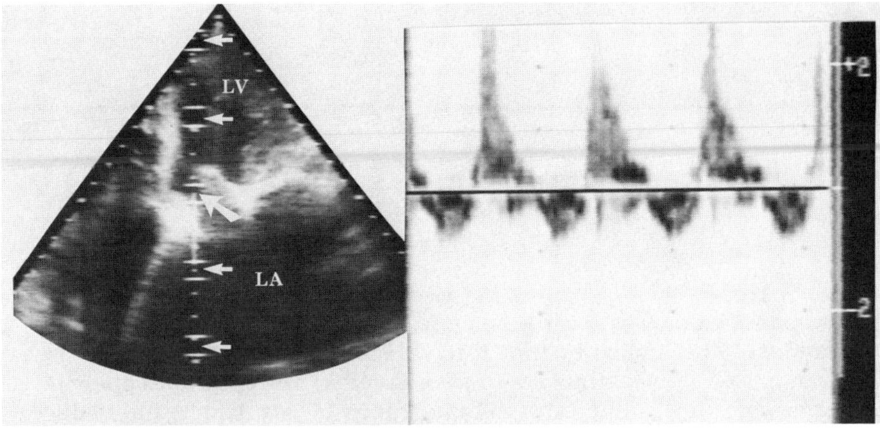

Figure 3.17
Apical four-chamber view obtained from a patient with mitral bioprosthesis with simultaneous HPRF Doppler recording. The arrows on the two-dimensional image point to the five sample volume locations from which the simultaneous Doppler tracing could have originated. The third sample volume is the most likely source of the simultaneous Doppler signal since it is closest to the valve prosthesis. LA = left atrium, LV = left ventricle.

sels. However, as was shown earlier, there are limitations to this technique for recording high velocities of flow due to frequency aliasing. Using the CW mode resolves the problem of aliasing at the cost of losing the advantage of range resolution.

Since aliasing occurs when the frequency shift exceeds the Nyquist limit of the system, it seemed logical to employ relatively high PRF (HPRF) in the PW mode to effectively increase the Nyquist limit. This new technique allows the recording of certain high velocities in the PW mode without the problem of aliasing; however, range ambiguity occurs since more than one ultrasound pulse is traveling within the heart at any point in time. Nevertheless, the judicious use of HPRF allows some degree of range resolution, which is better than the total lack of range resolution encountered with CW mode (Figure 3.17).

Doppler Signal Analysis

The reflected signals received by the transducer are not uniform and consist of a mixture of many signals superimposed on each other. Such complex signals are hard to interpret, especially in conditions of turbulent flow where many red blood cells are moving at various velocities and in different directions in relation to each other and to the ultrasound

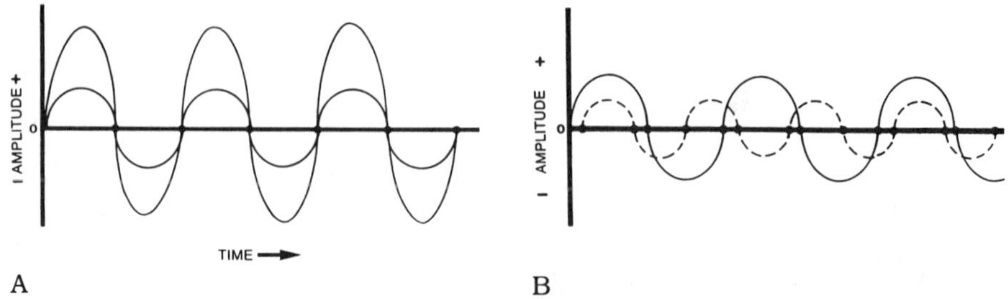

Figure 3.18
A. Two sinusoidal waves of the same frequency but different amplitudes cannot be distinguished by time interval histogram method of analysis. B. Summation of two sinusoidal waves of different frequencies alter the zero-crossing time. Time interval histogram analysis depicts the average zero-crossing time and cannot distinguish these waves from each other.

beam. Two general methods are employed to process these returning signals.

Time Interval Histogram

Examining a sinusoidal wave diagram, one realizes that the actual tracing periodically moves above and below the zero baseline. The distance between any two consecutive peaks is the wavelength. The height of each peak from the baseline represents the amplitude (Figure 3.18). By counting how many times such a sinusoidal wave crosses the zero-baseline, one can determine its frequency. This is referred to as the **zero-crossing time** or the **time interval histogram.** When two such waves of different frequencies are superimposed on each other, the resultant waveform is the sum of these two waveforms. Each of these sinusoidal waves has a different zero-crossing time. The overall signal will have another different zero-crossing time representing the average of the individual waves. By determining the shortest interval between any two adjacent zero-crossing points, such types of signal analysis can estimate the average frequency of the resultant complex waveform. The advantage of this type of signal analysis is that it is a very simple method that does not need complex electronic systems for analysis. However, major disadvantages occur. It is evident that there is no consideration for the amplitude of the sinusoidal wave in this type of analysis (Figure 3.18). Hence, time interval histogram can only define the frequency, but not the amplitude and, subsequently, the strength of the reflected signals. Moreover, since time interval histogram approximates the highest frequencies only, a potential source of error occurs when the signals with the highest frequencies are those of

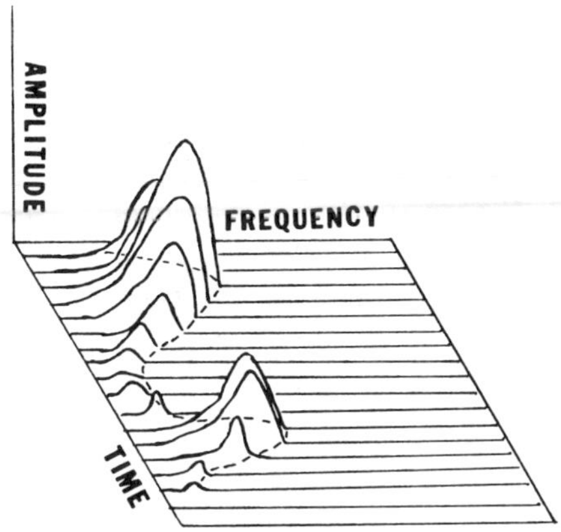

Figure 3.19
Transmitral Doppler flow signal with respect to frequency, amplitude, and time.

artifacts rather than true flow. Adequate adjustment in the gain setting is crucial in this mode of signal analysis. A high gain will detect artifacts, and a very low gain may not show any flow at all.

Discrete Fourier Analysis

Discrete Fourier analysis involves the separation of a composite signal into its component parts, thereby obtaining the frequency, amplitude, and phase interim of each of these component signals (Figure 3.19). The human ear is a good example of an analysis system using discrete Fourier analysis. Walking down a busy street, one can hear the different sounds of people talking, car horns, and music from a nearby restaurant. All of these sound signals arrive simultaneously to the ear, which then breaks this complex signal into its various components. If time interval histogram was used instead, all that could be recorded would be the sound with the highest frequency, reflecting the summation of all the component signals. There are three methods of discrete Fourier analysis in Doppler ultrasound.

1. Band pass filtering is when the signals are electronically processed to allow only certain predetermined frequencies to be displayed, with the remaining frequencies deleted.
2. Fast Fourier transform (FFT) involves using computers to assign numerical values to each signal in relation to amplitude, frequency, and phase in time (digitize the data), and then plotting this digitized image in a graphic presentation. This form of discrete Fourier analysis is most commonly

used in the Doppler units available commercially. Time is displayed on the x-axis (horizontal plane); velocity or frequency shift is displayed on the y-axis (vertical plane). A gray scale is used to represent the amplitude of the signal. The darkness or brightness of the spots on the tracings reflects the strength of the signal at that particular frequency (Figures 3.9, 3.12, 3.16).

3. Chirp-Z is a form of discrete Fourier analysis that allows rapid calculation time, which is needed for analysis of high velocities of flow. A minor disadvantage is some loss of resolution of certain frequencies.

Color Doppler Flow Imaging

M-mode echocardiography provides information along a single path of the ultrasound beam. The advent of two-dimensional echocardiography was a major step forward in cardiac ultrasound in as much as the whole heart could be examined in real time and in two dimensions rather than only one.

The conventional CW mode in Doppler ultrasound may be regarded as similar to conventional M-mode echocardiography. The information obtained by the CW mode reflects the flow along only one dimension and may not be an adequate reflection of true flows. This is a serious disadvantage in situations of eccentric flow patterns where the direction of flow cannot be predicted from simultaneous two-dimensional images. This is also a disadvantage since, occasionally, unexpected abnormal flow patterns can be easily missed without a prolonged search. The PW mode is a further disadvantage in these regards.

An ideal Doppler instrument should be capable of demonstrating flow in real time, similar to two-dimensional echocardiography, which demonstrates cardiac anatomy and motion in real time. Fortunately, advanced Doppler technology can now provide real-time imaging of flow. First, a two-dimensional image is recorded; then flow data obtained from many "sample volumes" within the viewed cardiac chamber are superimposed on the two-dimensional image and viewed in real time. Flow toward the transducer is displayed in red; flow away from the transducer is displayed in blue (Plate 1). Aliasing may also occur, whereby a high-velocity jet may produce orange and blue colors superimposed on each other (Plate 2). Turbulent flow is shown in green. Such color displays allow the observer to rapidly distinguish the direction of flow when viewed in real time. Depending on the clinical situation, mixed colors (mosaic) may be seen in high-velocity jets with turbulence (Plate 3). Similar to B-mode scans where the brightness of the signal reflects its amplitude, the brightness of colors reflects the amplitude of the frequency shifts. The reflected signals are processed by "autocorrelation," where there is continuous processing of these reflected signals in a manner similar to that performed in M-mode echocardiography.

This new approach in Doppler instrumentation provides rapid examination of the direction and velocity of flow within the cardiac chambers seen on the superimposed two-dimensional image. Once this flow information is obtained, the operator may switch to conventional CW or PW mode to record the highest velocities.

Moreover, color Doppler flow imaging is valuable in the identification of multiple abnormal flow patterns. This is best exemplified in patients with multiple valvular pathologic conditions. The abnormal jets of flow may be clearly distinguished from each other during the color Doppler flow examination.

4 Principles of Cardiac Imaging

Noninvasive cardiac imaging can be performed by using the principles of ultrasound outlined in the previous chapter. Ultrasound waves, emitted at the chest wall, travel through the thoracic cavity and are reflected at various tissue interfaces. The reflected ultrasound signals are received by the transducer and electronically processed to produce the final cardiac image.

Acoustic Windows

Because air is a poor medium for the transmission of ultrasound, a special gel should be used as an interface between the ultrasound transducer and the chest wall. In addition, part of the heart is usually covered by lung tissue filled with air. This is particularly important in many subjects with hyperinflated lungs as seen in patients with chronic lung disease. Moreover, the boney rib cage represents another obstacle to the transmission of ultrasound into the chest cavity. Proper imaging of the heart is thus limited to certain transducer locations that enable the ultrasound beam to bypass the lungs and ribs along its path to the heart. These transducer locations are referred to as acoustic windows. Routine echocardiographic examinations can be performed from several acoustic windows (Figure 4.1):

a. Suprasternal window, whereby the transducer is positioned at the suprasternal notch at the junction of the clavicles and sternum. With this approach, the ultrasound beam

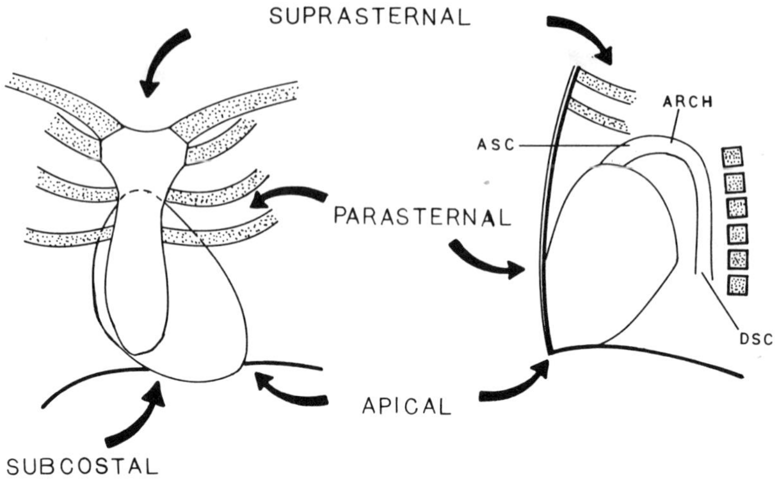

Figure 4.1
The standard acoustic windows. ASC = ascending aorta, DSC = descending aorta.

passes from under the boney rib cage and directly into the great vessels and base of the heart.

b. Parasternal window, whereby the transducer is positioned at the second or third intercostal space just to the left of the sternum. This allows the ultrasound beam to travel in between the ribs to the base of the heart. Moreover, there is usually no lung tissue overlying the heart at this location.

c. Apical window, whereby the transducer is positioned at or near the cardiac apex. The ultrasound beam can be maneuvered to travel in between the ribs directly to the apex of the heart with little interference by the lungs.

d. Subcostal window, whereby the transducer is positioned over the lower section of the chest just below the level of the sternal bone at the midline (the xyphoid). From this position, the ultrasound beam travels from under the boney rib cage and directly into the heart.

e. Recently, transesophageal echocardiography has been introduced. In this approach, a special transducer is introduced into the esophagus and advanced to a location behind the left atrium. The heart can be imaged with a high frequency transducer without interference by lung or bone. Such images are generally superior to conventional transthoracic imaging. Detailed discussion of this new imaging approach is not discussed in this book.

Patient Preparation

For reference, it is recommended to obtain an ECG tracing simultaneously with the echocardiographic recordings. This helps in the timing of the motion of various cardiac structures throughout the cardiac cycle. The ECG electrodes are usually placed on the patient's shoulders and lower part of the abdomen.

Cardiac imaging by ultrasound is usually performed with the patient in a supine position. This reduces patient discomfort and motion artifact. For best results, the patient's position should be adjusted to the acoustic window being employed.

The suprasternal approach necessitates that the patient be flat in bed, with the neck extended backward. This allows adequate maneuvering of the ultrasound transducer with minimal discomfort to the patient. At times, a small rolled towel placed under the patient's shoulders may allow better extension of the neck for adequate imaging.

Subcostal imaging is also performed with the patient flat in bed. Certain patients may tense their abdominal muscles during echocardiographic imaging with this approach, making the image more difficult to obtain. This may be avoided by asking the patient to slightly flex the knees and hips, thereby relaxing the abdominal muscles. The subcostal approach may be difficult to use in obese patients. The operator may have to exert mild pressure with the transducer in order to maneuver the ultrasound beam under the rib cage. The operator must be cautious not to exert too much pressure as this may cause patient discomfort.

By force of gravity, there is better contact of the heart with the inner surface of the chest wall when the patient's upper body is lifted to a 30- to 45-degree elevation in bed. This is further enhanced when the patient rotates slightly to the left. This position is useful during imaging from the parasternal and apical windows.

Maximum exhalation by thc patient forces more air out of the lung tissue surrounding the heart. This maneuver reduces air-tissue interface within the chest cavity and allows for better contact of the heart with the chest wall. Patients with heart disease may not be able to hold their breath. This maneuver can be repeated intermittently, keeping patient comfort in mind.

Although the procedure is virtually painless and requires minimal patient cooperation, it is important to perform the study within the shortest time possible. Many patients with heart disease are restless and may not be able to remain flat for extended periods of time. The usual complete M-mode and two-dimensional echocardiographic examination may be completed within 30 minutes.

Normal Echocardiographic Patterns

The complex three-dimensional structure of the heart cannot be adequately evaluated from one acoustic window. Routine evaluation is commonly performed through the four major acoustic windows so that the heart can be viewed from different angles. In addition, multiple cardiac images may be obtained from any standard location, simply by rotating or tilting the transducer in different directions.

Suprasternal Views

The ascending aorta lies anteriorly and to the right, and continues into the arch and then into the descending thoracic aorta, which lies posteriorly and to the left of the midline (Figure 4.1). Imaging of the aorta from the suprasternal window can be performed by positioning the transducer in a semioblique direction relative to the chest wall, with slight tilting anteriorly or posteriorly to maneuver the ultrasound beam along the major axis of the aorta. In this position, the aorta appears as two parallel linear echos that curve at the top of the monitor (Figure 4.2). From this view, the origins of the three major branches from the aortic arch may be identified. The innominate artery arises from the right side of the aortic arch, close to the ascending aorta, whereas the left carotid and subclavian arteries arise from the left side of the arch, and are closer to the descending aorta. These anatomic relations usually help to identify the ascending and descending segments of the aorta. By convention, the ascending aorta is displayed on the left side of the monitor, whereas the descending aorta is displayed on the right side. Rotating the transducer 180 degrees will reverse the image on the screen.

The main pulmonary artery divides into the right and left branches. The right branch of the pulmonary artery lies within the arch of the aorta. Its cross-sectional image can be identified as a circular structure at the center of the screen (Figure 4.2). Rotating the transducer 90 degrees, perpendicular to its previous orientation, alters the two-dimensional image so that the aortic arch is seen in cross section as a circle, whereas the right pulmonary artery appears as two parallel linear echos below the aortic arch.

These anatomic relations are very valuable for the diagnosis of various congenital cardiac abnormalities. The left atrial appendage is occasionally noted as an echo-free space distal to the right pulmonary artery in this view, particularly when it is enlarged.

Parasternal Long Axis View

To obtain the parasternal long axis view, the transducer is positioned in the left parasternal area with its reference point directed toward the right shoulder so that the plane of the two-dimensional image transects the heart along its long axis from the apex to the base (Figure 4.3). The resulting

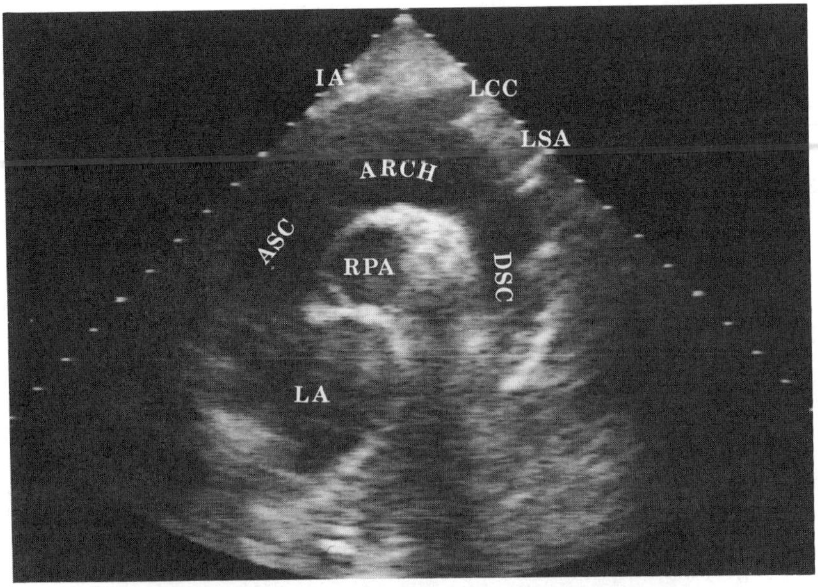

A

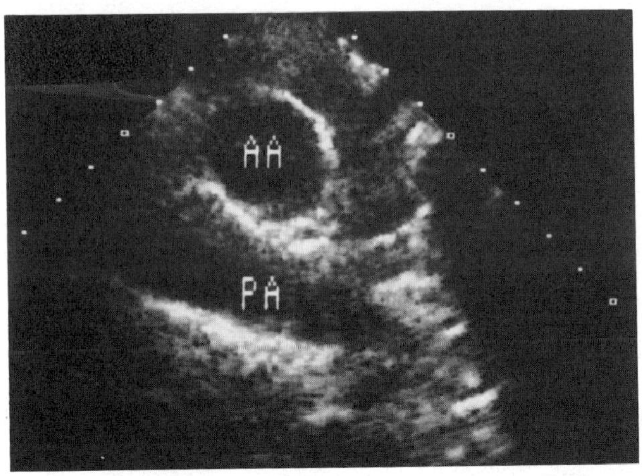

B

Figure 4.2
Suprasternal view of the aorta. A. Longitudinal cross section. B. Transverse cross section. The left atrium (LA) may be visualized in some individuals. The origin of the innominate artery (IA), left common carotid artery (LCC), and left subclavian artery (LSA) may be visualized. AA = aortic arch, ASC = ascending aorta, DSC = descending aorta, PA = pulmonary artery, RPA = right pulmonary artery.

image displays the heart at the center of the screen with the apex toward the left, and the base toward the right side of the monitor (Figure 4.4). If the parasternal window selected is too low, the transducer will be closer to the cardiac apex. The resulting image will be an oblique cross-sectional view of the heart and should be avoided because such distorted im-

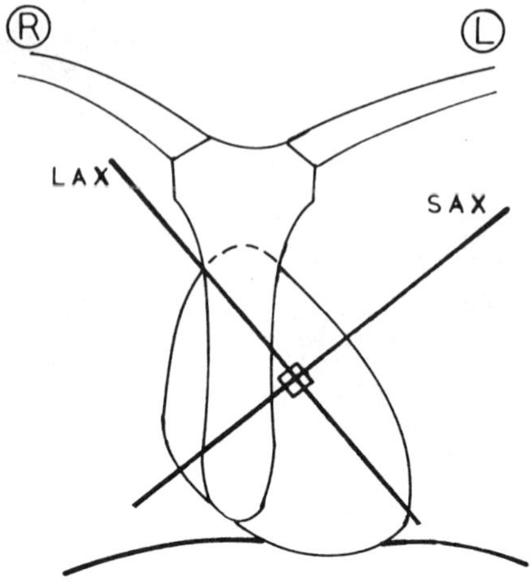

Figure 4.3
The plane of the ultrasound beam in the long axis view (LAX) and short axis view (SAX), relative to the heart. L = patient's left, R = patient's right.

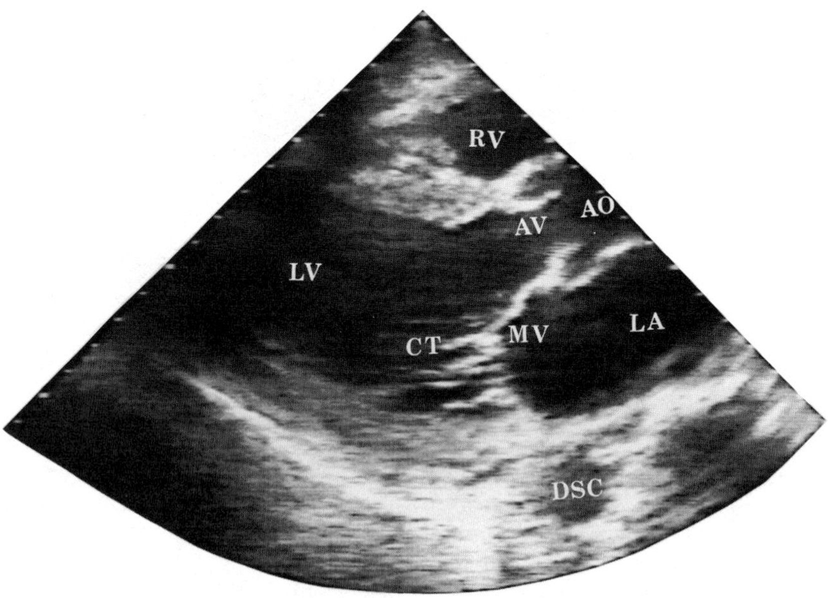

A

Figure 4.4
Two-dimensional cross-sectional image of the heart in the parasternal long axis view. A. In systole, the aortic valve (AV) is open and the mitral valve (MV) is closed. B. In diastole, the mitral valve is open and the aortic valve is closed. C. With the transducer in the parasternal long axis position, slight medial and inferior angulation allows the ultrasound beam to preferentially bisect the right atrium (RA) and ventricle only. This is the

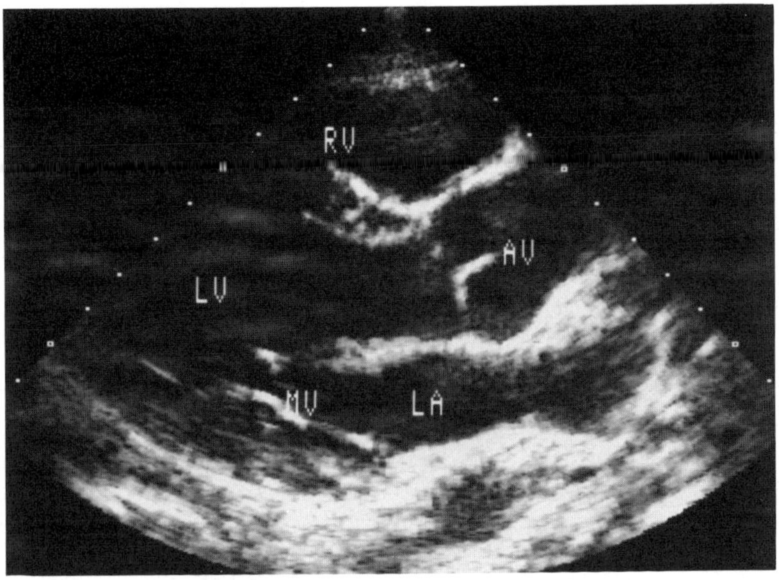

B

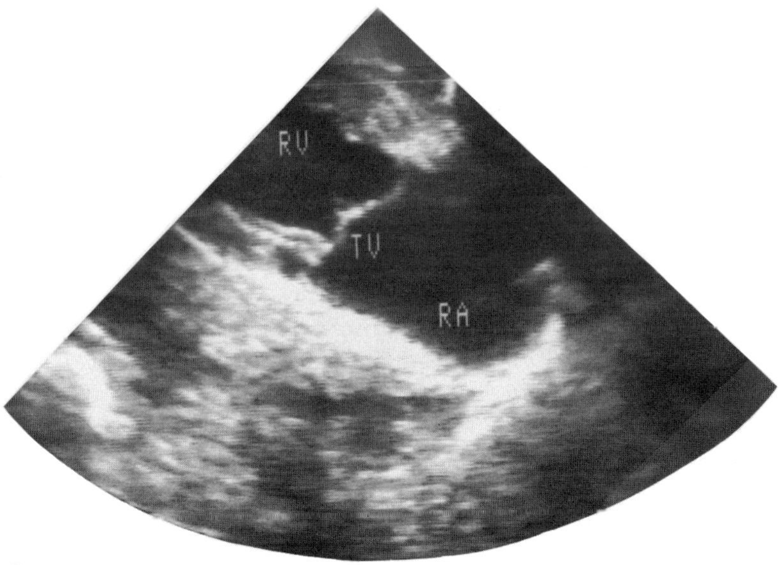

C

Figure 4.4 (continued)
right ventricular inflow tract view and is helpful in the evaluation of tricuspid valve (TV) disease and the right chambers. AO = aortic root, CT = chordae tendineae, DSC = descending aorta, LA = left atrium, LV = left ventricle, RV = right ventricle.

ages do not necessarily represent true cardiac function (Figure 4.5).

The most anterior cardiac chamber visualized in the parasternal long axis view is the right ventricle. The left ventricle lies posteriorly, with the interventricular septum separating these two chambers. The aorta arises from the left ventricle. The interventricular septum is continuous with the anterior wall of the aortic root, whereas the posterior wall of the aortic root is continuous with the anterior leaflet of the mitral valve. The left atrium lies posterior to the aortic root. One can also see the descending thoracic aorta as a circular structure outside the cardiac border, posterior to the left atrium at the atrioventricular groove (Figure 4.4).

Two-dimensional echocardiography provides real-time imaging of the heart as the myocardium contracts and relaxes and the valves open and close throughout the cardiac cycle. In systole, the interventricular septum and left ventricular posterior wall thicken and move toward each other, resulting in a decrease in the left ventricular internal dimension as blood is ejected into the aorta. During this phase of the cardiac cycle, the aortic valve opens, and its leaflets approximate the wall of the aorta. Only two leaflets can be seen at one time. These are the right and noncoronary cusps. The mitral valve opens in diastole and exhibits typical motion on the echocardiogram. The anterior leaflet moves anteriorly and the posterior leaflet moves posteriorly during the rapid filling period in early diastole. In diastasis, there is a decrease in the rate of transmitral blood flow, and the mitral leaflets slowly drift toward each other, assuming a semiopen position. Atrial contraction in late diastole reopens the valve for a brief interval, which is interrupted by left ventricular contraction, forcing the valve to close (Figures 4.4, 4.6).

Parasternal Short Axis View

Parasternal views of the heart can also be obtained by rotating the transducer 90 degress from the long axis orientation, so that the reference point is directed toward the patient's left shoulder. In this position, the two-dimensional ultrasound beam intersects the minor axis of the heart (Figure 4.3). Various cardiac structures can be viewed, depending on the direction of the ultrasound beam (Figure 4.7). Tilting the transducer superiorly and to the right causes the ultrasound beam to pass through the base of the heart. This view allows imaging of the chambers of the right side of the heart and pulmonary artery, including two of the three tricuspid valve leaflets and one or two of the three pulmonary valve leaflets (Figure 4.8). The three aortic leaflets can be

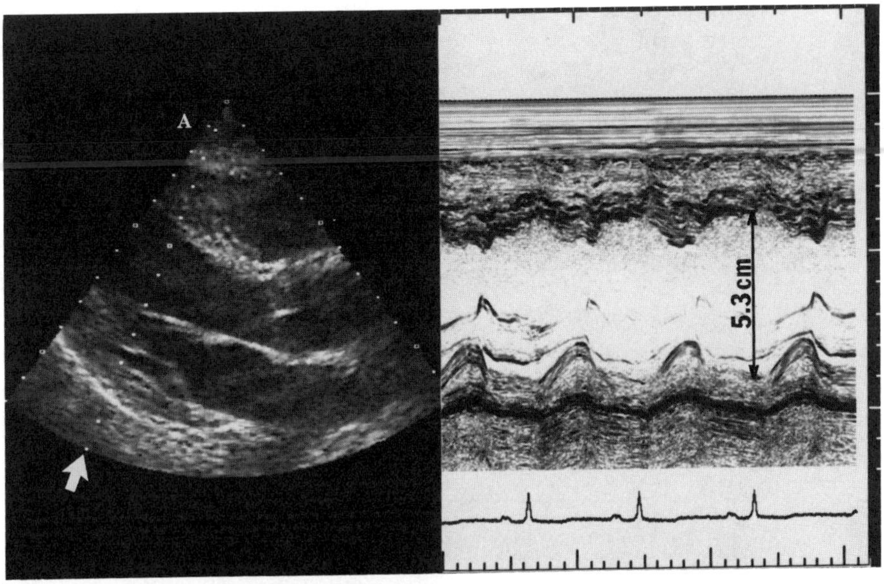

A

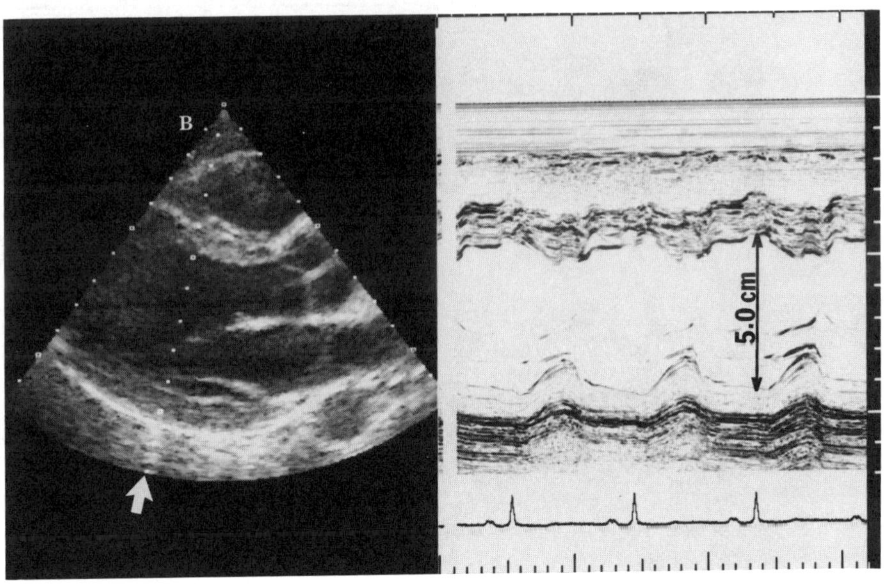

B

Figure 4.5
A. Parasternal long axis view with simultaneous M-mode recording of the left ventricle obtained from a low parasternal window. This is an oblique cross section of the left ventricle resulting in overestimation of left ventricular internal dimension. B. Similar view obtained from the proper parasternal window. The M-mode beam transects the left ventricle at a more perpendicular direction and results in a better estimate of its internal dimension. Note the relative position of the aortic root in B is closer to the transducer as compared to A. The arrows depict the path of the M-mode ultrasound beam.

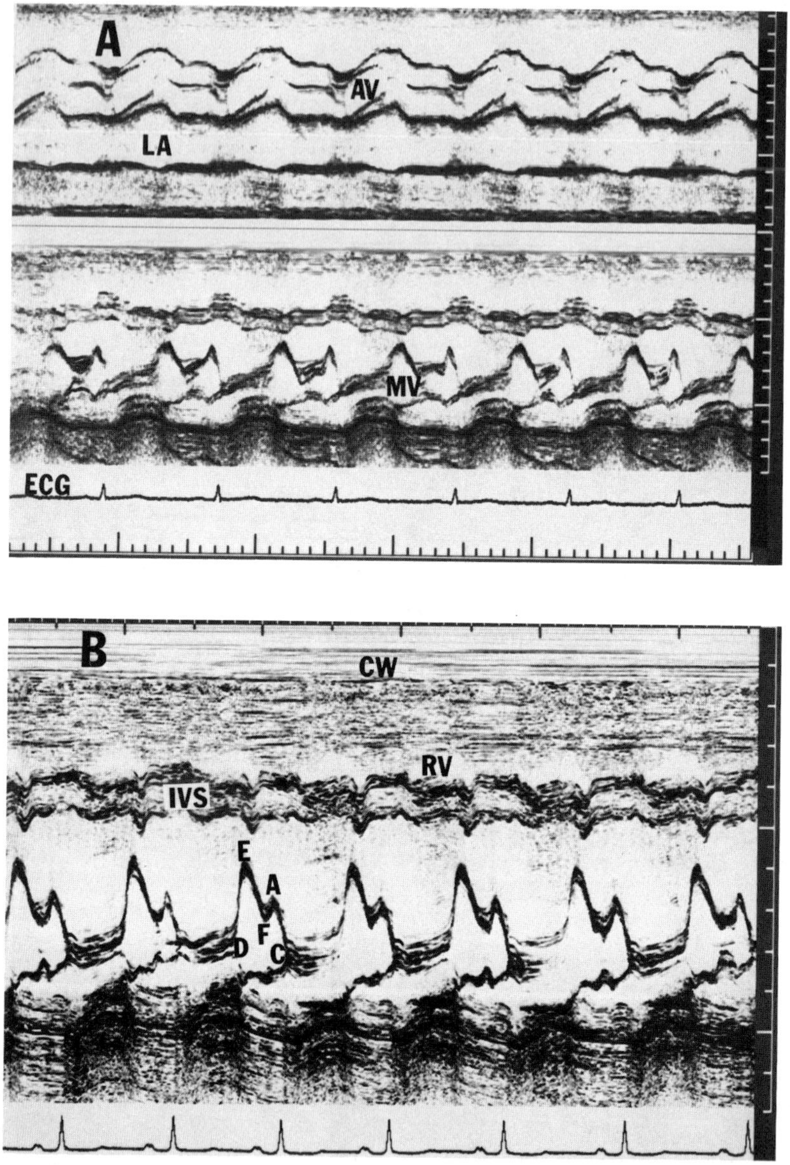

Figure 4.6
A. Simultaneous M-mode recording of the mitral and aortic valves showing opening and closure motion throughout the cardiac cycle. AV = aortic valve, ECG = electrocardiogram, LA = left atrium, MV = mitral valve. B. M-mode recording of the mitral valve motion in diastole. A = atrial contraction, C = leaflet closure, D = leaflet separation, E = peak leaflet excursion in early diastole, F = nadir of leaflet motion in diastasis, CW = chest wall, IVS = interventricular septum, RV = right ventricle.

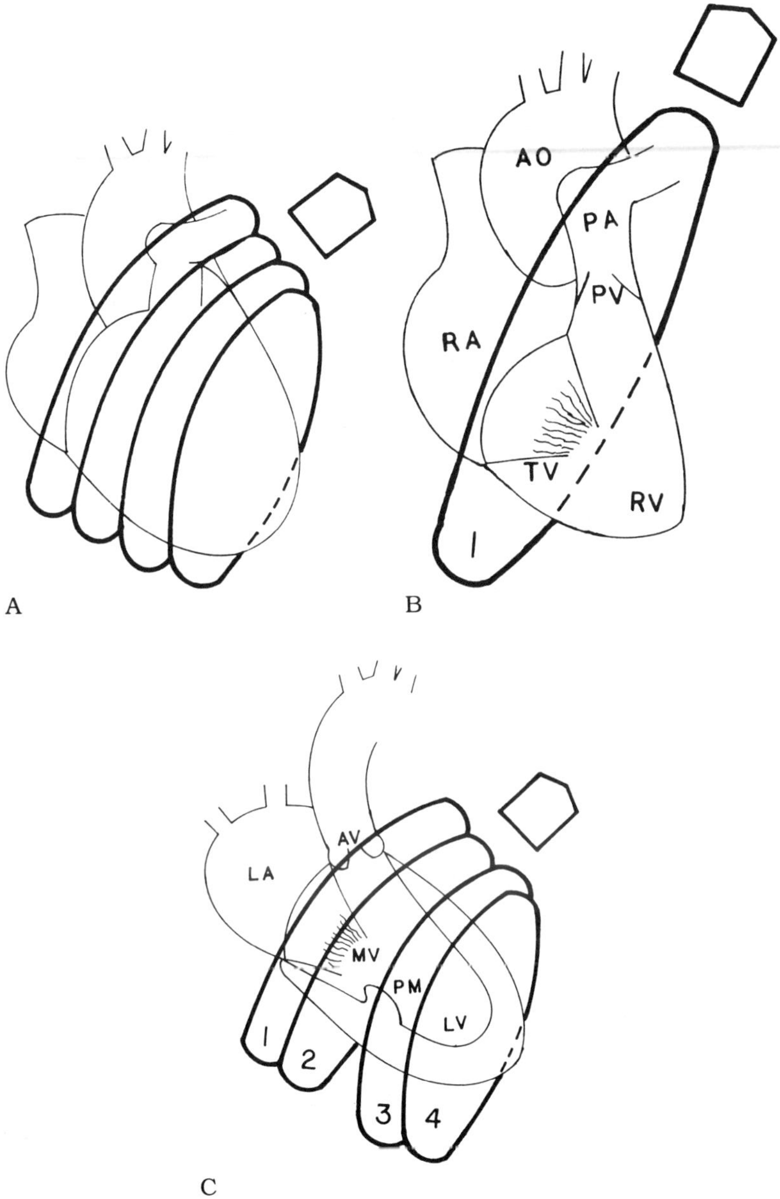

A B C

Figure 4.7
A. The transducer in the parasternal short axis view can be oriented to transect the heart at different imaging planes. B and C. Orienting the transducer at the base of the heart (plane 1), one can image the right chambers anteriorly and aortic valve (AV) and portion of the left atrium (LA), posteriorly. Imaging plane 2 transects the heart at the level of the mitral valve leaflets (MV). The left ventricle (LV) is imaged at the papillary muscle (PM) level in plane 3, and close to the apex in plane 4. AO = aorta, PA = pulmonary artery, PV = pulmonary valve, RA = right atrium, RV = right ventricle, TV = tricuspid valve.

seen within the circular cross section of the aortic root at the center of the monitor. In this view, the left atrial chamber is also seen posterior to the aortic root.

Motion of the cardiac valves can be observed throughout the cardiac cycle. In the open position, the three aortic leaflets approximate the inner wall of the aorta and form a triangle. In the closed position, the leaflet edges converge on each other, simulating the shape of the alphabet letter Y on the two-dimensional image (Figure 4.8).

Tilting the transducer in a position more perpendicular to the chest wall causes the plane of ultrasound beam to intersect the heart at the level of the mitral valve (Figures 4.7, 4.9). In this position, the right ventricle is visualized as a crescent shape at the top and to the left of the monitor. The mitral leaflets would be seen within the circular cross-sectional image of the left ventricular chamber. In the closed position, both mitral leaflets coapt, producing a linear horizontal echo. In the open position, the leaflets produce a typical fish-mouth appearance. The dimensions of the mitral valve orifice vary throughout the various phases of diastole.

When the transducer is tilted inferiorly and toward the

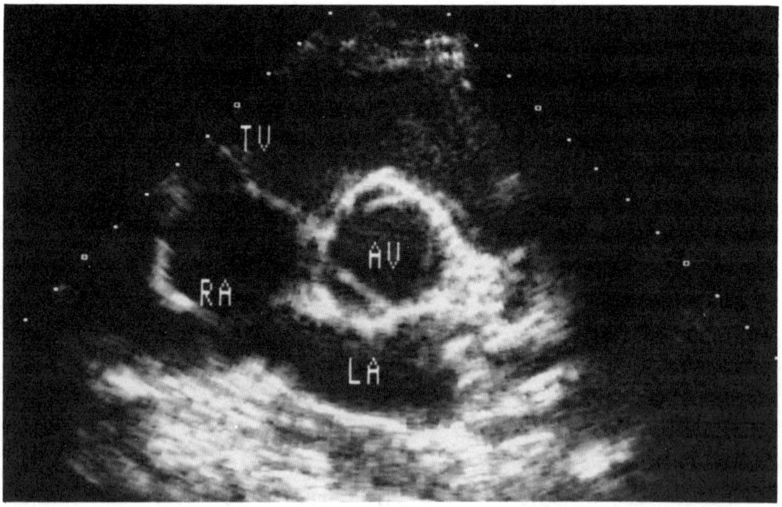

A

Figure 4.8
Systolic (A) and diastolic (B) frames of a short axis view at the base of the heart. C. Extensive medial angulation of the transducer allows imaging of the bifurcation of the pulmonary artery. AO = aorta; AV = aortic valve; LA = left atrium; MPA = main pulmonary artery; LPA, RPA = left and right pulmonary arteries, respectively; PV = pulmonary valve; RA, RV = right atrium and ventricle, respectively; TV = tricuspid valve.

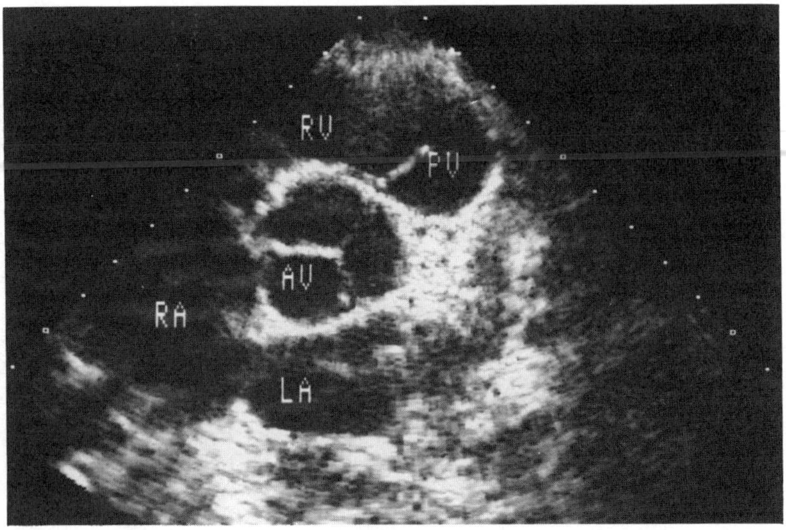

B

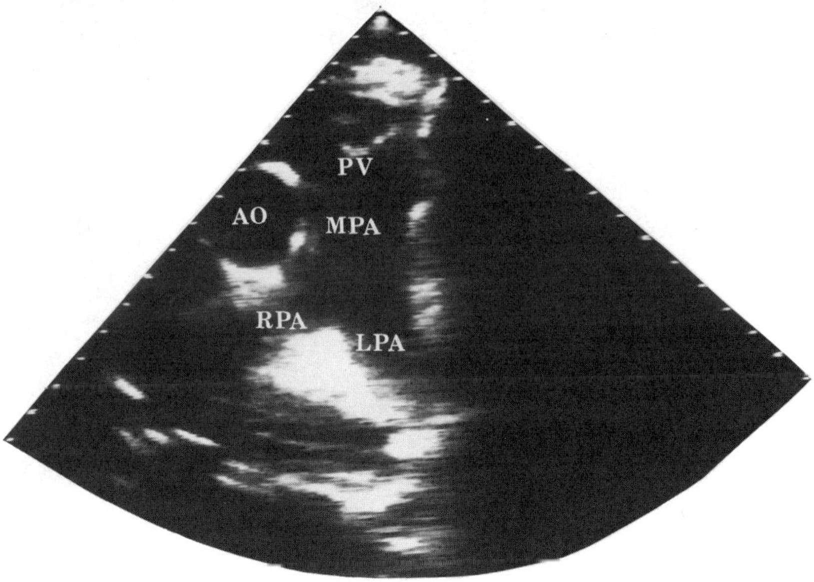

C

Figure 4.8 (continued)

apex of the heart, the two-dimensional plane of ultrasound bisects the midportion of the left ventricular chamber (Figures 4.7, 4.10). With this angulation of the transducer, the papillary muscles can be seen in the left ventricular cavity. The parasternal short axis view, at the level of the papillary muscles, is best suited to evaluate left ventricular contractile performance and segmental wall motion (Figure 4.11). In

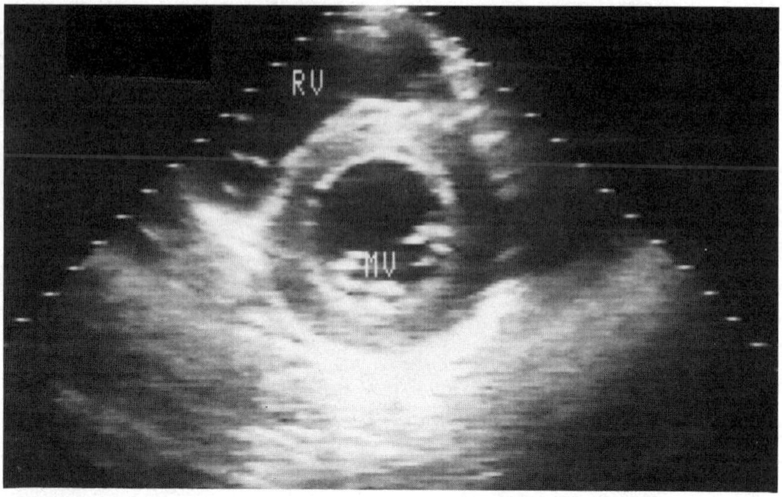

A

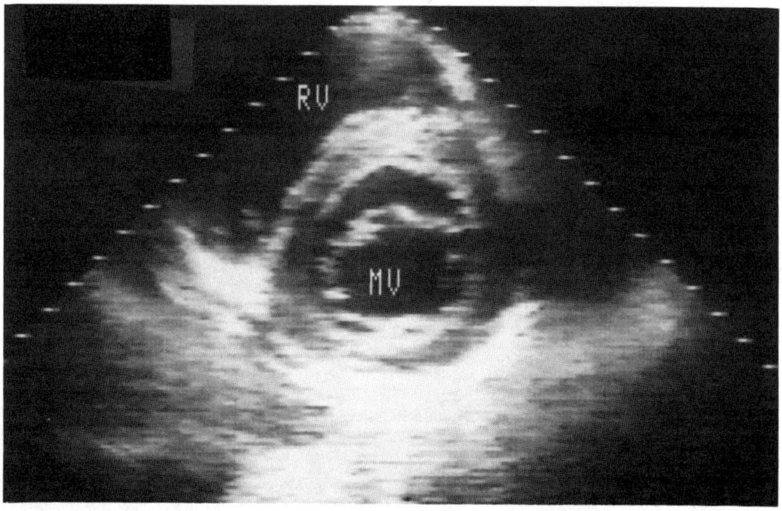

B

Figure 4.9
A. Systolic and B. Diastolic frames of a short axis view at the level of the mitral valve (MV). RV = right ventricle.

systole, left ventricular contraction causes a decrease in the internal diameter with thickening of the walls of the ventricle. The opposite happens in diastole. Hence, continuous imaging of the left ventricular chamber in this view will exhibit the cyclical changes in the dimensions of the left ventricle between systole and diastole. Further tilting of the transducer inferiorly directs the plane of imaging closer to the left ventricular apex.

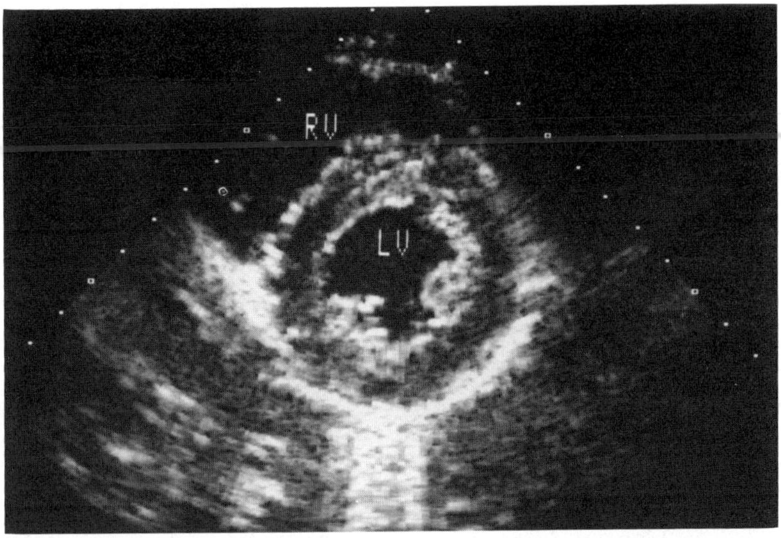

A

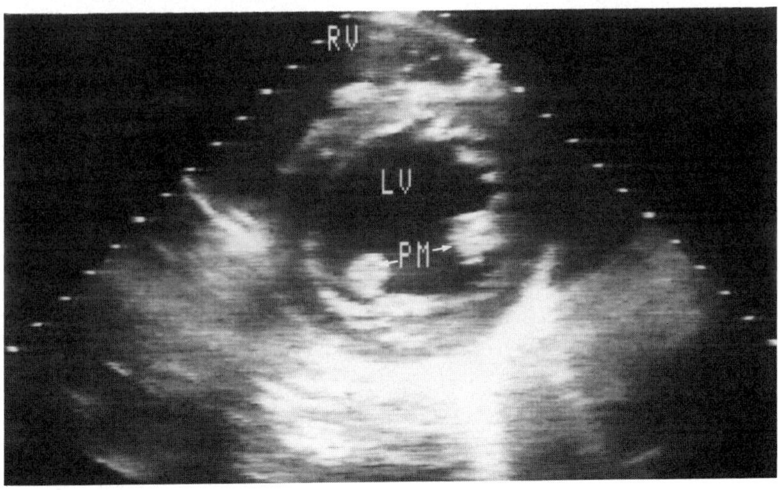

B

Figure 4.10
A. Systolic and B. Diastolic frames of a parasternal short axis view at the level of the papillary muscles (PM). RV = right ventricle, LV = left ventricle.

Apical Views

To obtain these views, the transducer is positioned at the cardiac apex and angulated superiorly toward the right shoulder (Figures 4.1, 4.12). The apical long axis view is obtained by orienting the reference point on the transducer superiorly toward the patient's right shoulder. The ul-

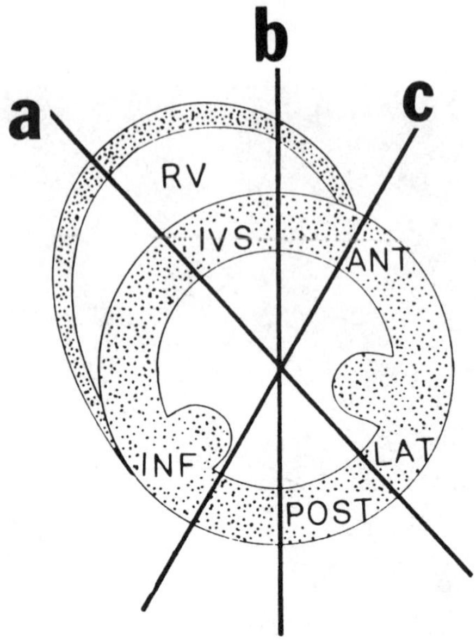

Figure 4.11
A short axis view at the level of the papillary muscle, depicting the various segments of the left ventricular walls. In the apical four-chamber view, the direction of the ultrasound beam (a) bisects the left ventricle through the interventrical septum (IVS) and lateral wall (LAT). In the apical or parasternal long axis view, the ultrasound beam (b) bisects the left ventricle through the interventricular septum and posterior wall (POST). In the apical two-chamber view, the ultrasound beam (c) bisects the left ventricle through the anterior (ANT) and inferior (INF) walls.

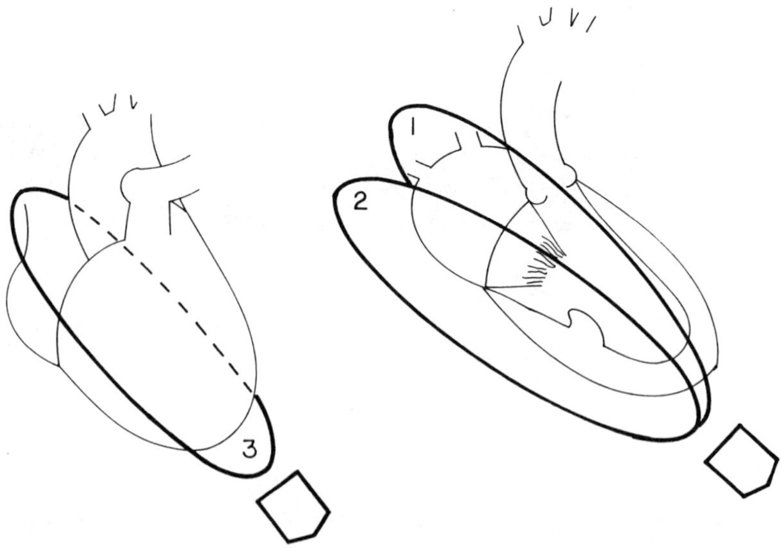

Figure 4.12
The transducer at an apical window can be oriented to transect the heart at different imaging planes. Imaging plane 1 results in the apical long axis view. Imaging planes 2 and 3 result in the apical two-chamber and four-chamber views, respectively.

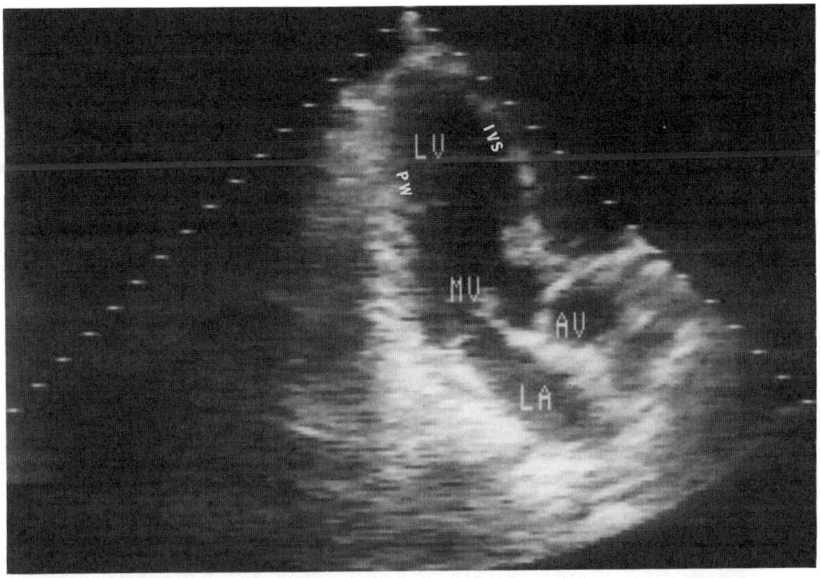

Figure 4.13
Apical long axis view. This plane transects the interventricular septum (IVS) and left ventricular posterior wall (PW). (See Figure 4.11.) AV = aortic valve, LA = left atrium, LV = left ventricle, MV = mitral valve.

trasound beam traverses the heart in the same plane as that observed for the parasternal long axis view (Figure 4.3). However, since the transducer is positioned at the cardiac apex, the resulting image displays the heart upside down so that the apex is at the top of the monitor and the base is at the bottom (Figures 4.12, 4.13).

Rotating the transducer so that the reference point is directed toward the patient's left side of the neck causes the ultrasound beam to bisect the chambers on the left side of the heart only. This is the apical two-chamber view, which allows visualization of the left atrium and left ventricle (Figure 4.14). This view allows visualization of the anterior and inferior walls of the left ventricle, and it is important in the evaluation of segmental wall motion abnormalities. (Figure 4.11).

All four cardiac chambers can also be imaged from the apical window by orienting the reference point on the transducer toward the patient's left shoulder (Figure 4.12). This is the apical four-chamber view, which images both ventricles and atria simultaneously (Figure 4.15). This view is useful in the evaluation of the left ventricular lateral wall (Figure 4.11), right ventricular anterior wall, and the mitral and tricuspid valves. The interventricular and interatrial septae can be observed in this view as well.

The apical five-chamber view is a variant of the apical four-

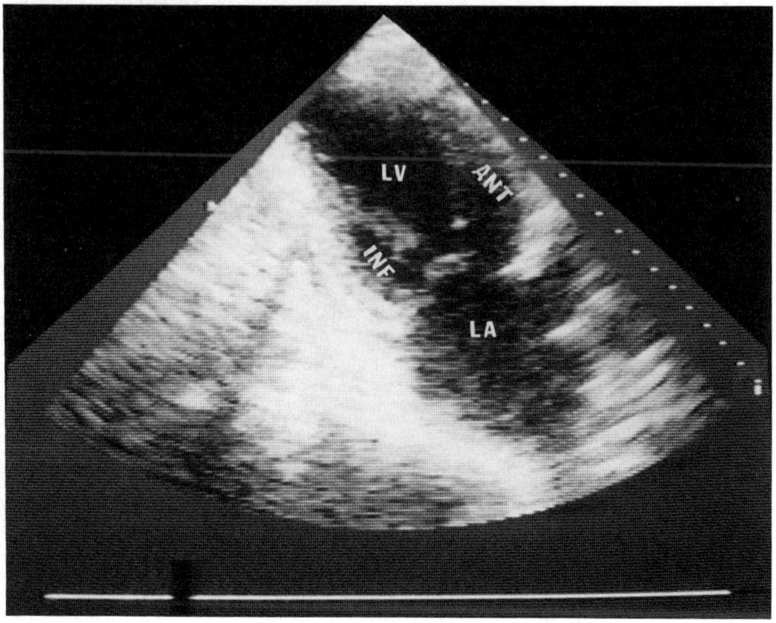

Figure 4.14
The apical two-chamber view depicts the left chambers only. This plane transects the left ventricular anterior (ANT) and inferior (INF) walls. (See Figure 4.11.) LV = left ventricle, LA = left atrium.

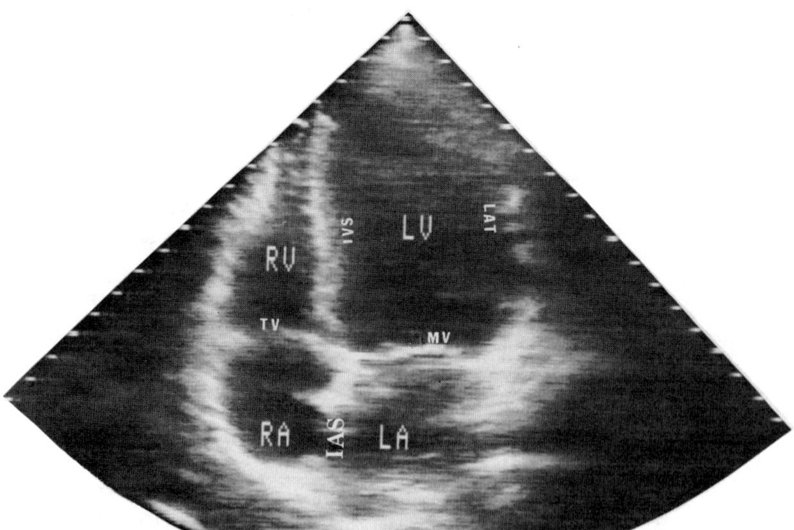

Figure 4.15
The apical four-chamber view depicts the four cardiac chambers. This plane transects the interventricular septum (IVS) and left ventricular lateral wall (LAT). RV = right ventricle, LV = left ventricle, RA = right atrium, LA = left atrium, IAS = interatrial septum, MV = mitral valve, TV = tricuspid valve.

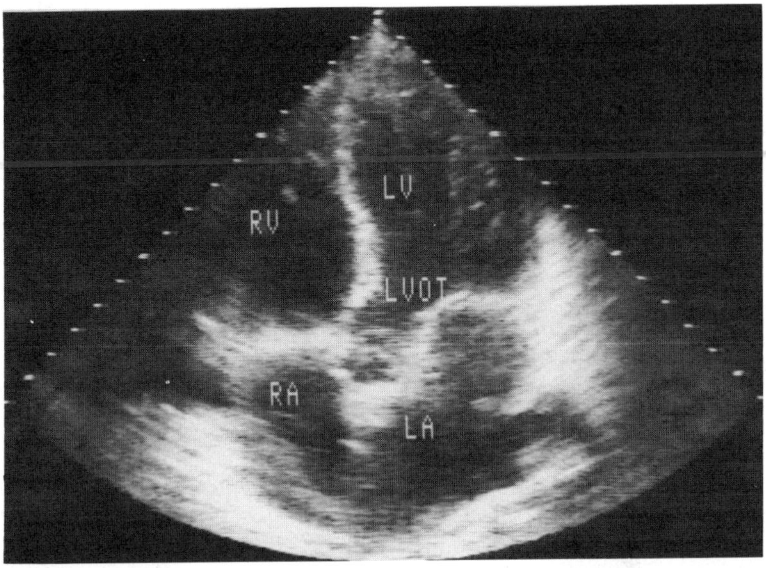

Figure 4.16
The apical five-chamber view is angulated anteriorly to visualize the four cardiac chambers and the left ventricular outflow tract (LVOT). LA = left atrium, LV = left ventricle, RA = right atrium, RV = right ventricle.

chamber view, in which the transducer is tilted more anteriorly so that the ultrasound beam traverses the left ventricular outflow tract and aortic valve (Figure 4.16).

Subcostal Views

In the subcostal approach to cardiac imaging, the ultrasound beam travels through the abdominal wall, a portion of the liver, and the diaphragm before it arrives at the heart (Figure 4.1). This approach produces angulated images of the heart and is a suitable alternative to the other standard acoustic windows, particularly in patients with chronic lung disease in whom the hyperinflated lungs obstruct the path of the ultrasound beam from the standard parasternal views.

Similar to the apical four-chamber view, the subcostal four-chamber view allows visualization of both ventricles and atria, as well as the atrioventricular valves. This view is obtained by directing the reference point on the ultrasound transducer toward the right shoulder, with anterior and superior angulation of the transducer (Figures 4.17, 4.18). Frequently, gentle pressure must be applied on the transducer to allow the ultrasound beam to pass from under the boney rib cage. From this transducer location, the base of the heart is displayed to the left of the monitor and the apex

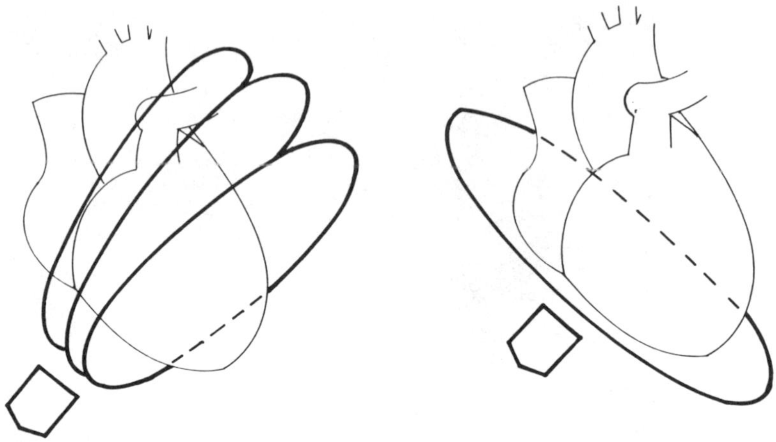

Figure 4.17
The transducer at the subcostal window can be oriented to image the heart at different planes.

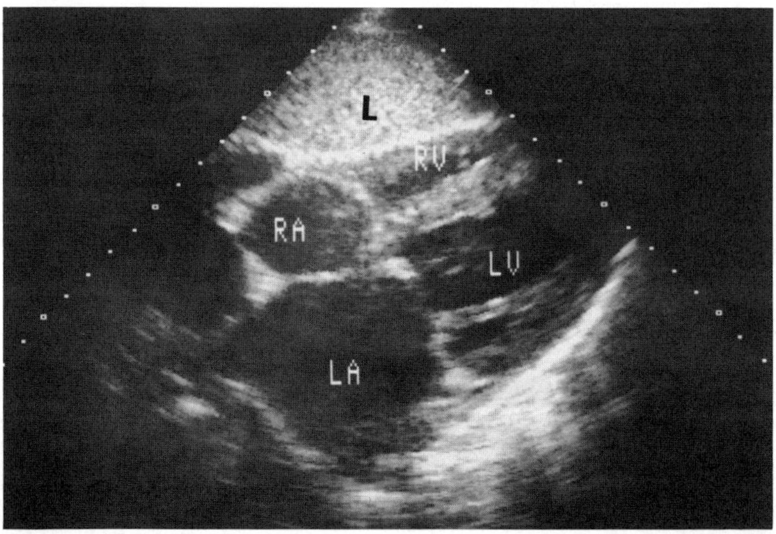

Figure 4.18
Subcostal four-chamber view. L = liver, RA = right atrium, LA = left atrium, LV = left ventricle, RV = right ventricle.

is displayed to the right, pointing upward. The chambers on the right side of the heart are closer to the transducer and are displayed anterior to the left chambers.

Because of its anatomic location, the plane of the interatrial septum is almost perpendicular to the path of the ultrasound beam. This produces better echocardiographic images of this structure than those obtained from the apical four-chamber view because, from the apex, the ultrasound beam travels a path parallel to the interatrial septum (Figure 4.15). The anatomic relation of the plane of the interatrial septum to the path of the ultrasound beam is of particular importance when patients with suspected atrial septal defect are being evaluated, as will be discussed in Chapter 12.

Short axis views of the heart can be obtained from the subcostal window by rotating the transducer so that the reference point is directed toward the left side of the neck (Figure 4.17). By varying the direction of the ultrasound beam, images almost similar to those obtained from the parasternal short axis view can be obtained (Figure 4.19A). The inferior vena cava is best visualized by the subcostal approach (Figure 4.19B).

M-mode Echocardiography

M-mode recordings of the cardiac structures are best obtained from the parasternal window. From this location, the ultrasound beam can be maneuvered to examine all cardiac valves and the basal portion of the cardiac chambers. Most current ultrasound equipment is capable of performing M-mode and two-dimensional echocardiography with the same transducer. This has proved to be a valuable feature that greatly enhances the ease and rapidity of obtaining M-mode recordings. From a parasternal two-dimensional view, the operator can electronically maneuver the M-mode cursor to pass through the various cardiac structures and obtain the required M-mode echocardiographic images (Figure 4.6).

Aortic Root and Aortic Valve

M-mode recordings of the aortic root and aortic valve can be obtained from the parasternal long axis two-dimensional view or the parasternal short axis view at the level of the aortic root. The path of the M-mode cursor on the two-dimensional image delineates the section of the aortic root and valve being recorded on M-mode echocardiography. Echoes reflected from the anterior and posterior walls of the aortic root appear as two parallel lines. In systole, ventricular contraction causes the aortic root to move anteriorly, closer to the chest wall; during diastolic relaxation the aortic root moves posteriorly, away from the chest wall. Hence, the M-mode recording typically shows two parallel echoes that exhibit wavy motion patterns throughout the cardiac cycle (Figure 4.6).

Two of the three aortic valve leaflets can be seen within the aortic root. In diastole, these leaflets coapt and produce a

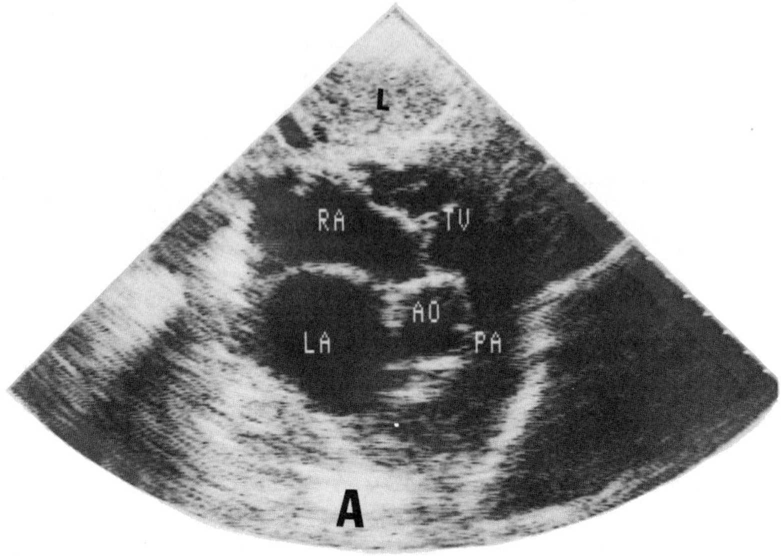

A

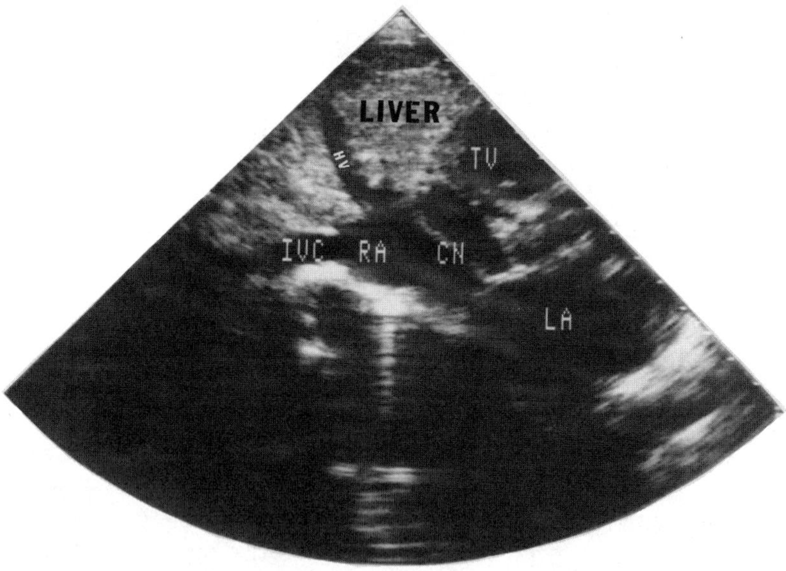

B

Figure 4.19
A. Subcostal short axis view at the base of the heart. Note the similarity of this view to the standard parasternal short axis view at the same level. B. Angulated subcostal view depicting the inferior vena cava (IVC) draining into the right atrium (RA). CN = chiari network (see Chapter 14), HV = hepatic vein, LA = left atrium, TV = tricuspid valve, AO = aortic root, PA = pulmonary artery.

linear echo at the center of the aortic root. In systole, ventricular ejection forces the leaflets to separate; the right coronary cusp moves anteriorly and approximates the anterior aortic wall, and the noncoronary cusp moves toward the posterior wall of the aorta. The aortic valve remains open throughout the ejection phase in systole, and promptly closes at end systole–beginning diastole.

The left atrium appears as an echo-free space situated posterior to the aortic root. The posterior wall of the left atrium is depicted as a dense linear echo that exhibits minimal undulating motion throughout the cardiac cycle (Figure 4.6).

Mitral Valve

M-mode recordings of the mitral valve can be obtained from the parasternal long axis view by moving the cursor through this valve (Figure 4.6). As the M-mode ultrasound beam travels through the chest wall, the right ventricular outflow tract is seen anteriorly. The basal portion of the interventricular septum is reflected as thick echoes that exhibit anterior and posterior motion throughout the cardiac cycle. As the ultrasound beam traverses the mitral valve, motion of the anterior and posterior leaflets can be recorded. In systole, both leaflets coapt, producing multiple linear echoes. Early in diastole, during the rapid filling phase, the leaflets separate; one leaflet moves anteriorly and the other leaflet posteriorly. Echoes reflected from the anterior leaflet rapidly approach the left ventricular side of the interventricular septum, then gradually move posteriorly in diastasis into a semiopen positon. Left atrial contraction in late diastole forces the valve to reopen so that the anterior leaflet moves again anteriorly. Finally, ventricular systolic contraction causes rapid posterior motion into the closed position. This series of anterior and posterior motion of the anterior mitral leaflet exhibits a characteristic M-shaped pattern on the M-mode echocardiograms. The smaller posterior leaflet of the mitral valve also exhibits similar motion but in the opposite direction, so that the M-mode recordings simulate a W-shaped pattern in diastole.

Posterior to the mitral valve, the ultrasound beam traverses the basal portion of the left ventricular posterior wall and mitral annulus. These structures produce thick echoes with variable motion throughout the cardiac cycle.

The Left Ventricle

From the same parasternal long axis two-dimensional view, moving the M-mode cursor inferior to the mitral valve allows

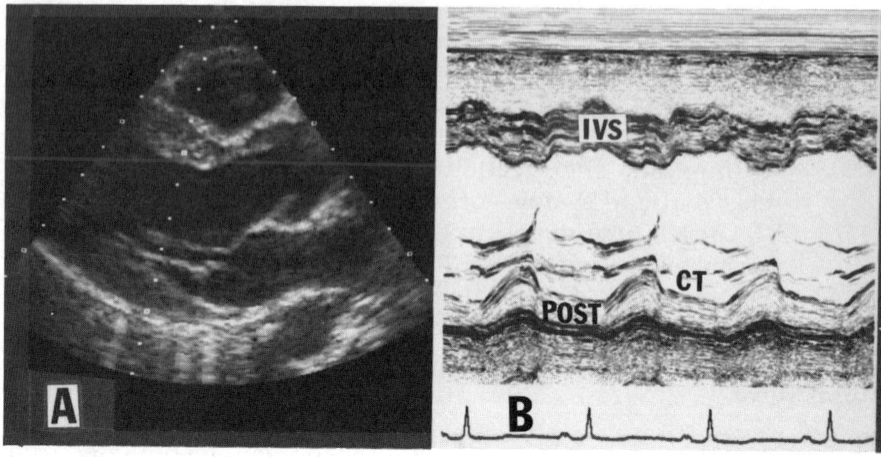

Figure 4.20
A. Parasternal long axis view. The vertical dotted line depicts the path of the ultrasound beam employed for M-mode imaging of the left ventricle. B. M-mode of the left ventricle showing the motion of the interventricular septum (IVS) and posterior wall (POST) throughout the cardiac cycle. CT = chordae tendineae.

the ultrasound beam to traverse the right ventricular chamber, interventricular septum, and the left ventricular posterior wall (Figure 4.20). Systolic contraction and diastolic relaxation of the left ventricular myocardium can be easily appreciated from these recordings. In systole, the interventricular septum thickens and moves into the left ventricular cavity away from the transducer, whereas the left ventricular posterior wall thickens and moves into the left ventricular cavity, toward the transducer. In diastole, the interventricular septum and left ventricular posterior wall become thinner and move back to a more neutral position. In diastole, the opened mitral valve allows the left ventricle to fill with blood, which is later ejected into the aorta in systole. Thus, the opposing motion of the interventricular septum and left ventricular posterior wall throughout the cardiac cycle reflects the instantaneous changes in size of the left ventricular chamber. One can estimate these changes by measuring the distance between the interventricular septum and left ventricular posterior wall at end diastole and end systole. The degree of change of left ventricular internal dimension, as well as the degree of motion of the interventricular septum and posterior wall, represents a measure of left ventricular contractile performance. This will be discussed in Chapter 19.

The chordae tendineae that attach the mitral leaflets to the papillary muscles are often recorded on the M-mode echocardiogram. These appear as multiple thin linear echoes in close proximity to the left ventricular posterior wall, and should be distinguished from the true endocardial echoes originating from the posterior wall itself (Figures 4.4, 4.20).

If the M-mode cursor is moved further inferiorly, it may pass through the posterior papillary muscle situated at the midventricular level. The resulting M-mode recordings are similar to those obtained from the left ventricular chamber already described. However, the left ventricular internal dimension would be smaller and the echoes reflected from the posterior wall would be thicker. Estimates of left ventricular contractile performance from these M-mode recordings should be avoided since they do not reflect ventricular size and function adequately.

Tricuspid Valve

From a parasternal short axis two-dimensional view, the M-mode cursor can be directed to pass through the tricuspid valve (Figure 4.21). The tricuspid valve exhibits a motion pattern similar to that described for the anterior mitral leaflet. However, because of its location in the heart, closer to the chest wall, usually only one leaflet can be visualized on M-mode echocardiography at any one time.

Pulmonary Valve

The pulmonary valve can be recorded from the parasternal short axis two-dimensional view (Figure 4.21). Since the pulmonary valve is situated anteriorly, just below the sternum, usually only the posterior leaflet can bc rccorded. In diastole, this leaflet causes oblique linear echoes with a small notch (A wave) caused by a forceful contraction of the right atrium. Right ventricular contraction forces the pulmonary valve to open so that the posterior leaflet exhibits rapid posterior motion on the M-mode tracing in early systole, followed by gradual return to a more neutral position in late systole.

The M-mode Sweep

From a parasternal long axis two-dimensional view, the M-mode cursor positioned at either edge of the image can be slowly moved to the other side of the monitor during continuous recording of the M-mode echocardiogram. This allows M-mode recordings of the left ventricular chamber, mitral valve, and aortic root in continuous succession, without interruption of the recording process (Figure 2.7). This maneuver is helpful in delineating the continuity of various

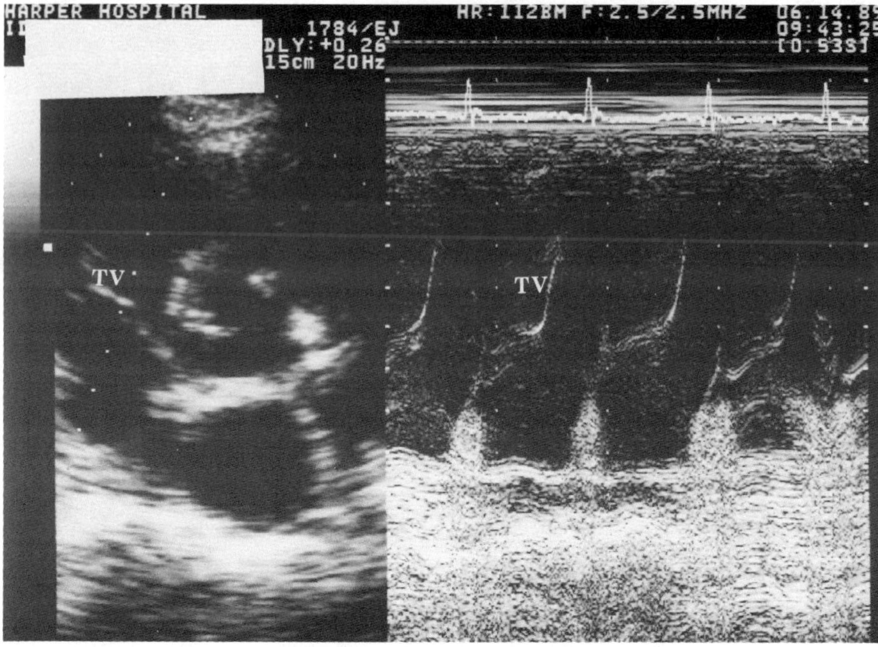

A

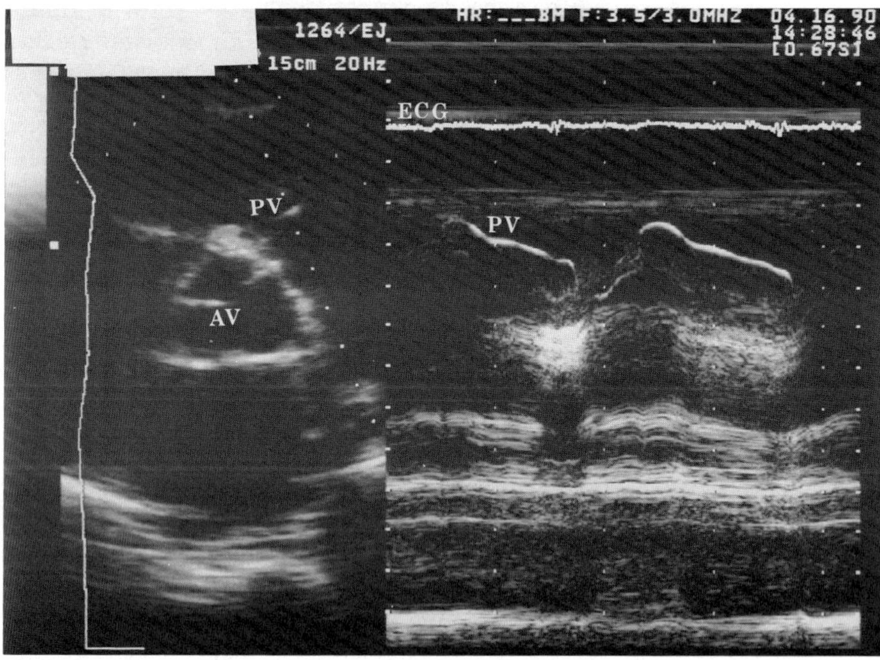

B

Figure 4.21

A. Short axis view at the base of the heart showing the path of the ultrasound beam employed for imaging the tricuspid valve (TV) and pulmonary valve. B. Parasternal short axis view in diastole showing the posterior leaflet of the pulmonic valve (PV). The dotted line on the 2-dimensional image depicts the path of the M-mode ultrasound beam with simultaneous M-mode image of the posterior PV leaflet. AV = aortic valve, ECG = electrocardiogram.

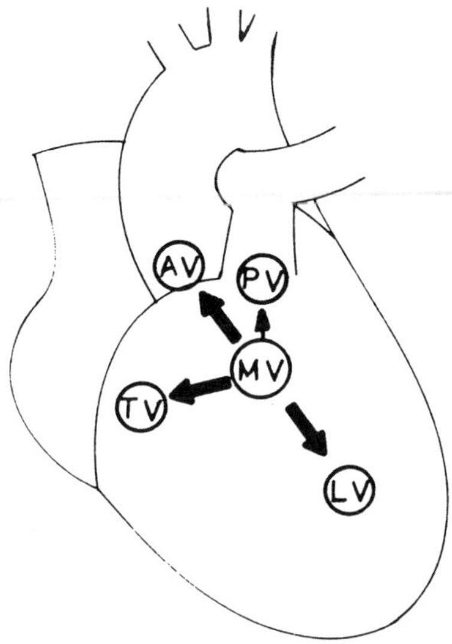

Figure 4.22
The position of various cardiac structures relative to the mitral valve (MV). PV = pulmonary valve, LV = left ventricle, TV = tricuspid valve, AV = aortic valve.

cardiac structures, particularly in patients with suspected congenital heart disease or pericardial effusion.

Independent M-mode Recordings

M-mode echocardiography was prevalent during the early years of cardiac imaging by ultrasound, prior to the development of two-dimensional echocardiography. One can still find a few such ultrasound units capable of performing M-mode echocardiography only. The technique of M-mode recording without the assistance of simultaneous two-dimensional imaging depends on adequate operator knowledge of cardiac anatomy. Instead of an electronically steered M-mode cursor, the operator has to manually tilt the transducer to direct the ultrasound beam toward the cardiac structures to be recorded.

The M-mode recording is usually started by positioning the transducer at the second or third left parasternal window. Keeping the transducer perpendicular to the chest wall, the mitral valve can be easily recorded. The aortic valve is recorded by tilting the transducer medially and superiorly toward the right shoulder, whereas tilting the transducer in the opposite direction, inferiorly and laterally, allows recording of the left ventricular chamber. The tricuspid valve is recorded by tilting the transducer medially and inferiorly.

Tilting the transducer superiorly and medially allows recording of the pulmonary valve (Figure 4.22).

Adequate recording of various cardiac structures requires skillful maneuvering that only comes with practice. The procedure is further complicated by cardiac pathologic conditions with alterations of its anatomy relative to the chest wall. Fortunately, two-dimensional echocardiography has significantly simplified the technique of M-mode echocardiography so that independent M-mode recording has been largely abandoned.

5 Cardiac Doppler Ultrasonography

Normal flow across the cardiac valves is pulsatile and occurs at different time intervals within the cardiac cycle. Moreover, flow occurs in different directions, depending on the cardiac valve being examined.

Normal Directions of Blood Flow

Normal Mitral Flow

The normal flow pattern across the mitral valve closely resembles the normal M-mode echocardiographic appearance of the anterior leaflet of the mitral valve (Figure 5.1). This is expected because opening of the mitral valve is dependent on the amount of flow across it. As has been described earlier regarding the diastolic events in the cardiac cycle (Figure 1.7), there is no flow across the mitral valve during the isovolumic relaxation period. As soon as the left ventricular diastolic pressure drops below the left atrial pressure, the mitral leaflets separate and flow starts from the left atrium into the left ventricle. Inertial forces cause a minimal time delay between opening of the valve and beginning of flow. The rapid filling phase shows an initial increase of blood flow velocity followed by a sharp deceleration during diastasis (Figure 5.1). The atrial kick is forceful enough to push more blood across the valve, hence causing a second rise in blood flow velocity toward the end of diastole. Flow does not stop with the onset of the next QRS complex; however, flow stops shortly afterward when ventricular contraction has gener-

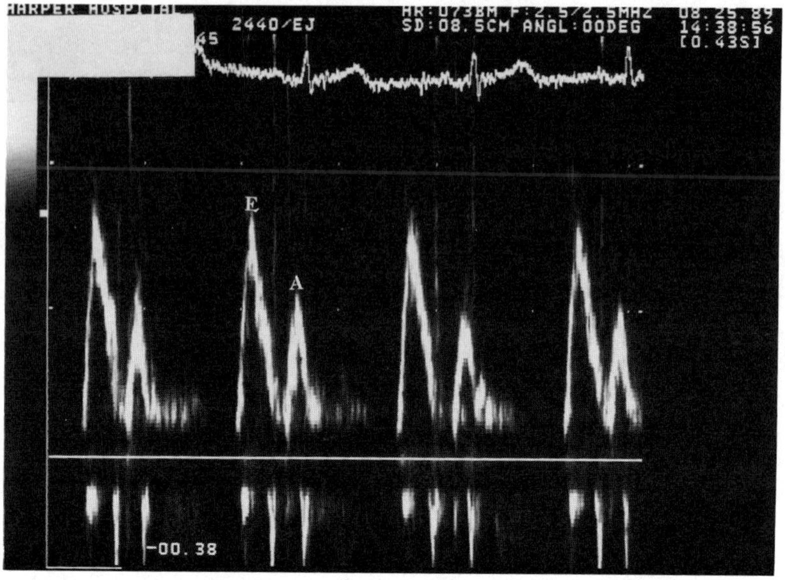

Figure 5.1
Normal transmitral flow recorded with the transducer in an apical location. Blood flows in diastole from the left atrium into the left ventricle, toward the Doppler transducer. Blood flow peaks in early diastole (E), slows in diastasis, and peaks again after atrial contraction (A). Note that peak E velocity is higher than peak A velocity.

ated enough pressure to exceed left atrial pressure and close the mitral valve (Figure 5.1).

Normal Aortic Flow

As soon as the left ventricle generates sufficient pressure to exceed aortic diastolic pressure, the aortic valve opens and ejection begins. Hence, there is no aortic flow during the preejection period in early systole (Figure 1.7). Blood flows from the left ventricle to the ascending aorta. The velocity of blood flow demonstrates fast acceleration during early systole, reaching a peak before midsystole, then a slow deceleration until flow ceases at end systole (Figure 5.2). Minimal retrograde flow may be recorded immediately after the end of ejection. There is no flow across the aortic valve in diastole.

Normal Tricuspid Flow

Normal flow across the tricuspid valve resembles that across the mitral valve, except that peak velocities of flow across the

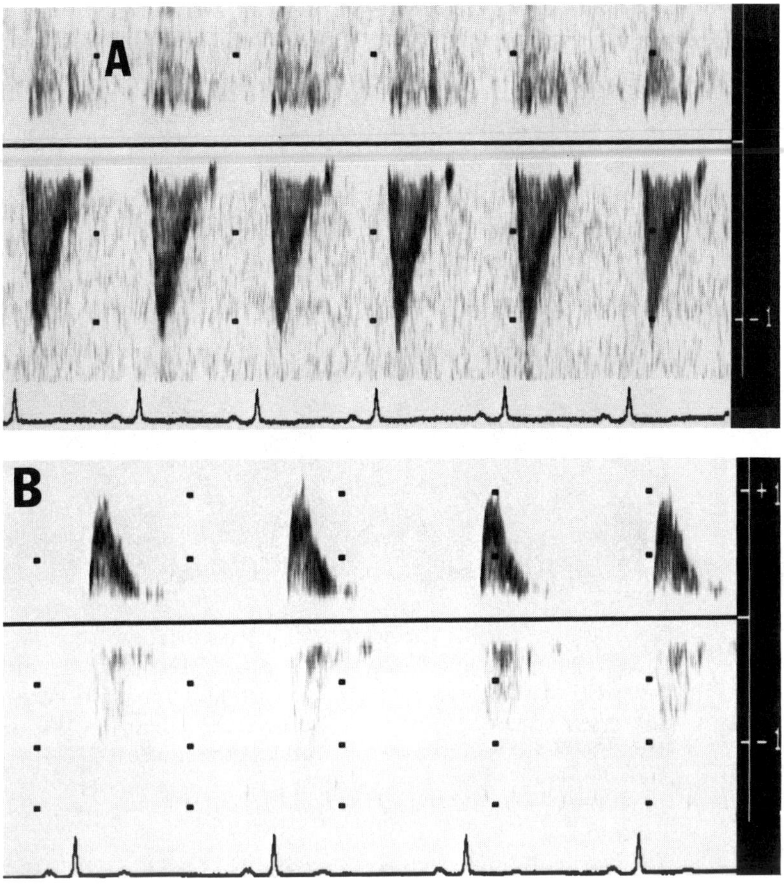

Figure 5.2
A. Normal transaortic flow recorded with the transducer in an apical location. Blood flows in systole from the left ventricle into the aorta, away from the Doppler transducer. B. Normal transaortic flow recorded from a suprasternal location. Blood flows in systole toward the Doppler transducer.

tricuspid valve are generally less than the corresponding values across the mitral valve (Figure 5.3) (Table 5.1).

Normal Pulmonary Flow

Blood flow across the pulmonary valve is similar to that across the aortic valve (Figure 5.4). However, right ventricular ejection time and, thus, the duration of pulmonary flow is longer than left ventricular ejection time. Also, peak velocities of pulmonary flow occur in midsystole with gradual acceleration and deceleration.

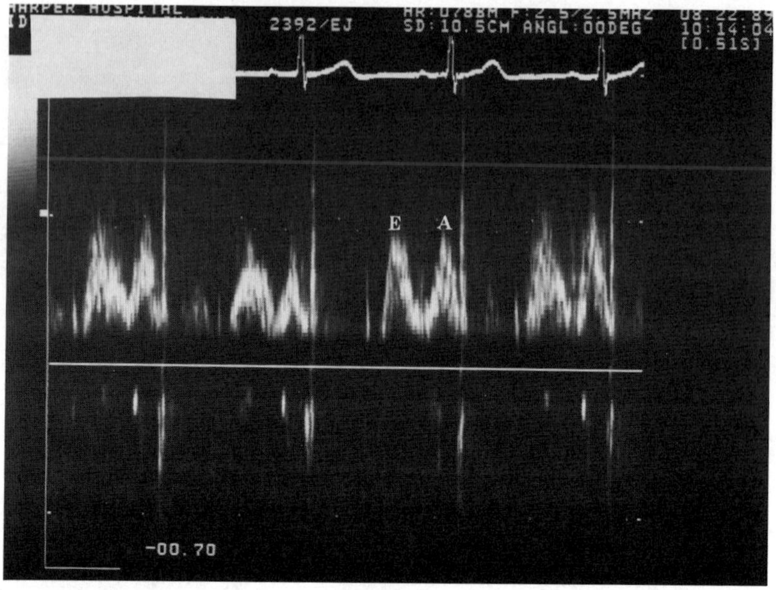

Figure 5.3
Normal flow across the tricuspid valve recorded from an apical location. Note the similarity of this flow pattern to transmitral flow except that the peak velocities across the tricuspid valve are usually lower than the corresponding velocities across the mitral valve. E = early diastole, A = atrial contraction.

Table 5.1
Normal peak flow velocities across the cardiac valves in adults[a]

	Average (cm/sec)	Range (cm/sec)
Mitral valve[b]	90	60–130
Aortic valve	135	100–170
Tricuspid valve[b]	50	30–70
Pulmonary valve	75	60–90

[a]These values may differ slightly depending on the source of reference.
[b]There are no published data on the peak velocities of flow after the atrial kick. However, they are normally less than the peak velocities of flow in early diastole.

Superior and Inferior Venae Cavae

Flow in the superior and inferior venae cavae is triphasic (Figure 5.5). Flow is toward the right atrium during early diastole. The atrial kick generates enough pressure so that flow either stops or becomes temporarily reversed. Flow then resumes toward the right atrium during ventricular systole.

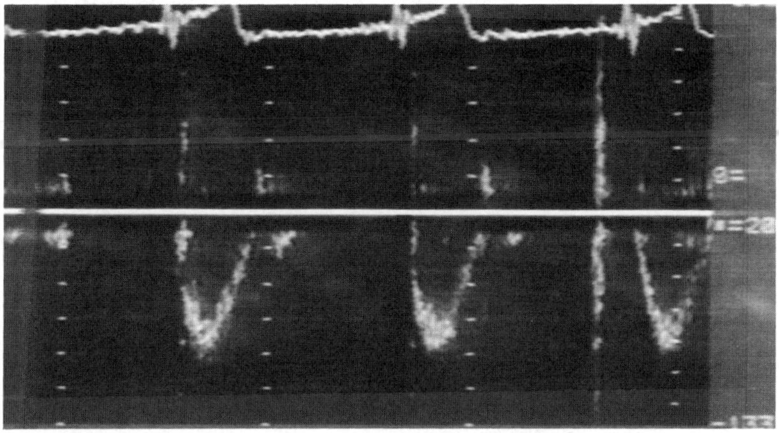

Figure 5.4
Normal flow across the pulmonary valve recorded with the transducer in a parasternal location. Flow is in systole, away from the Doppler transducer. Note that peak velocity of flow is not as sharply delineated as that of transaortic flow, and occurs in midsystole.

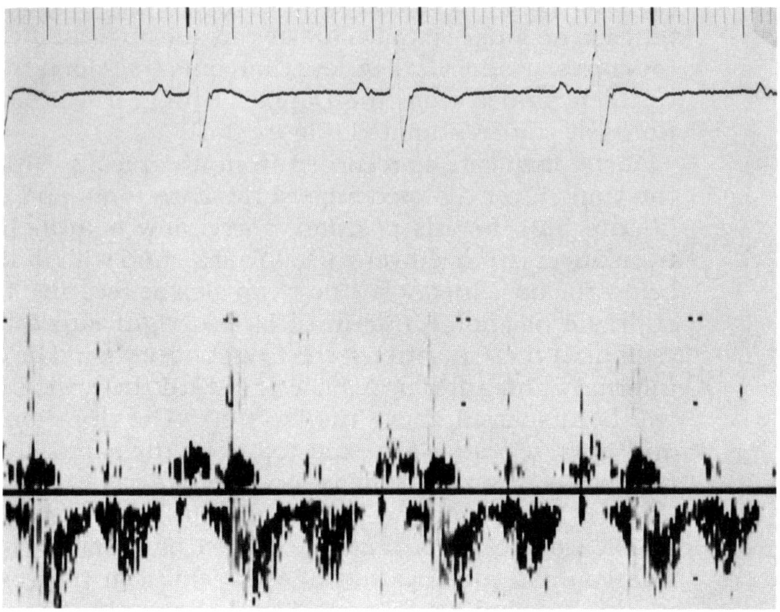

Figure 5.5
Normal flow pattern in the superior vena cava recorded from a suprasternal window. Flow is away from the Doppler transducer throughout the cardiac cycle, with temporary reversal of flow after right atrial contraction.

Flow in the pulmonary veins is similar to flow in the venae cavae.

Techniques in Cardiac Doppler Recordings

Positioning of the Transducer

Once the directions of the various flow patterns within the heart are understood, it becomes easier to predict the transducer position over the chest wall that will produce the best Doppler recordings. By convention, flow toward the transducer is displayed above the baseline, and flow away from the transducer is displayed below the baseline on the Doppler recordings.

When recording flow across the mitral valve, one should recall that blood flows from the left atrium to the left ventricle. Hence, the apical position is the best location for the transducer, where the ultrasound beam will be parallel to the direction of blood flow (Figure 5.1). The transducer should be directed superiorly and posteriorly. In this location, blood flow is toward the apex of the left ventricle and is displayed above the baseline on the Doppler recording.

Mitral flow may also be recorded with the transducer in the parasternal or subcostal position; however, the ultrasound beam is no longer parallel to flow. As the angle of incidence θ increases, cosine θ will be less than one; therefore, the velocities determined from the Doppler equation will be proportionately underestimated (Figure 3.4).

Aortic flow can be recorded from an apical position with the transducer directed superiorly, anteriorly, and medially (Figure 5.2). In this position, aortic flow is away from the transducer (from left ventricle to aorta) and will be displayed below the baseline. Aortic flow can also be recorded from the suprasternal notch (Figure 4.1) and right supraclavicular region. In these positions, the transducer should be directed inferiorly and anteriorly. Flow is toward the transducer and will be displayed above the baseline. The duration of flow and peak velocities are expected to be the same whether or not flow is recorded from an apical or suprasternal position. The only difference would be the mode of signal display on the Doppler recordings, i.e., above or below the baseline. The suprasternal location is also helpful in recording flow in the descending thoracic aorta where the flow is away from the transducer and is displayed below the baseline. The parasternal and subcostal positions for the transducer are not adequate since the angle θ is high, causing underestimation of the true velocities. However, these positions may be helpful in visualizing aortic stenosis. This will be discussed later.

Flow across the pulmonary valve can be recorded from a parasternal or subcostal location. In general, the parasternal position gives easier access to recording pulmonic flow. Since blood flow is from the right ventricle to the pulmonary artery, flow will be away from the transducer and will be displayed below the baseline (Figure 5.4).

Flow across the tricuspid valve can be recorded from an apical position, with the ultrasound beam directed superiorly and medially (Figure 5.3). In this position, flow is toward the transducer and will be displayed above the baseline. Tricuspid flow can also be recorded from a parasternal location, with the ultrasound beam directed inferiorly and medially.

Flow in the superior vena cava is easily recorded from the suprasternal or right supraclavicular areas. It can also be recorded at times from the subcostal position. Flow in the inferior vena cava may be recorded from a parasternal position; however, it is best recorded from the subcostal location. Flow in the pulmonary veins is difficult to record in normal conditions, because these structures are located far from the chest wall and may be beyond the range of the Doppler ultrasound beam.

Doppler Recordings with Echocardiographic Guidance

Earlier Doppler research utilized M-mode echocardiography for proper orientation of the Doppler ultrasound beam within the cardiac chambers. However, as has become evident from the preceding discussion, the parasternal location for the transducer, which is best suited for M-mode echocardiography, is the least useful for Doppler recordings, as mitral and aortic flows are usually at a large angle from the direction of the M-mode ultrasound beam.

Advances in Doppler technology have provided the opportunity to combine two-dimensional echocardiography with Doppler (PW mode, CW mode, or both). Two-dimensional echocardiography can provide orientation for the correct positioning of the Doppler cursor within cardiac chambers and great vessels. This is important for the examination of diseased hearts with abnormal flow patterns. It is important to realize that the two-dimensional image does not account for the third dimension in space, referred to as the azimuthal plane. This plane projects outside the plane of the two-dimensional image. It is not uncommon to record an excellent four-chamber apical view of the heart while the

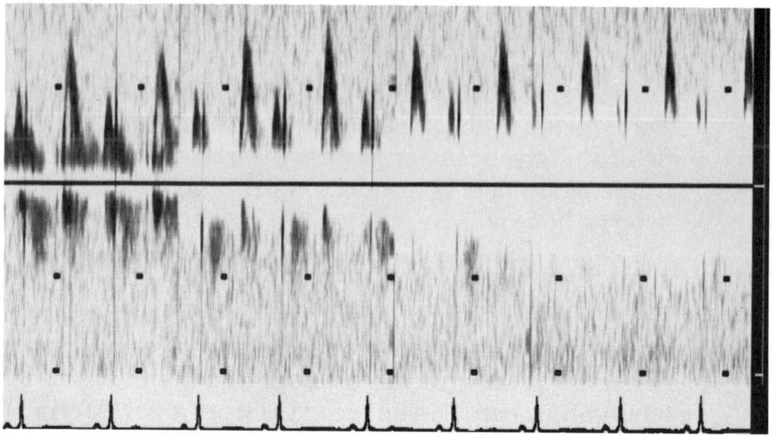

Figure 5.6
Incremental increase in the Doppler velocity filter eliminates low-frequency shift artifacts, as shown in this recording of transmitral flow. A high filter setting eliminates a portion of the true velocity signal.

Doppler recordings of mitral flow are inadequate, despite the Doppler cursor appearing to be parallel to the expected direction of blood flow. In these situations, one should account for the azimuthal plane and maneuver the transducer more posteriorly or more anteriorly to obtain a small angle θ and improve the quality of the Doppler recordings. Obviously, this maneuvering will distort the two-dimensional image and make it suboptimal. One should remember that the main purpose of the Doppler study is to record flow and not two-dimensional echo images.

Doppler Velocity Filter

The Doppler unit detects frequency shifts caused by any moving structure in the heart. The cardiac valves as well as the chamber walls also move throughout the cardiac cycle, although the velocities of motion of these structures are usually less than the velocity of blood flow. Nevertheless, cardiac valves and chambers are highly echogenic and may produce high-intensity signals that interfere with the normal recordings of blood flow velocities.

Most Doppler units allow the operator to filter all frequency shifts below a certain value and eliminate artifacts originating from wall motion (Figure 5.6). However, one should be careful not to use too high a filter that could eliminate certain low-frequency shifts caused by blood moving at slow velocities such as in conditions of low cardiac output.

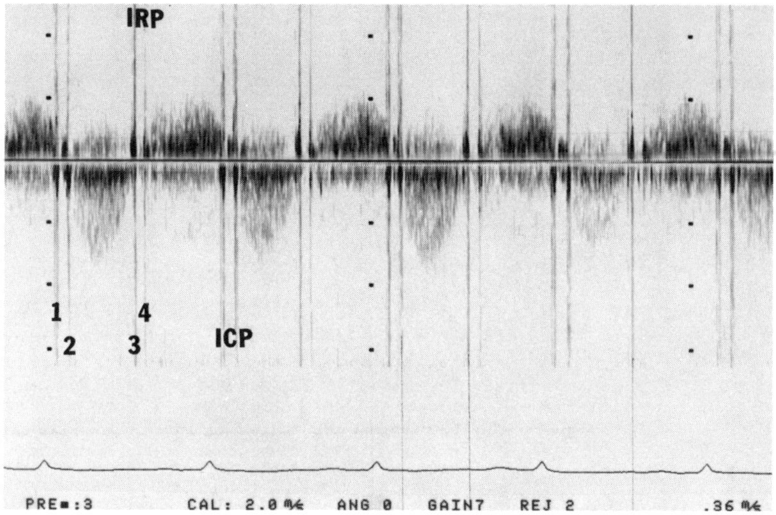

Figure 5.7
This Doppler recording was obtained from a patient with mitral and aortic valve prostheses. The vertical lines in this recording represent the opening and closure clicks of the prosthetic valves throughout the cardiac cycle. Lines 1 and 4 represent the closure and opening signals of the mitral prosthesis, respectively. Lines 2 and 3 represent the opening and closure signals of the aortic prosthesis, respectively. ICP = isovolumic contraction period, the time interval between signals 1 and 2; IRP = isovolumic relaxation period, the time interval between signals 3 and 4.

Doppler Amplitude Signal

Similar to artifacts produced by wall motion, valvular leaflet motion may be recorded with Doppler ultrasound. These are most commonly recorded during valve opening and closure. These high-intensity signals appear as dark lines extending vertically along the Doppler spectral analysis recording (Figures 5.7, 5.8). Although these amplitude signals are considered artifacts, they can occasionally be used to an advantage during routine Doppler recordings.

Zero-Baseline Shift

The baseline that indicates zero velocity, or no flow, is usually positioned at the center of the Doppler tracing. Velocities above this baseline represent flow toward the transducer, and velocities below the baseline represent flow away from the transducer. When frequency aliasing occurs in the PW mode, the Doppler recording will show the velocity in one direction starting at the baseline and extending all the way toward the edge of the Doppler recording, and then appear-

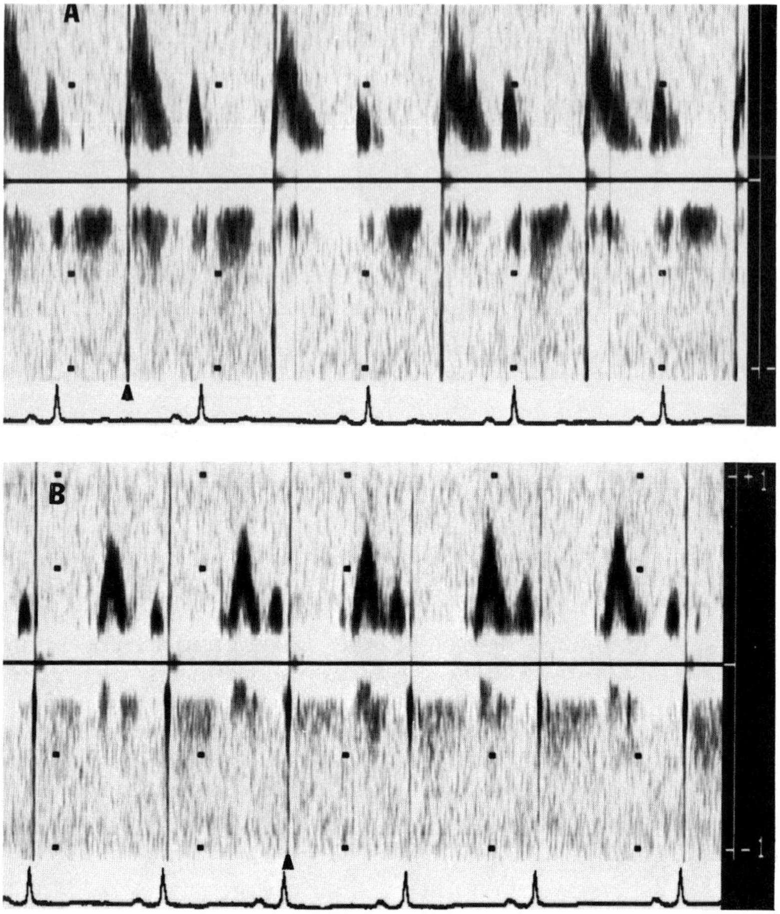

Figure 5.8
A. With the sample volume situated downstream to flow, the amplitude signal (arrowhead) of the mitral valve opening is depicted. B. Positioning the sample volume upstream to flow, just behind the mitral valve, depicts the amplitude signal (arrowhead) of valve closure, at the end of flow.

ing as if it is originating from the opposite extreme edge of the tracing. One way to avoid this artifactual recording is to move the zero baseline (up or down the scale) in the opposite direction of the true flow (Figure 3.16). In simple terms, this maneuver allows extension of the range of the scale so as to accommodate the recording of high velocities on one side of the baseline. Obviously, this maneuver will significantly limit the scale for recording velocities in the other direction. When recording very high velocities in the PW mode, severe frequency aliasing may occur. In this situation, both components of the velocity recording (above and below the baseline) may overlap. Thus, shifting the zero baseline cannot correct this artifactual recording, and CW mode or HPRF must be used instead.

Positioning the Sample Volume

In the CW mode, there is no depth resolution and all returning signals are processed. However, in the PW mode depth resolution is possible. Therefore, one should determine the optimal depth location of the sample volume that will produce the best Doppler recording. If simultaneous two-dimensional imaging is available, then the associated image will help the operator in positioning the sample volume close to the valve being insonated and thereby obtain the highest velocities possible. However, the sample volume as displayed on the two-dimensional image may not faithfully disclose the position of the true sample volume within the heart. This is because the sample volume has finite dimensions that are dependent on the nature of the transducer and the pulse width. These dimensions are not necessarily similar to the square-shaped or longitudinal sample volume display seen on the two-dimensional image. Furthermore, one also has to account for the azimuthal plane. This problem becomes more important when independent PW mode Doppler is used without two-dimensional imaging.

The amplitude signal has been shown to be very useful in resolving this issue. Earlier studies have shown that in the PW mode, positioning the sample volume downstream to flow across a certain valve will record the forward flow velocities as well as the high-intensity signals from valve opening. Positioning the sample volume upstream to flow across the same valve will record forward flow of lower velocities and the high-intensity signals from valve closure (Figure 5.8). The optimal sample volume location is just downstream to flow across the respective valve. Hence, when recording flow with PW mode, one should attempt to position the sample volume in the location that demonstrates the high-intensity signals of valve opening with minimal signals of valve closure. This applies to Doppler recordings across all cardiac valves.

Vortices within the left ventricular outflow tract may occasionally be recorded with Doppler ultrasound. These will appear as flow in diastole going away from the transducer in an apical position (Figure 5.9). It is important to understand that such flow patterns, if present, are normal (Plate 1).

Doppler Signal Recording

As discussed in Chapter 3, several methods can be employed for recording the Doppler shift. In the fast Fourier transform

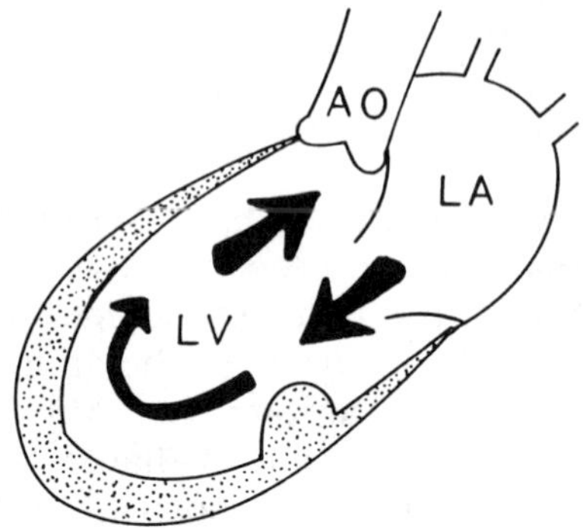

Figure 5.9
Blood entering the left ventricular (LV) cavity in diastole swirls at the apex and turns toward the left ventricular outflow tract. This may be recorded by Doppler ultrasonography as low-velocity flow away from the Doppler transducer in late diastole, with the sample volume positioned in the left ventricular outflow tract. AO = aorta, LA = left atrium.

method of recording, the Doppler signal is recorded on the video screen or hard copy (Figures 5.1, 5.2). One can either record the frequency shift (in Hz) or the velocity (in cm/sec or m/sec) as a function of time. A gain switch and reject switch are standard on most Doppler instruments. Compression to change the gray scale may be available in some instruments. The operator should adjust these parameters to record the best possible signals with the least amount of artifact. The time of onset and end of flow should be easily identifiable. Moreover, since not all red blood cells may be moving at the same velocity, it is not uncommon to encounter situations where the fastest moving particles have a low signal intensity; therefore, if a low gain or high reject setting is employed, these high velocities may not be recorded.

In conditions of laminar flow at normal velocities, most red blood cells will be moving at the same velocity, so the spectral analysis signal will show one thick dark line throughout the period of flow with a relatively clear center within the boundaries of the velocity recording. There may be some spectral broadening, i.e., widening of the spectral analysis signal, indicating a higher proportion of red blood cells moving at different velocities. This may be seen during deceleration of flow or if the ultrasound beam is not closely parallel to the direction of blood flow (Figure 5.10). Adjustment of this angle of incidence may correct this problem. However, in turbulent flow, spectral broadening is common and efforts to correct for the angle will not alter the recording significantly.

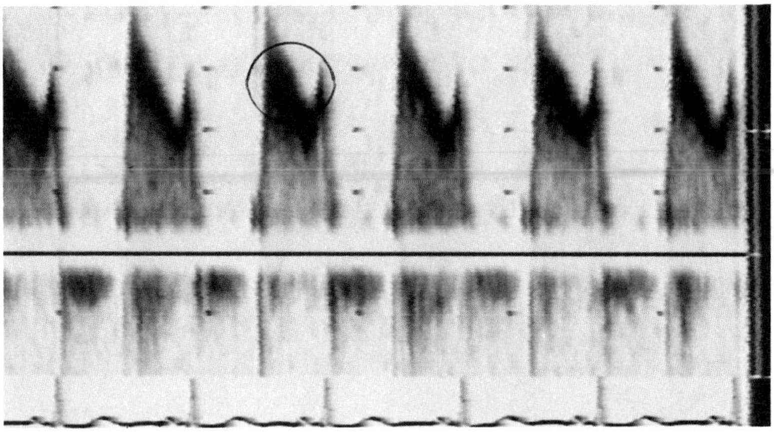

Figure 5.10
Spectral broadening is noted in this Doppler tracing of mitral flow obtained from a patient with mild mitral stenosis. Turbulence of blood creates multiple frequency shifts, which are most clearly noted in diastole, during deceleration. Note the wide dark spectral recordings highlighted within the circle.

Moreover, turbulent flow will demonstrate velocities above and below the baseline since the motion of red blood cells is more chaotic.

The time interval histogram, as referred to earlier, can record the highest velocities only. Thus, gain adjustments are very crucial in determining the highest velocity. A very low gain setting may seriously underestimate the velocity, while a very high gain setting may do the opposite and record the artifacts with overestimation of the true velocities. This problem is compounded when frequency aliasing occurs in the PW mode, where the aliasing signals will distort the time interval histogram recordings. For these reasons, time interval histograms are not commonly employed any longer.

Doppler Audio Signal

The frequency shifts usually have a magnitude within the hearing range of the human ear. These audible signals are very helpful to align the Doppler ultrasound beam parallel to flow. Similar to the spectral analysis signal, a smaller angle θ will produce a louder and clearer audible signal. This is particularly helpful while performing Doppler examinations of abnormal flow patterns where the two-dimensional image may not adequately reflect the true direction of flow. One should realize that frequency aliasing may alter the audio signal.

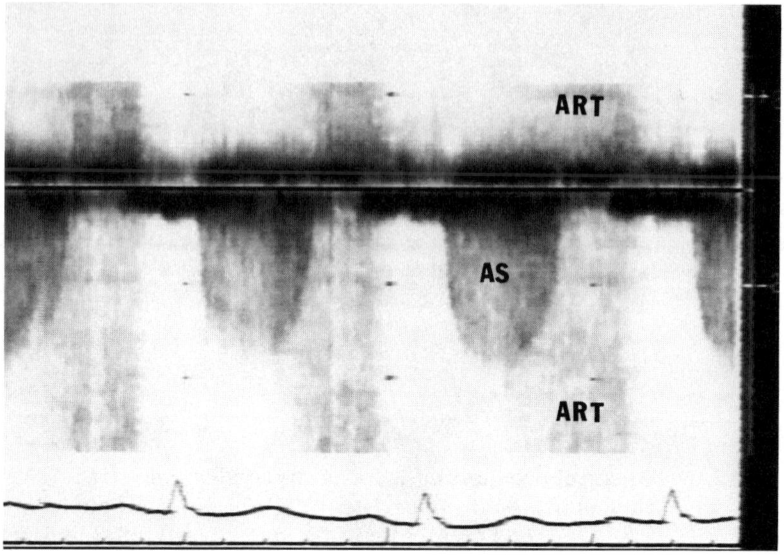

Figure 5.11
High-velocity jet of aortic stenosis (AS) has a high-intensity signal. The effect of automatic gain control in this setting exhibits artifactual recording, simulating high-velocity recording in late systole–early diastole. ART = artifact.

Automatic Gain Control

Most Doppler instruments have automatic gain control capabilities. However, if a signal of unusually high intensity is encountered while the manually controlled gain setting is also high, the built-in automatic gain control may alter the displayed recording and may confuse the inexperienced operator. A typical recording, shown in Figure 5.11, demonstrates the effect of the automatic gain control, which suggests very high velocity with aliasing, when in fact, there is no flow at all during that period; it is simply an artifact of high intensity.

Doppler Recording of Vibratory Motion

Typically, the frequency shifts recorded by the Doppler instrument represent velocities of flow. However, certain abnormal conditions exist where the frequency shifts do not represent velocities. Rather they actually depict the frequency and its harmonics of a vibrating structure along the ultrasound beam (Figure 5.12). Such frequency shifts typically produce musical sounds and should not be confused with actual flow.

Air Flow in the Trachea

If the transducer is positioned in the supraclavicular or suprasternal area and the Doppler ultrasound beam directed medially and posteriorly, one may record the velocity of air flow in the trachea. This velocity has no relationship to the cardiac cycle and will increase on deep inspiration.

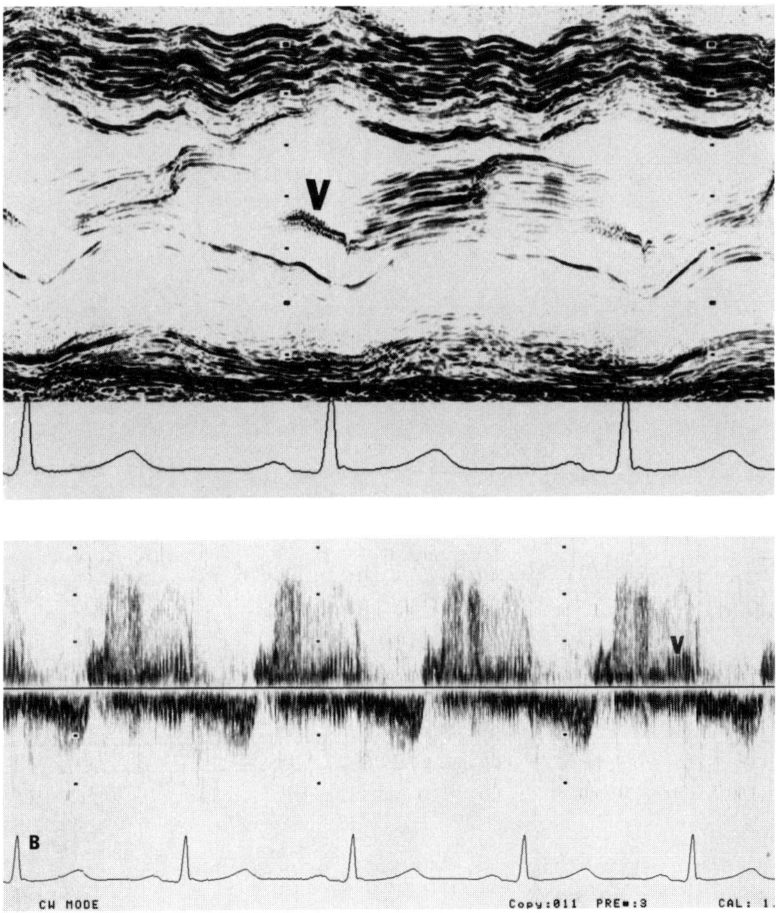

Figure 5.12
A. M-mode recording of mitral valve stenosis, with the ultrasound beam angulated to show high-frequency vibratory motion of the mitral valve apparatus (V). B. Doppler recording across the mitral valve showing high-velocity flow in diastole. Note the multiple dense vertical lines at end diastole (V), representing the effect of vibratory motion on the Doppler spectral analysis signal. C and D. Another form of vibratory motion recorded by Doppler from a patient with aortic regurgitation, with high-frequency vibrations of the aortic valve. Note the multiple dense horizontal and oblique lines (V) above and below the zero baseline recorded by continuous wave (CW) and pulsed wave (PW) modes.

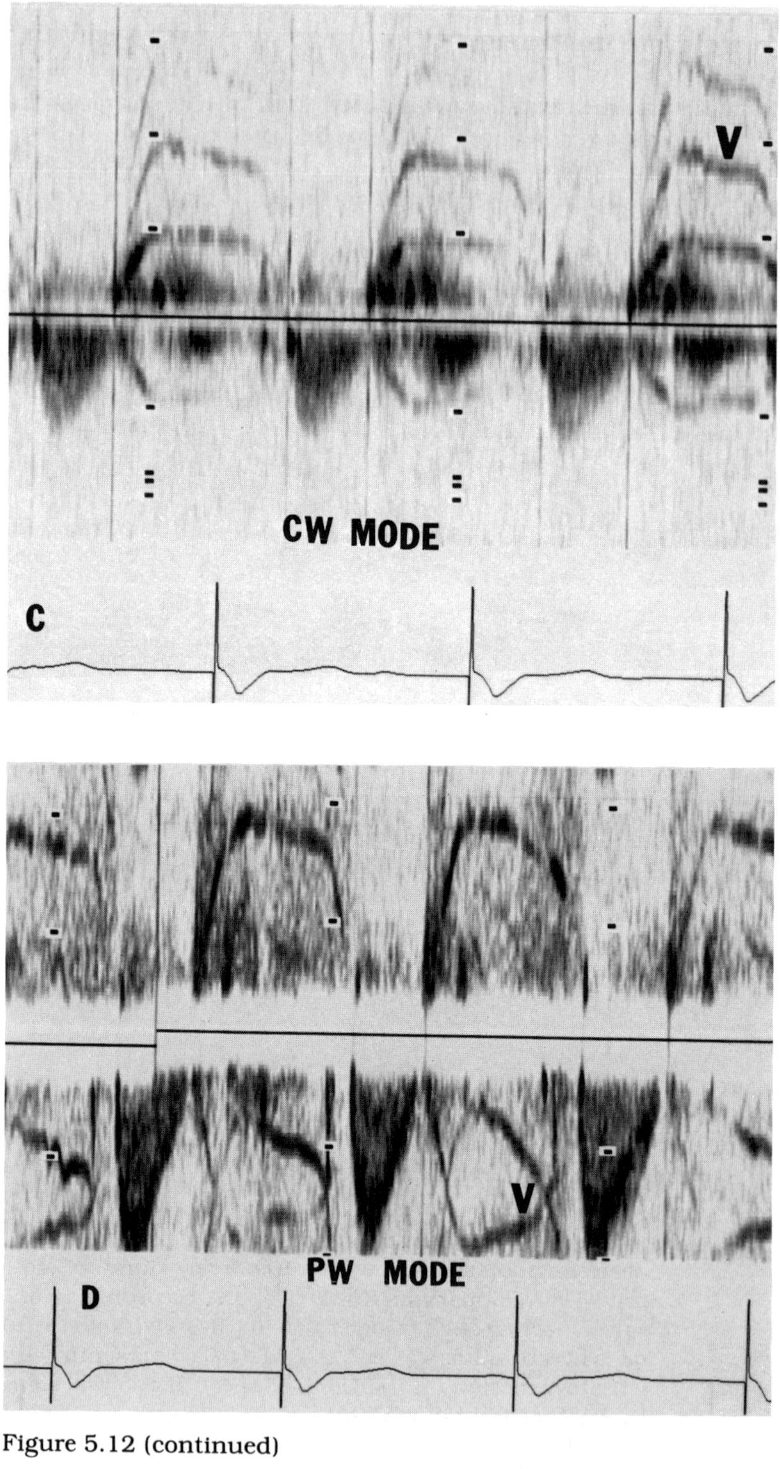

Figure 5.12 (continued)

II Abnormal Cardiac Anatomy and Function

6 Coronary Artery Disease

The coronary arteries supply blood to the myocardium. If the blood supply is inadequate for myocardial oxygen demand, ischemia of the muscle wall occurs. Total loss of blood supply results in myocardial infarction and cell death. The hallmark of coronary artery occlusion is the loss of normal contraction of the portion of myocardium supplied by the occluded artery. Brief periods of myocardial ischemia without infarction will also lead to contraction abnormalities that are usually transient.

Abnormalities in Wall Motion

Myocardial ischemia leads to loss of normal contractile performance of the affected muscle, initially exhibiting hypokinesia (decreased contractility). Worsening ischemia will cause further abnormalities in wall motion leading to akinesia (absence of wall motion) (Figure 6.1) and finally dyskinesia (paradoxical wall motion). The ischemic myocardium cannot contract and generate wall tension, whereas the nonischemic areas will contract normally and generate pressure within the left ventricular cavity. This increasing cavity tension leads to distension of the ischemic myocardial segment, which passively retracts and moves in a direction opposite to the expected normal pattern (Figure 6.2).

Abnormalities in Wall Thickness

In contrast to normal muscle that thickens during systolic contraction, ischemic muscle does not contract adequately

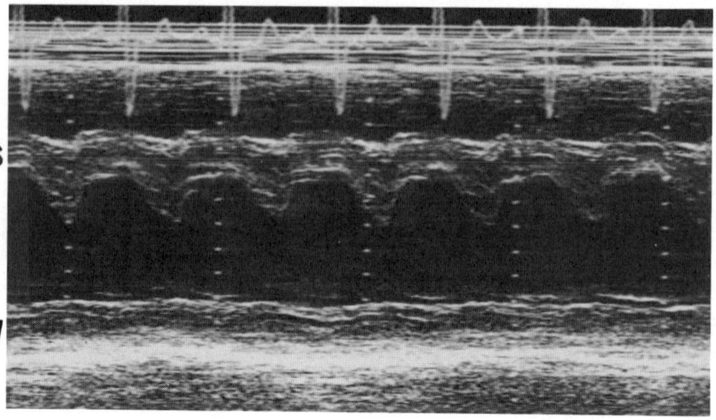

Figure 6.1
M-mode recording from a patient with myocardial infarction of the left ventricular posterior wall (LVPW), showing virtual akinesis of the infarcted segment. Note the vigorous contractions of the interventricular septum (IVS) in systole.

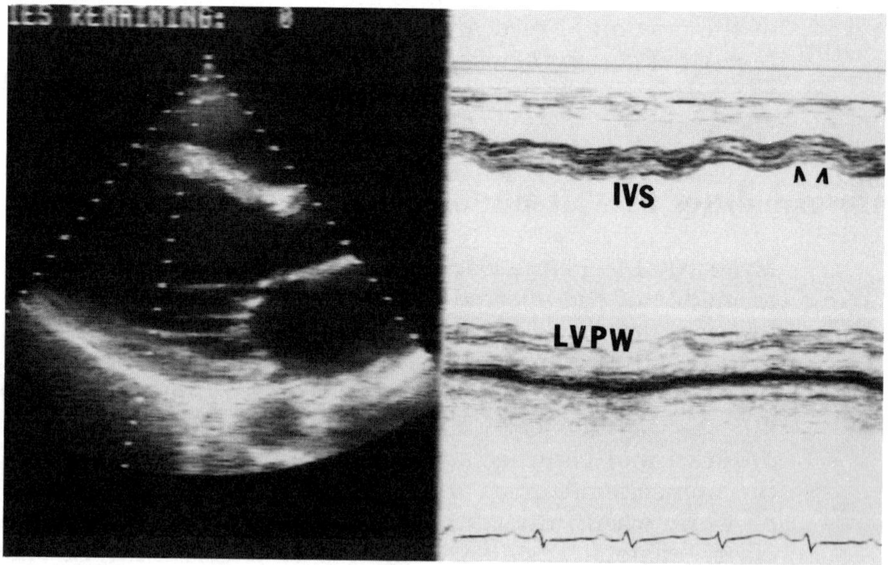

Figure 6.2
Parasternal long axis two-dimensional view with simultaneous M-mode recording of the left ventricle, showing a dilated left ventricle in a patient with multiple myocardial infarctions. Note the akinetic left ventricular posterior wall (LVPW) and dyskinetic motion of the interventricular septum (IVS) (open arrowheads). Also note the increased echo density of the interventricular septum due to the formation of scar tissue after infarction.

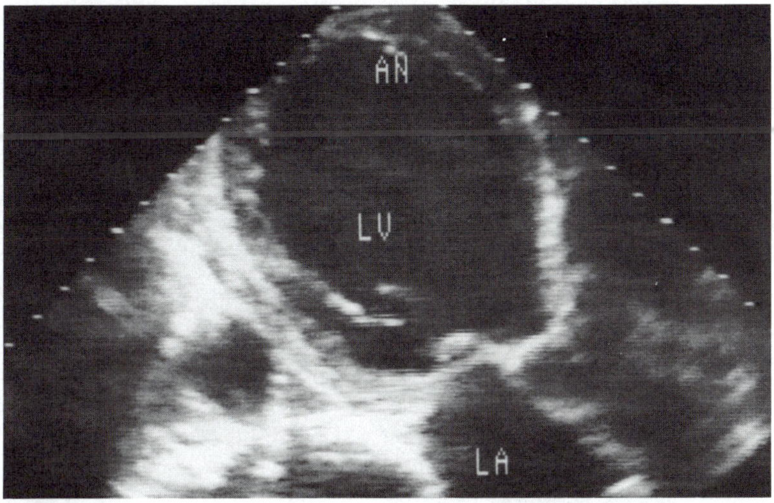

Figure 6.3
Aneurysmal dilatation (AN) of the left ventricular apex secondary to myocardial infarction. Note marked dilatation of the apex relative to the base of the left ventricle (LV). LA = left atrium.

and wall thickness does not change significantly (Figures 6.1, 6.2). In fact, if the ischemia is severe, or if infarction ensues, the affected muscle will be distended and actually become thinner due to the passive stretch effect generated by the rising left ventricular pressure and tension.

Formation of Myocardial Scar

After the initial injury phase, healing begins. The necrotic myocardium is replaced within a few weeks by a scar of fibrous tissue. The resulting echocardiographic appearance is that of a thin akinetic myocardial wall that is more echogenic than the surrounding healthy myocardium (Figure 6.2).

A large scar may continuously stretch because of the relatively high ventricular pressure and wall tension. At times, such large scars may balloon out, resulting in formation of an aneurysm. This is clearly seen on the echocardiogram as a large outpouching of the dead myocardial wall, most commonly seen along the left ventricular apex (Figures 6.3, 6.4).

Impaired Pumping Action

Depending on the size of the infarcted muscle, the heart, as a pump, attempts to compensate for the loss of contractile

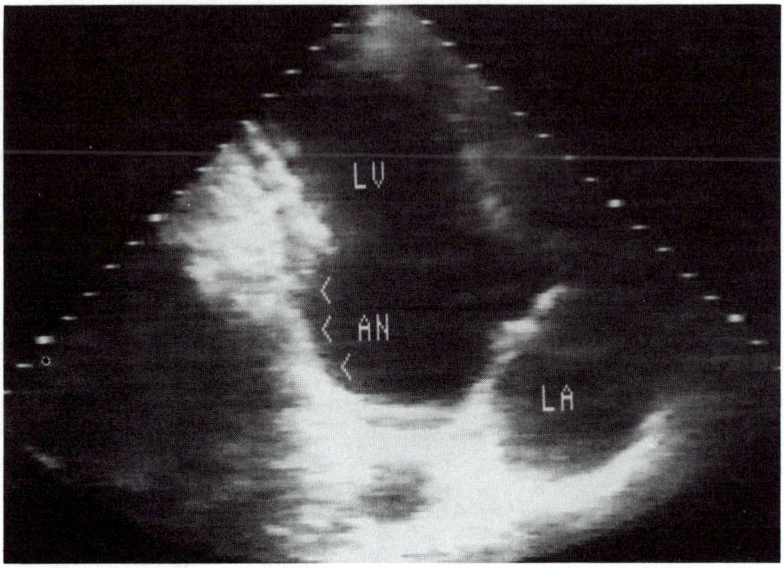

Figure 6.4
Apical long axis view showing aneurysmal dilatation (AN) of the left ventricular posterior wall. Note the ballooning of this segment of left ventricular wall, with thinning of its wall relative to the normal segments of the left ventricle (LV). LA = left atrium.

function. The remaining healthy tissue may be hyperdynamic (super normal contractile performance) (Figure 6.1); however, this is rarely adequate to restore normal pumping action. The left ventricular cavity may dilate, with resulting impairment of overall contractile performance. The degree of dilatation and the abnormal contractility are commensurate with the severity and size of infarction.

Formation of Thrombus

As a result of infarction, the smooth endocardial surface of the left ventricular cavity is denuded and replaced by fibrous tissue with a relatively rough surface. This leads to activation of platelets that start the coagulation process whereby clot formation occurs. It is not uncommon to observe such clots on the echocardiogram, usually adherent to the muscle wall at the site of the infarction (Figure 6.5). The larger the scar in the left ventricular wall is, the higher the chance for thrombus formation is. The thrombus is composed of platelet aggregates with fibrinous material and trapped red blood cells. Normally, blood does not reflect ultrasound, partly because of the speed with which the small red blood cells move in and out of the path of the ultrasound beam.

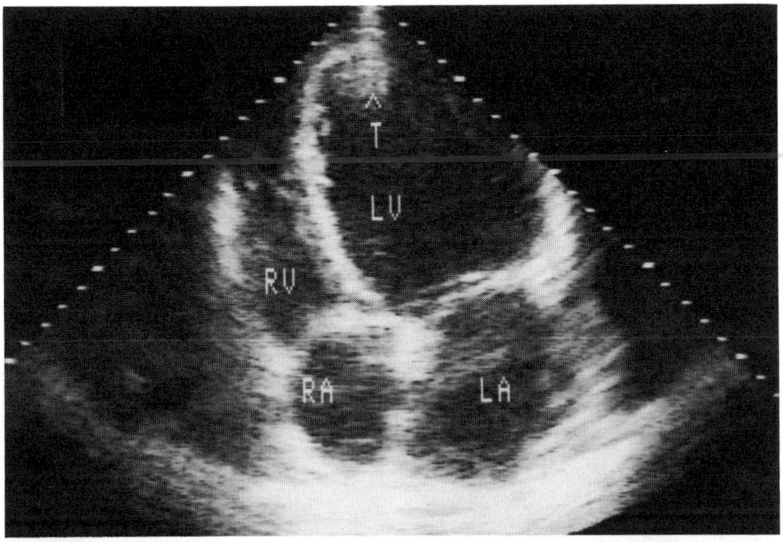

A

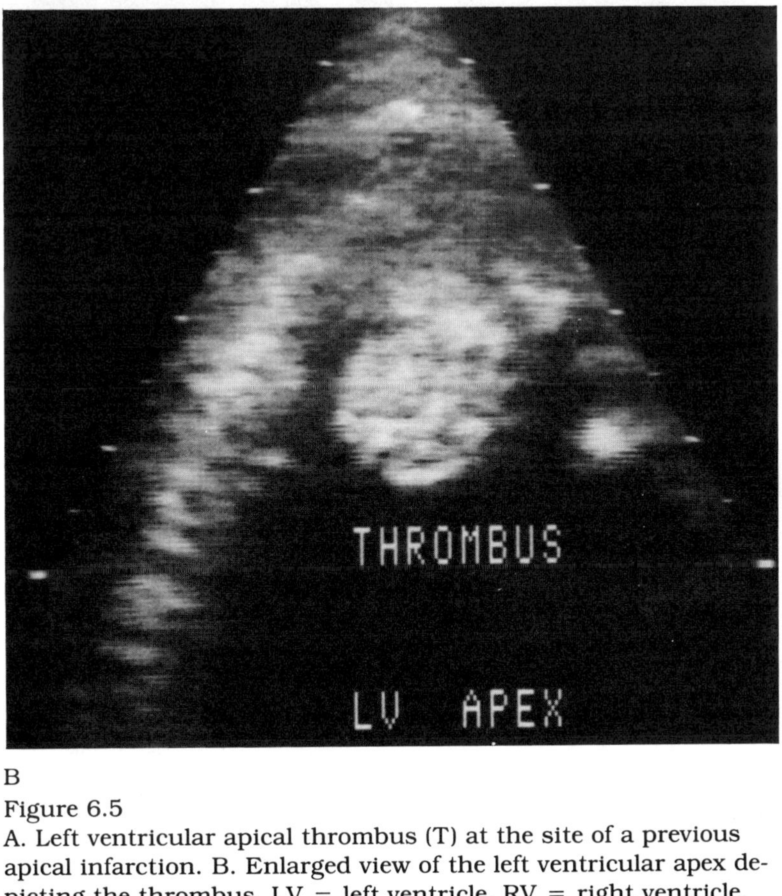

B

Figure 6.5
A. Left ventricular apical thrombus (T) at the site of a previous apical infarction. B. Enlarged view of the left ventricular apex depicting the thrombus. LV = left ventricle, RV = right ventricle, LA = left atrium, RA = right atrium.

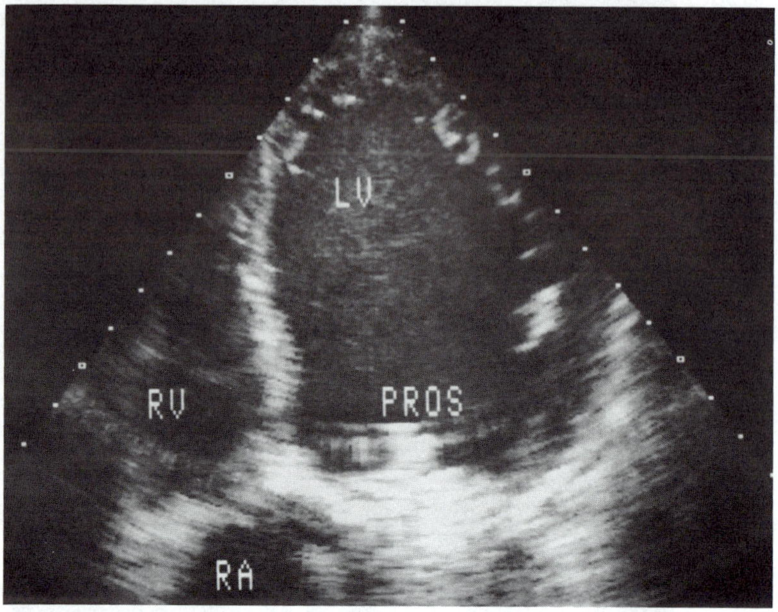

Figure 6.6
Apical four-chamber view from a patient with prosthetic mitral valve (PROS) who sustained a perioperative myocardial infarction. The ill-defined hazy echoes within the left ventricle (LV) are not artifacts. These are ghost echoes that are not uncommonly noted in patients with severely impaired ventricular function and low flow. RA = right atrium, RV = right ventricle.

However, a dense thrombus acts as a tissue interface with blood, and is more echogenic and becomes readily identifiable on the echocardiogram. Moreover, when the infarct size is large enough, overall left ventricular contractile performance can be severely impaired. There is significant decrease of the cardiac output, with relative blood stasis within the ventricular cavity. Blood stasis potentiates the coagulation process, and thus allows the thrombus to grow in size.

As was mentioned earlier, moving red blood cells do not reflect ultrasound adequately (echolucent). However, in the presence of a low flow state with relative blood stasis, it is not uncommon to observe ghost echoes, commonly referred to as "smoke," within the left ventricular chamber. These echoes primarily represent red blood cells clumped together, resulting in a weak interface that reflects ultrasound (Figure 6.6). Since these ghost structures are not well adhered to the muscle wall, they continuously swirl within the left ventricular chamber, and by continuously moving in and out of the ultrasound path, the echocardiographic image is faint with ill-defined borders.

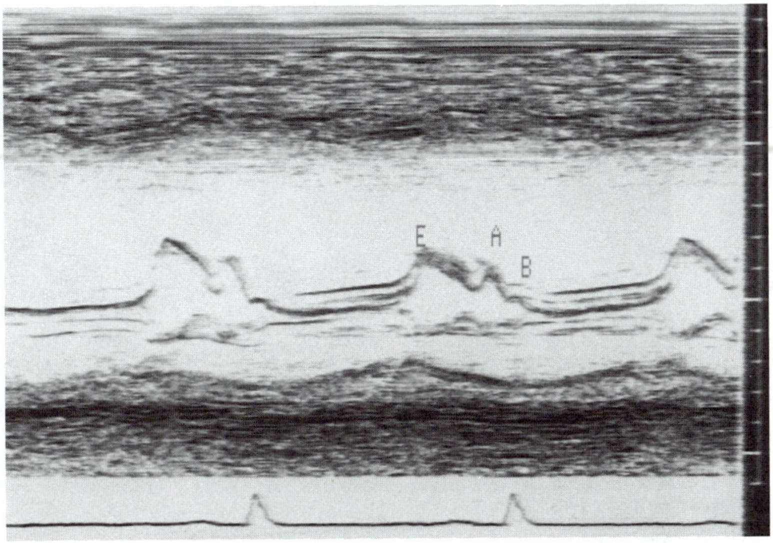

Figure 6.7
M-mode recording of the mitral valve in a patient with coronary artery disease and elevated left ventricular end diastolic pressure. Following the usual E and A waves, note the notching of the anterior mitral leaflet (B wave) prior to valve closure. Also note the diminished excursion of the anterior mitral leaflet due to reduced stroke volume and cardiac output. These findings are discussed in more detail in Chapter 19.

Abnormalities in Diastolic Relaxation

Abnormal relaxation is thought to be the earliest abnormality in myocardial ischemia. This is usually transient and returns to normal after the ischemia subsides.

In myocardial infarction, with significant loss of myocardial cells and impaired contractility, the left ventricle tries to compensate by dilatation. Moreover, the ischemic myocardial cells become stiff with loss of their elasticity and compliance. This leads to elevation of left ventricular filling pressures with associated elevation of left atrial pressures as well. Chronic elevation of left atrial pressure leads to gradual dilatation of the left atrium. The M-mode echocardiogram may demonstrate abnormal mitral leaflet motion suggestive of elevated left ventricular end diastolic pressure (Figure 6.7).

The Echocardiogram in Acute Myocardial Infarction

As a result of the acute muscle injury, the echocardiogram reflects the various degrees of abnormal wall motion and

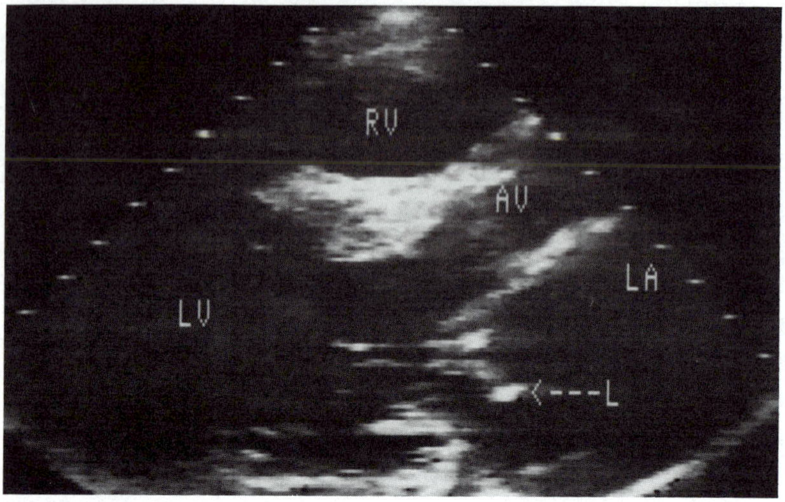

Figure 6.8
Parasternal long axis view depicting a flail mitral leaflet (L) extruding into the left atrial cavity (LA) in systole, due to ruptured papillary muscle in a patient with extensive acute myocardial infarction. Note the dilated left chambers. AV = aortic valve, LV = left ventricle, RV = right ventricle.

impairment of overall contractile performance. Cardiogenic shock refers to massive myocardial damage resulting in hypotension and pulmonary congestion and edema. Left ventricular size may not be significantly increased during this acute phase.

If the myocardial infarction extends to the right ventricular muscle as well, right ventricular failure ensues. Abnormal motions of the right ventricular free wall are not uncommon in this condition.

Severe left or right ventricular failure secondary to acute myocardial infarction often leads to low cardiac output. This may be suspected on the echocardiogram by demonstrating diminished excursion of the mitral or aortic valve leaflets, or both, consistent with diminished volume of blood flow across these valves (Figure 6.7).

Extensive damage to the myocardium leads to weak and friable tissue that may rupture due to high left ventricular tension in systole. Rupture of the papillary muscle head leads to severe acute mitral regurgitation. Rupture of the posteromedial papillary muscle is more common than rupture of the anterolateral muscle group (Figure 6.8). Rupture of the interventricular septum usually occurs at the muscular portion, near the apex. This condition will also lead to severe left ventricular failure secondary to the acute volume overload on an already compromised ventricular function.

This complication is occasionally noted on the echocardiogram if the rupture is large enough.

Acute Pericarditis in Myocardial Infarction

It is not uncommon for patients with acute myocardial infarction to develop acute pericarditis within a few days of the heart attack. Chest pains secondary to acute pericarditis may be confused with persistent anginal pain caused by myocardial ischemia. The echocardiogram may demonstrate pericardial effusion, thereby pointing to pericarditis as the possible cause of the chest pain (Figure 13.2).

Doppler Ultrasound in Coronary Artery Disease

Ischemia, with or without infarction of the papillary muscles, predisposes to abnormal systolic contraction. This leads to incomplete coaptation of the mitral valve leaflets, allowing blood to regurgitate into the left atrium during systole. This abnormal flow pattern may be detected by Doppler. Rupture of a papillary muscle may cause more severe mitral regurgitation that can be recorded by Doppler ultrasound

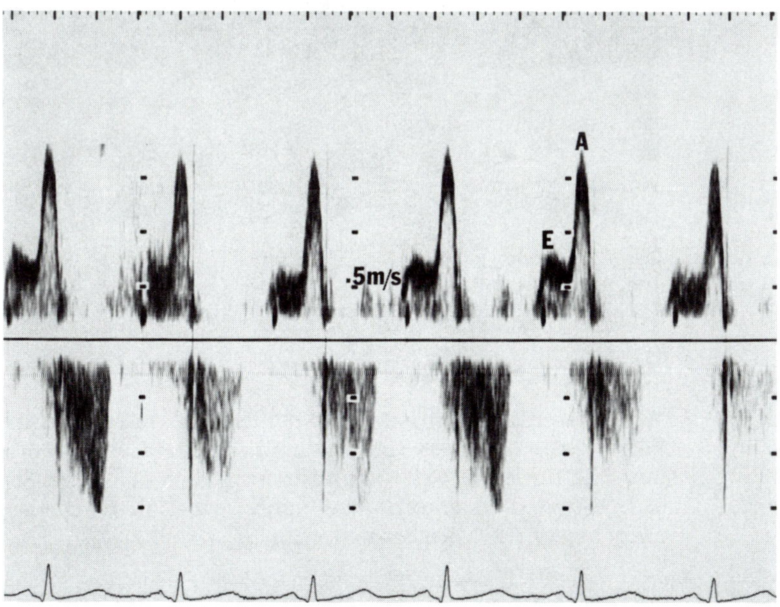

Figure 6.9
Transmitral flow in a patient with severe coronary artery disease, impaired systolic contractility, and diastolic relaxation. Note the prominent A velocity and low E velocity.

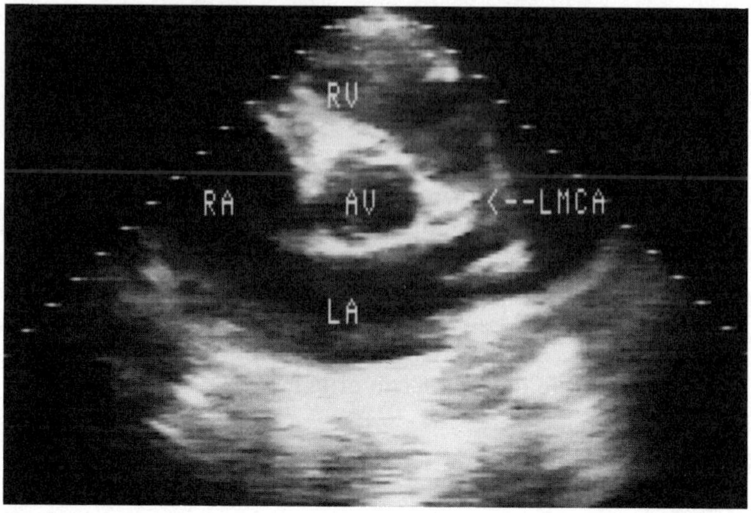

A

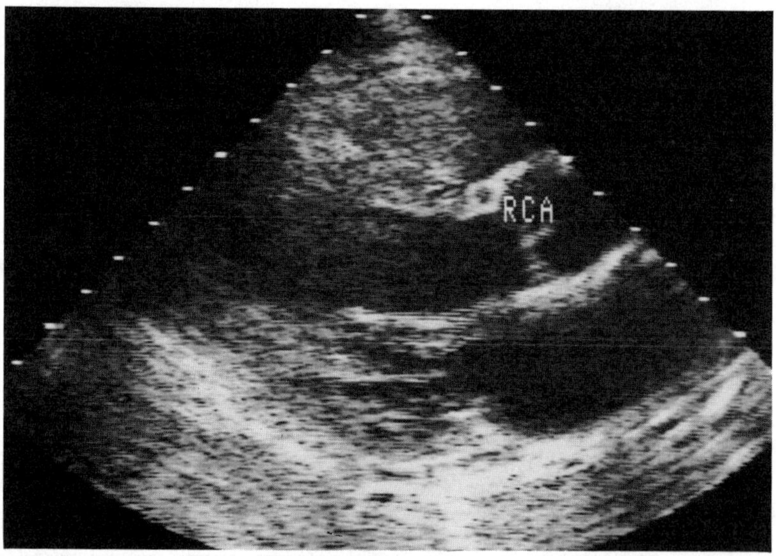

B

Figure 6.10
A. Parasternal short axis view depicting the origin of the left main coronary artery (LMCA) from the aorta. AV = aortic valve, LA = left atrium, RA = right atrium, RV = right ventricle.
B. Angulated parasternal long axis view showing the right coronary artery (RCA) in cross section.

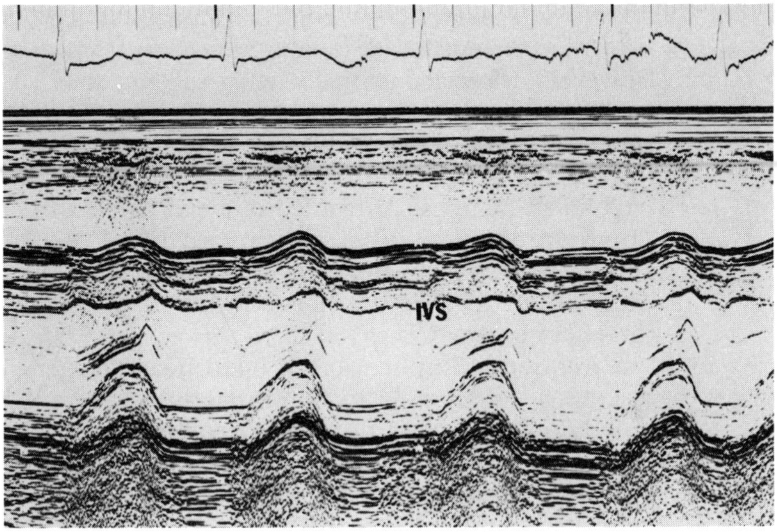

Figure 6.11
M-mode recording of the left ventricular chamber from a patient who underwent recent coronary bypass graft surgery. Note increased wall thickness in systole relative to diastole, indicating normal systolic contraction. However, the motion of the interventricular septum (IVS) is atypical, as expected after open heart surgery.

and can be differentiated from the abnormal flow that occurs due to rupture of the interventricular septum.

Severe impairment of left ventricular function resulting in low cardiac output may be reflected in the Doppler recordings across the mitral and aortic valves, typically demonstrating low velocities of flow (Figure 6.9). Finally, impaired left ventricular relaxation may alter the normal pattern of transmitral flow so that the velocity after the atrial kick exceeds the velocity in early diastole (Figure 6.9).

Echocardiography after Coronary Artery Bypass Graft Surgery

Coronary revascularization utilizes vein grafts harvested from the lower limbs to create a conduit from the ascending aorta to the coronary artery, distal to the site of the occlusion or stenosis. More recently, the internal mammary artery has been used in coronary bypass surgery. Echocardiographic visualization of the coronary arteries is difficult. Occasionally, one may observe the origin of the left main coronary artery or the right coronary artery (Figure 6.10). Visualization of the bypass vein grafts is not possible.

After successful revascularization of the coronary arteries, the contractility of ischemic myocardium may improve. However, infarcted muscle will not improve. A common finding after open heart surgery is paradoxical motion of the interventricular septum (Figure 6.11). Most commonly, this finding is not related to new muscle damage if the interventricular septum exhibits adequate wall thickening in systole. This paradoxical motion is thought to be related to adhesions between the anterior border of the heart and the chest wall, which restrict the normal motion of the heart within the chest cavity.

A frequent complication of open heart surgery is the formation of small pericardial effusions. These are frequently noted on the echocardiogram. Occasionally, intrapericardial bleeding occurs and, if the blood is not promptly drained, may lead to pericardial tamponade (this is discussed in more detail in Chapter 13).

Unfortunately, technical problems are not infrequent during the echocardiographic examination immediately after open heart surgery. Discomfort and pain at the site of incision prevent adequate cooperation during the procedure or adequate positioning of the patient in the left lateral position. Bandages over the incision or drainage catheters may prevent optimal positioning of the transducer on the patient's chest wall. Nevertheless, echocardiographic recordings of a fair quality can be obtained in most cases.

Exercise Echocardiography

Frequently, a resting echocardiogram may not demonstrate any significant wall motion abnormalities since the limited blood supply may be adequate at rest. Ischemia may become evident only during exercise. An echocardiogram is performed at rest and repeated immediately post treadmill or bicycle ergometry. The pre- and postexercise echocardiograms are digitized on a computer and viewed in a continuous loop for qualitative and quantitative assessment of wall motion and contractility. On the Doppler study, ischemia is suspected when new-onset mitral regurgitation or reversal of the E-A ratio occurs post exercise. Decrease of peak, aortic, systolic flow velocity or reduction of the acceleration rate of transaortic-flow postexercise values, as compared to preexercise values, suggests impaired systolic performance due to ischemia.

7 Echocardiography in Valvular Heart Disease

The cardiac valves are strategically located within the heart to allow blood flow in only one direction. They are also designed to provide minimal resistance to flow. Valvular malfunction allows either retrograde blood flow (an incompetent valve causing regurgitation of blood), increased resistance to forward flow (stenosis), or both.

Echocardiography is the best noninvasive method to delineate the anatomy of the cardiac valves. Cardiac adaptations to the hemodynamic overload caused by valvular malfunction can also be identified. Doppler ultrasound recordings of transvalvular velocities of flow provide the best noninvasive method to confirm and quantify the severity of the valvular abnormality. This chapter deals with the echocardiographic features of valvular heart disease. The next chapter describes the Doppler findings associated with valvular pathologic states.

A practical approach to evaluating cardiac valve function is to search the echocardiogram for answers to the following questions:

1. How many valve leaflets are present?
2. Are there any abnormal masses, thickening, or calcification attached to the valve leaflets?
3. Is leaflet mobility normal, restricted, or hypermobile?
4. What are the associated abnormalities of the cardiac chambers and other cardiac valves?

Aortic Valve

Aortic Stenosis

The primary abnormality in aortic stenosis is restriction of leaflet mobility and diminished opening of the aortic valve in systole during left ventricular ejection (Figure 7.1). The left ventricle is required to generate higher than normal systolic pressure to overcome the increased resistance to emptying during the ejection phase in systole. It adapts to this chronic pressure overload by inducing hypertrophy of its muscle wall.

Valve Anatomy

The echocardiogram typically demonstrates various degrees of leaflet thickening with or without fusion of their edges (commissures). Bright echoes are reflected from these leaflets at the site of calcium deposition. Depending on the cause and severity of the stenosis, the restricted leaflets typically demonstrate a "doming" appearance in systole whereby the body of the leaflet bulges into the aortic root (Figure 7.2).

In mild to moderate stenosis, it may be possible to identify each of the aortic valve leaflets. However, this may not be possible if the stenosis is severe with marked calcification and fusion of the leaflets (Figure 7.1).

Determining the Severity of Stenosis

In addition to defining the anatomy of the diseased aortic valve, the echocardiogram provides clues as to the severity of the lesion. Mild stenosis causes less restriction of mobility than does severe stenosis, where the leaflets hardly open in systole (Figure 7.3). Systolic leaflet separation can be measured on the M-mode echocardiogram. In general, cusp separation smaller than 12 mm indicates significant obstruction. Unfortunately, the M-mode echocardiogram is not very accurate in determining the severity of stenosis. This is because the narrowed aortic valve orifice has irregular borders. Hence, variable cusp separation will be noted on the M-mode recordings, depending on the direction of the ultrasound beam across the diseased aortic valve (Figure 7.4). Moreover, if the ultrasound beam passes across the body instead of the tips of the aortic leaflet, the severity of obstruction may be underestimated. This is particularly important in patients with congenital aortic stenosis, especially when calcium deposition is minimal during the early stages of the disease (Figure 7.5).

Two-dimensional echocardiography provides better evalu-

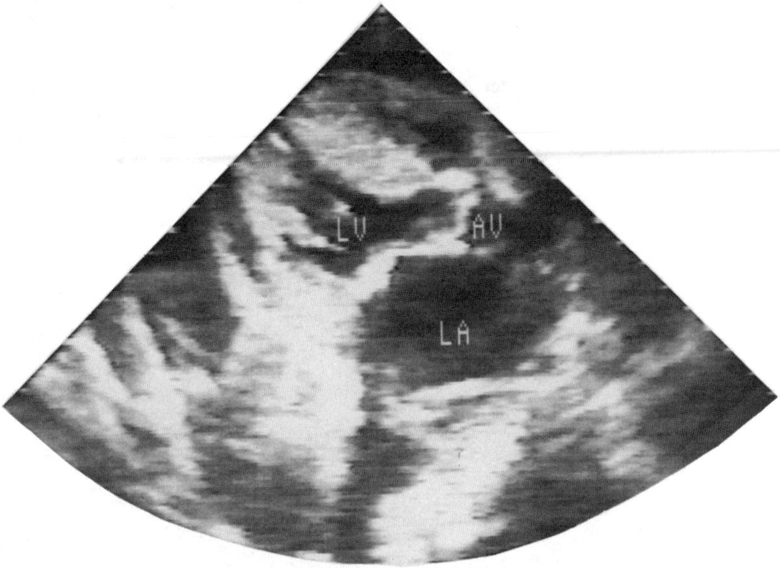

A

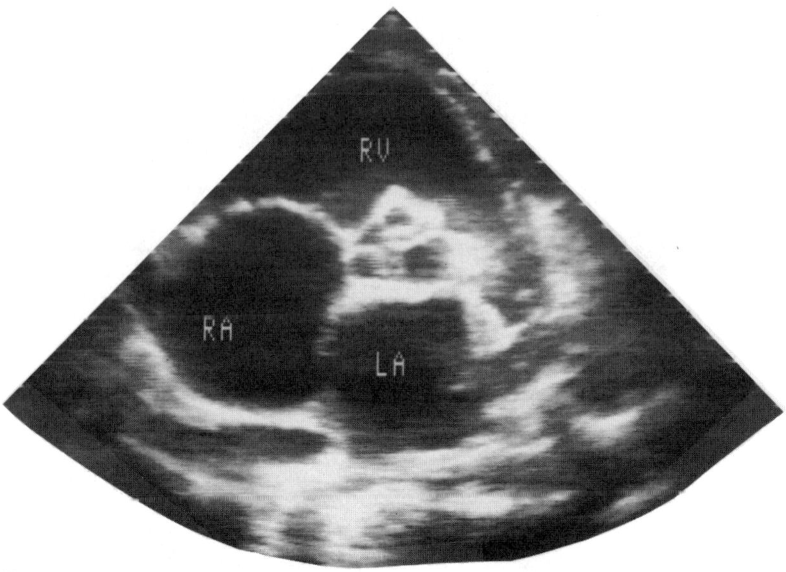

B

Figure 7.1
A. Parasternal long axis view obtained from a patient with aortic valve stenosis. Note the thickened aortic valve leaflets (AV) with slitlike opening in this systolic frame. Associated echocardiographic findings in aortic stenosis include hypertrophied left ventricle (LV) and dilated left atrium (LA). B. Parasternal short axis view of the aortic valve with slitlike opening in systole in this patient with rheumatic heart disease and aortic valve stenosis. RA = right atrium, RV = right ventricle.

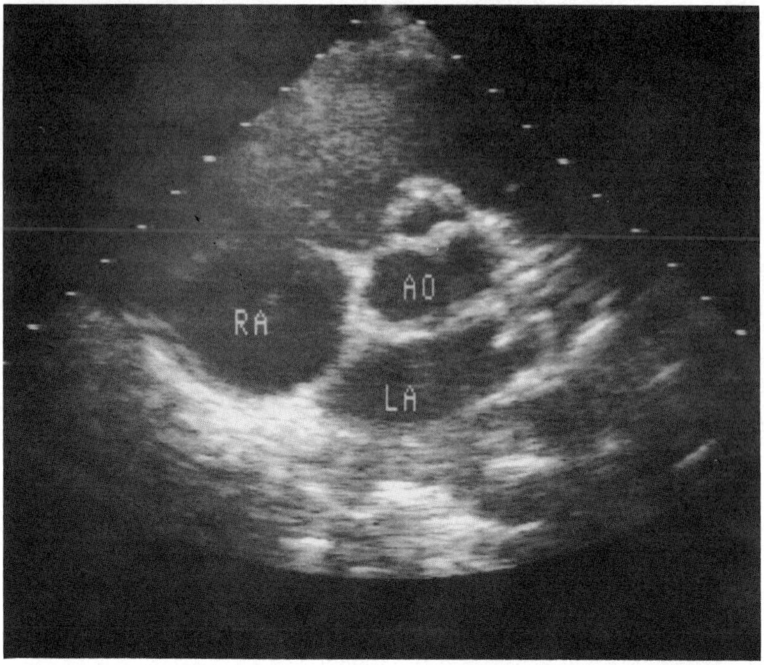

A

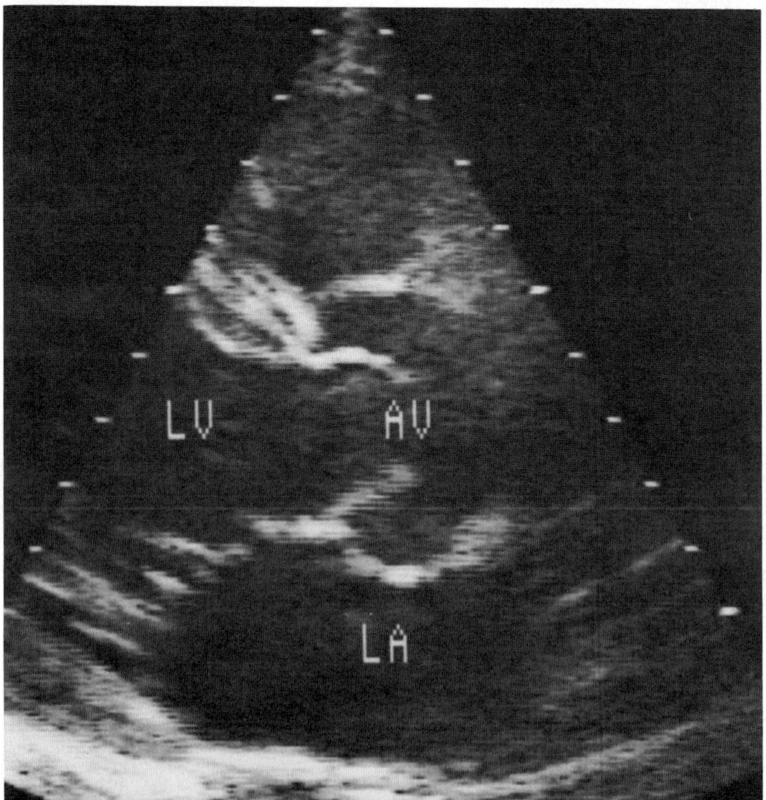

B

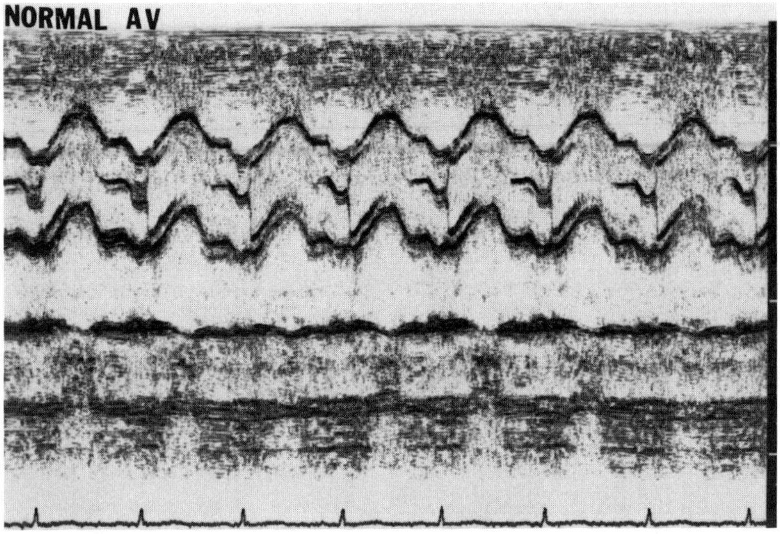

A

Figure 7.3
M-mode recordings. A. Normal aortic valve (AV). B. Mild aortic stenosis (AS). C. Severe aortic stenosis (AS). Note increased echoes in B with adequate systolic separation, whereas in C, cusp separation is hardly noticeable, with prominent echoes within the aortic root.

ation of the severity of stenosis (Figure 7.1). The parasternal long axis view delineates the restricted opening of the tips of the aortic leaflets. The parasternal short axis view, at the level of the aortic valve, may show the true orifice of the stenotic valve, and its anatomic area can be measured. Unfortunately, this method is not very accurate either. The heavily calcified leaflets cause bright echoes with ill-defined borders that limit the ability to truly define the margins of the valve orifice. Moreover, it is difficult at times to obtain good short axis views perpendicular to the leaflet edges; a portion of the valve orifice may lie outside the plane of the ultrasound beam, thus preventing accurate measurements. One may observe variable degrees of calcification and leaflet

---

Figure 7.2
A. Parasternal short axis view of the aortic valve (AO) in a patient with bicuspid aortic valve, showing two leaflets only, of unequal size and irregular commissures. B. Parasternal long axis view of the same aortic valve. Note the doming effect whereby commissural fusion restricts full leaflet opening with bulging of the body of the leaflet into the aortic root simulating a domelike appearance. RA = right atrium, LA = left atrium, LV = left ventricle.

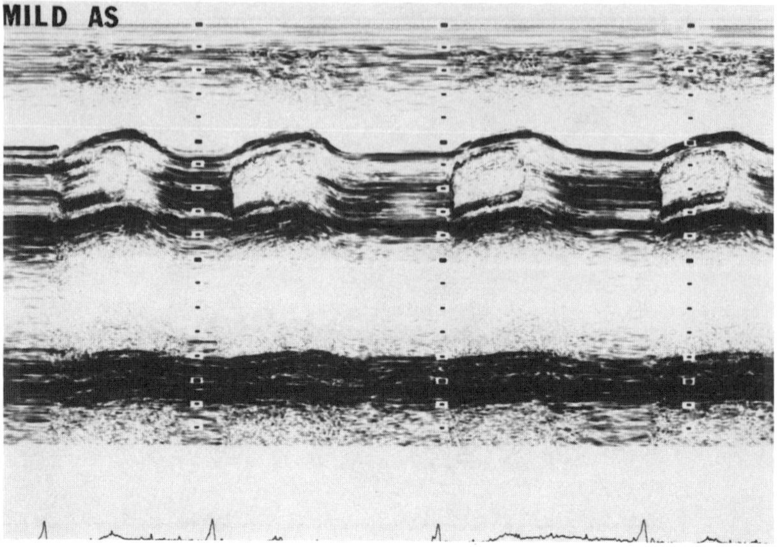

B

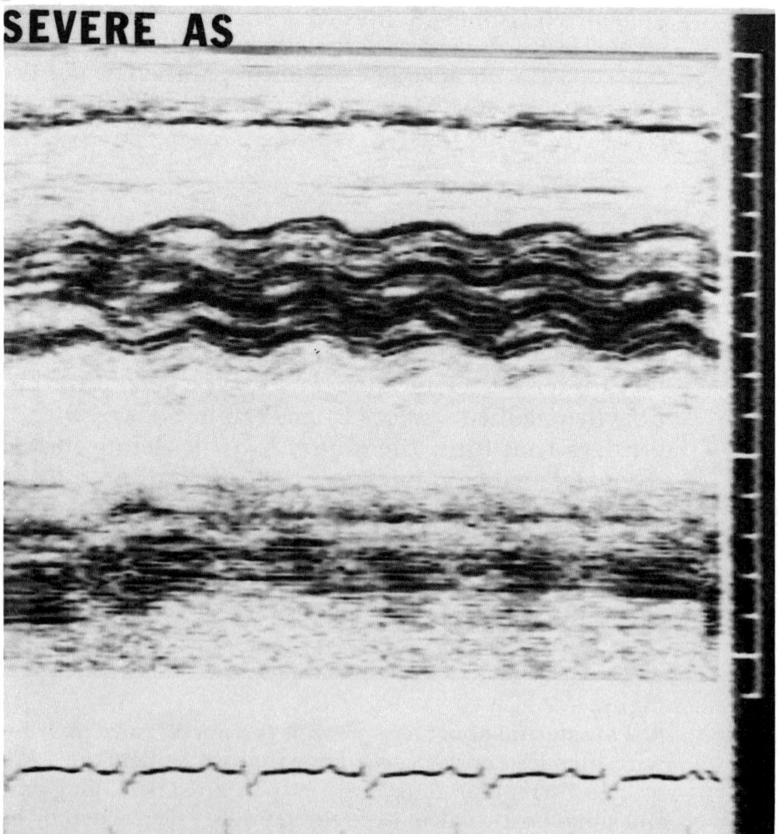

C

Figure 7.3 (continued)

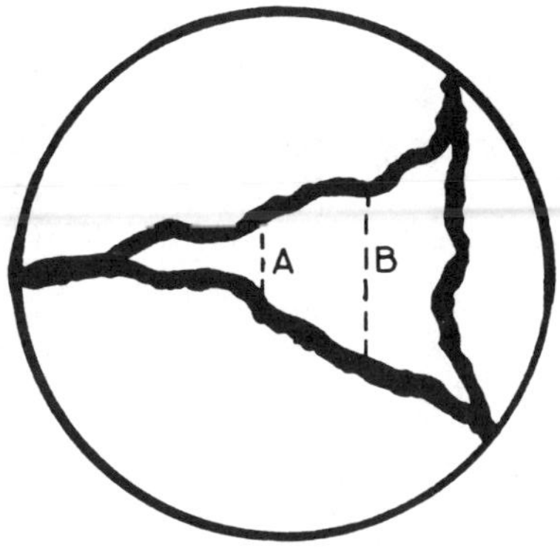

Figure 7.4
A cross-sectional image of the aortic valve in aortic stenosis with irregular orifice. Cusp separation measured from an M-mode ultrasound beam traversing this valve at A will be significantly smaller as compared to cusp separation measured from an ultrasound beam traversing the valve at B. Thus, M-mode estimates of the severity of aortic valve stenosis are generally unreliable.

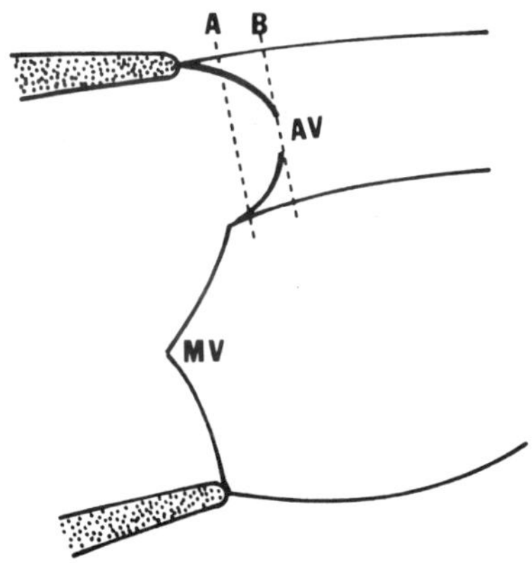

Figure 7.5
A long axis cross-sectional image of a bicuspid aortic valve (AV) with doming effect. Cusp separation measured from an M-mode ultrasound beam traversing the body of the leaflets at A will underestimate the severity of stenosis. The correct ultrasound path should be at the tips of the leaflets, at B. MV = mitral valve.

fusion. In general, the presence of at least one leaflet with adequate mobility excludes severe stenosis.

Associated Abnormalities

In the absence of any other cause for left ventricular hypertrophy, the degree of wall thickening indirectly reflects the severity of the obstruction (Figure 7.1). In general, worsen-

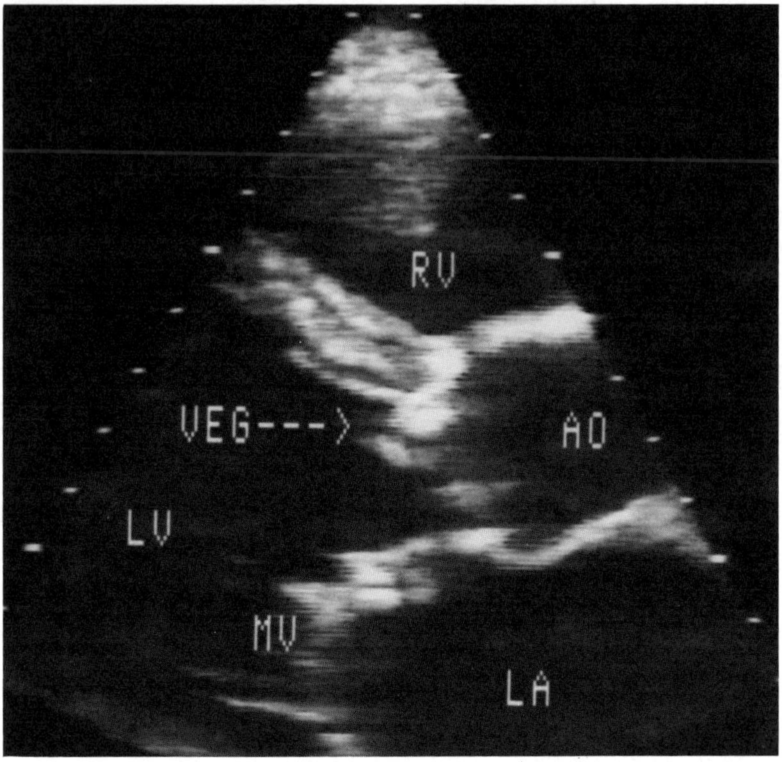

A

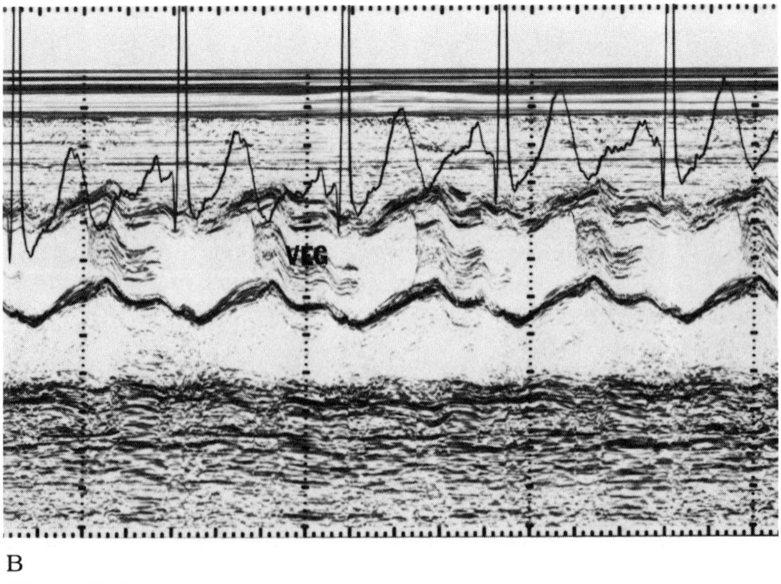

B
Figure 7.6

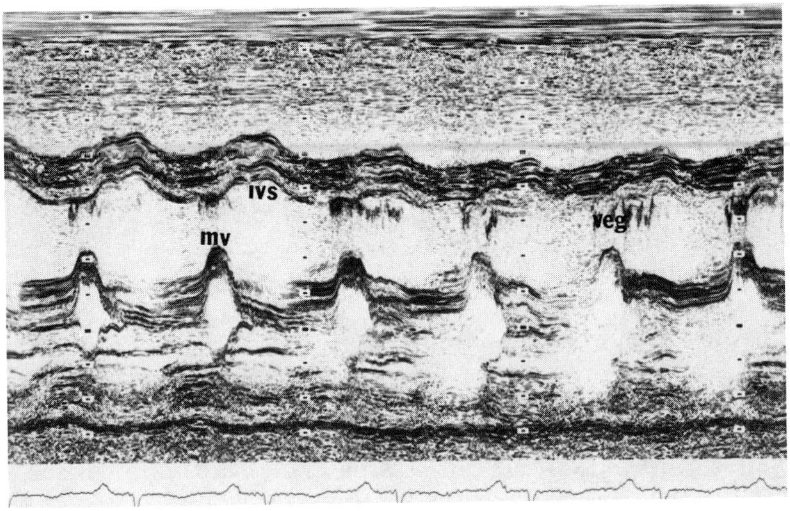

C

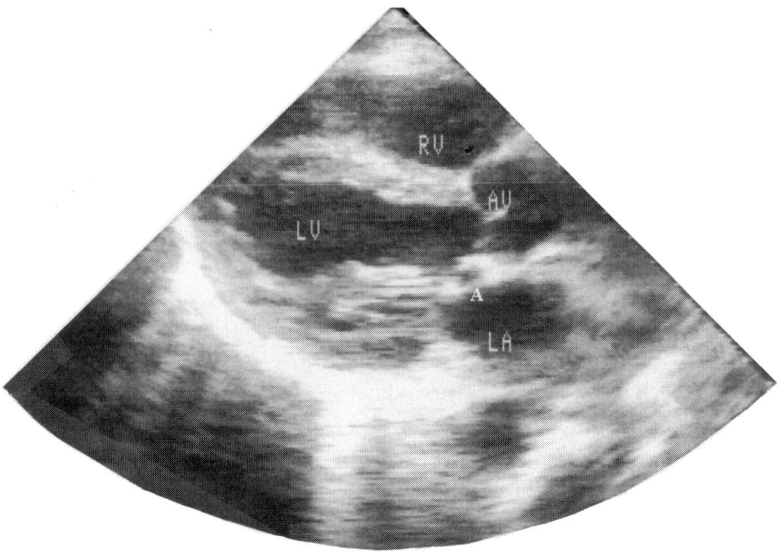

D

Figure 7.6

A. Parasternal long axis view of the aortic valve with vegetation (VEG) protruding into the left ventricular outflow tract. MV = mitral valve. B. M-mode recording of the aortic valve showing multiple linear echoes in diastole, representing the vegetation. C. M-mode recording at the left ventricular outflow tract showing ill-defined echo densities between the anterior mitral leaflet (mv) and interventricular septum (IVS) only in diastole. These echoes represent the vegetation (veg) prolapsing into the left ventricular outflow tract in diastole. D. Parasternal long axis view from a patient with abscess (A) situated at the aortic valve (AV) annulus. AO = aorta; LA = left atrium, LV = left ventricle, RV = right ventricle.

ing obstruction to left ventricular emptying induces more hypertrophy. Occasionally, severe aortic stenosis may be accompanied by inadequate hypertrophy so that the degree of wall thickening does not reliably reflect the severity of obstruction. It is not unusual to observe some widening of the aortic root. This poststenotic dilatation is thought to be secondary to the eccentric jet of blood flow hitting the wall of the aorta at high velocity, in association with turbulence of blood distal to the obstruction.

Chronic Aortic Regurgitation

The primary abnormality in this disorder is inadequate leaflet coaptation, which allows blood to leak backward into the left ventricle in diastole. There are many causes for aortic valve incompetency leading to various degrees of regurgitation. A ruptured aortic leaflet or the presence of a large vegetation on one or more leaflets present clear-cut evidence of the presence of regurgitation (Figure 7.6). However, such gross valvular pathologic states may be lacking, making the echocardiographic diagnosis of aortic regurgitation more subtle. One has to rely on indirect evidence to establish the diagnosis.

Valve Anatomy

The anatomy of the aortic valve varies according to the original pathologic condition leading to regurgitation. Diseases of the aorta indirectly cause aortic incompetence by dilatation of the valve annulus. This leads to valve incompetency without any demonstrable leaflet pathologic state (Figure 7.7). Bacterial endocarditis involving the aortic valve leaflets causes inadequate coaptation, leaflet fenestration, and occasionally rupture. Associated formation of abscess in the aortic valve annulus may also occur.

Fibrosis with or without calcification of the aortic valve leaflets (aortic valve sclerosis) may occur secondary to degenerative disease in elderly patients (Figure 7.8). Various degrees of regurgitation are not uncommon in these situations. Rheumatic aortic valve disease may cause thickening and fusion of the leaflets, leading to various degrees of regurgitation, stenosis, or both.

Indirect Echocardiographic Findings of Aortic Regurgitation

Depending on the cause and severity of the aortic incompetency, the echocardiogram may be completely normal or show nonspecific findings. If the aortic regurgitation is

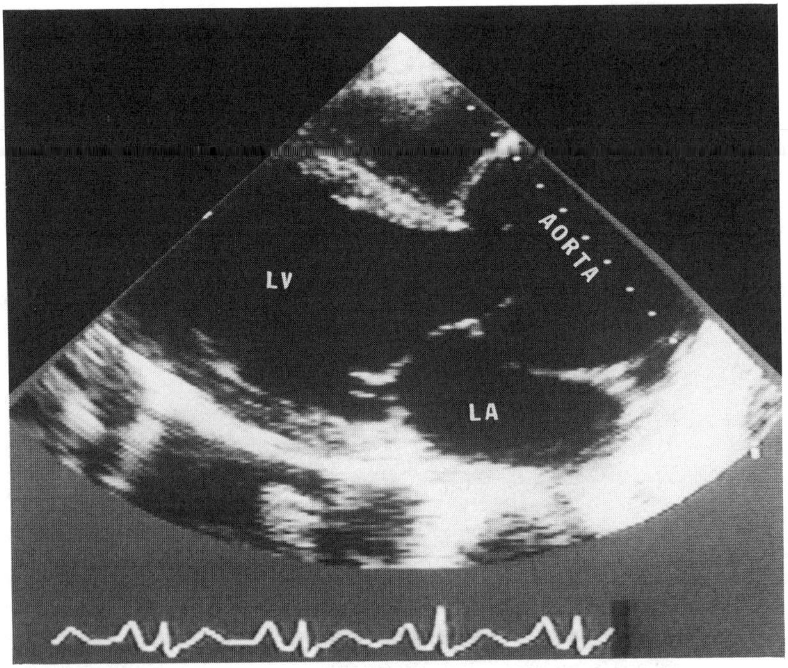

Figure 7.7
Parasternal long axis view from a patient with Marfan's syndrome. Note the markedly dilated aorta measuring approximately 75 mm in diameter. Aortic regurgitation was also noted on Doppler. Note the dilated left ventricle (LV) due to significant volume overload. LA = left atrium.

significant, the regurgitant jet of blood may hit the left ventricular surface of the interventricular septum. This may be observed on the M-mode echocardiogram as fine fluttering or vibrations in diastole. This is a very specific sign of this disease, but unfortunately is rarely evident. It is more common to observe fine diastolic fluttering of the anterior mitral leaflet, which vibrates under the influence of two jets of blood flow (Figures 7.9, 7.10). One jet is that of the normal transmitral flow from under the leaflet, and the second jet is that of the regurgitant flow above. It is important to note that diastolic fluttering of the anterior mitral leaflet may occur secondary to causes other than aortic regurgitation. Fluttering of a flail mitral leaflet is more coarse and chaotic as compared to the fine fluttering in aortic regurgitation (Figure 7.10).

The two-dimensional echocardiogram is less sensitive in detecting the fluttering of the anterior mitral valve leaflet; however, two-dimensional recordings may show another sign characteristic of aortic regurgitation. When the regurgitant jet hits the anterior mitral leaflet, it causes an inden-

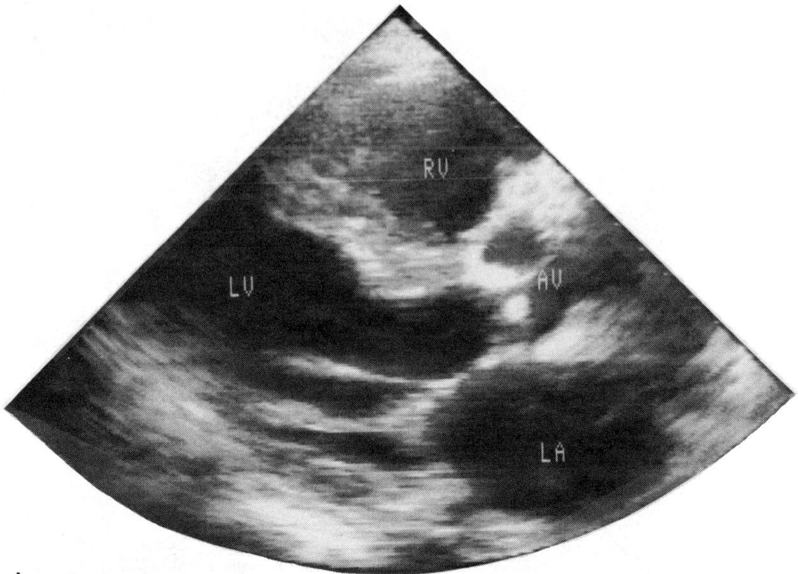

A

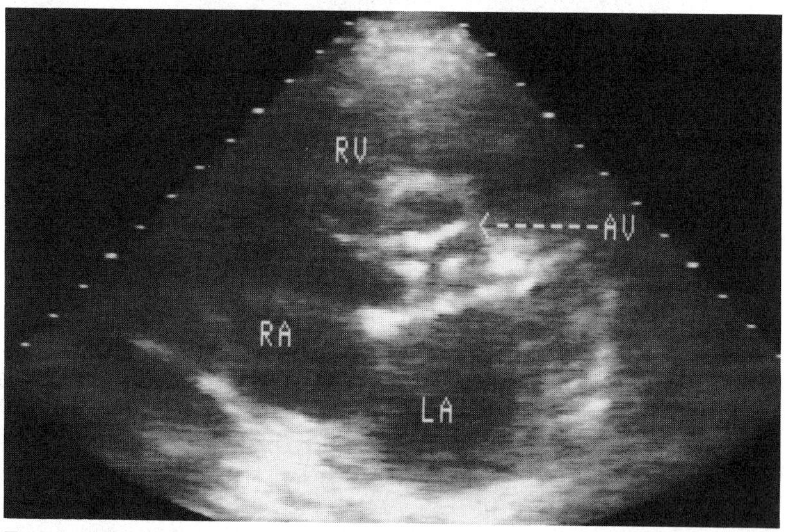

B

Figure 7.8
A. Long axis, and B. Short axis views showing thickened aortic valve leaflets (AV) with slightly diminished valve opening, commonly noted in elderly patients with aortic valve sclerosis and insignificant stenosis. LA = left atrium, LV = left ventricle, RA = right atrium, RV = right ventricle.

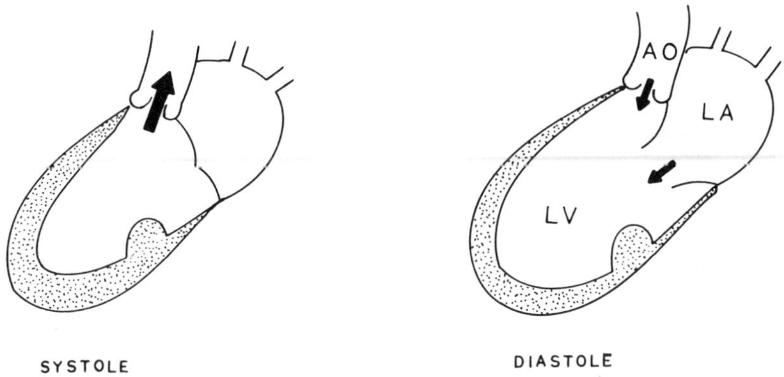

Figure 7.9
The anterior mitral leaflet lies within two jets of flow in diastole. This may cause the anterior leaflet to exhibit fine fluttering in diastole, which may be observed on the M-mode tracing and less often on the two-dimensional tracing. AO = aorta, LV = left ventricle, LA = left atrium.

tation on this leaflet that assumes a concave configuration. This is best observed on the short axis view at the level of the body of the mitral leaflet (Figure 7.11). At times, it can be seen on the four-chamber view also.

Determining the Severity

Depending on its severity, chronic aortic regurgitation imposes volume overload on the left ventricle. The adaptive response of the left ventricle is to dilate in order to accommodate the regurgitant blood volume, in addition to the normal stroke volume coming across the mitral valve. During the early stages of the disease, the left ventricle is hyperdynamic with exaggerated motion of its walls. Prolonged and severe volume overload causes marked dilatation of the left ventricle. This ultimately leads to significant myocardial stretching with gradual impairment of contractility.

Dilatation of the aortic root may cause aortic regurgitation by stretching and widening of the aortic valve, which becomes incompetent. However, aortic root dilatation may occur secondary to intrinsic aortic valve disease with severe regurgitation. This is because the left ventricle ejects a greater volume of blood in systole with secondary passive dilatation of the aortic root.

Acute Aortic Regurgitation

Acute disruption of the normal aortic valve leads to sudden onset of severe regurgitation. The echocardiogram may de-

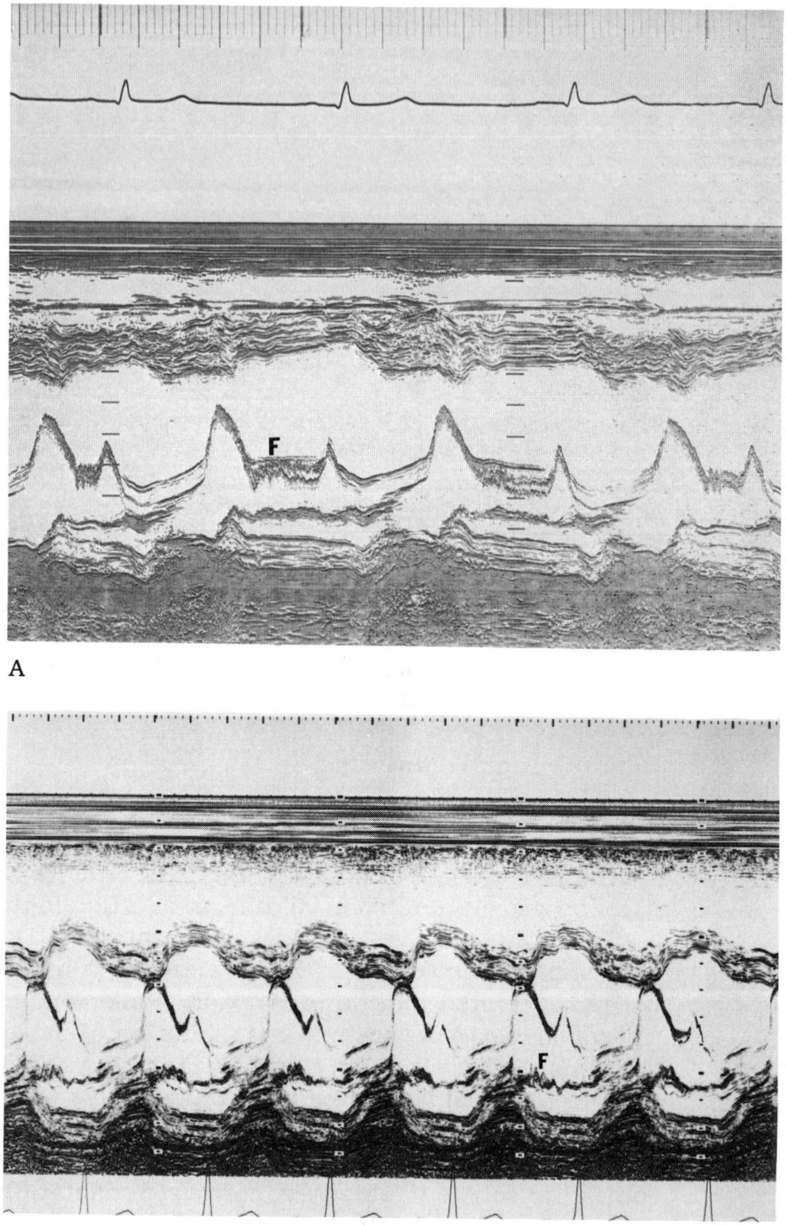

Figure 7.10
A. High-frequency diastolic fluttering (F) of the anterior leaflet secondary to aortic regurgitation. B. Flail posterior mitral valve leaflet causes coarse diastolic fluttering (F), which at times is also noted in systole.

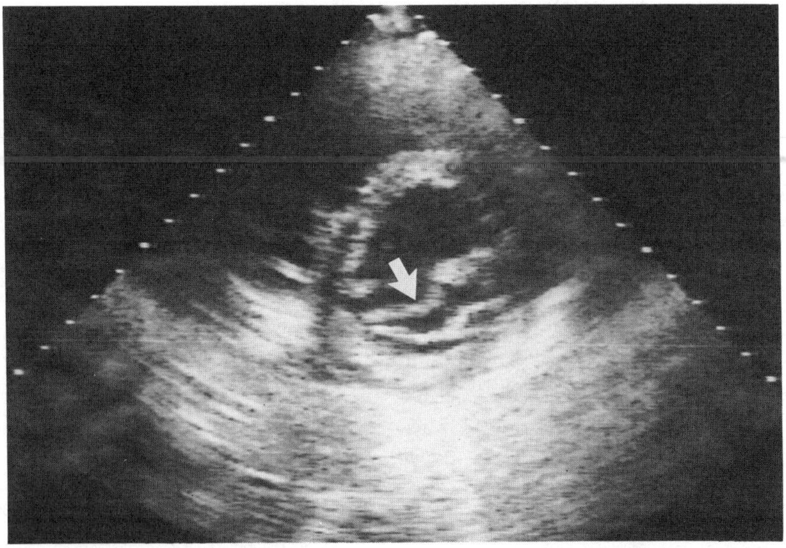

Figure 7.11
Short axis view of the left ventricle and mitral valve in a patient with aortic regurgitation. Note the indentation (arrow) on the anterior mitral leaflet, whereby the aortic regurgitant jet restricts full excursion of the anterior mitral leaflet in diastole.

tect a flail aortic leaflet, with associated findings leading to the diagnosis of the cause of the acute valve malfunction (Figure 7.6). Because of the acute nature of the volume overload, the left ventricle may be normal in size and vigorously contract. Clinical heart failure may be present despite good left ventricular function. In this context, diastolic fluttering of the anterior mitral valve may not be evident. However, the acute volume overload in the normal-sized left ventricle frequently causes significant elevation of left ventricular diastolic pressure, which may exceed left atrial pressure and cause premature closure of the mitral valve in late diastole (Figure 7.12).

Mitral Valve

Mitral Stenosis

Congenital stenosis of the mitral valve is rare. Occasionally, calcification of the mitral annulus secondary to degenerative disease may extend into the mitral valve leaflets and cause stenosis. Most commonly, mitral stenosis is acquired secondary to rheumatic heart disease.

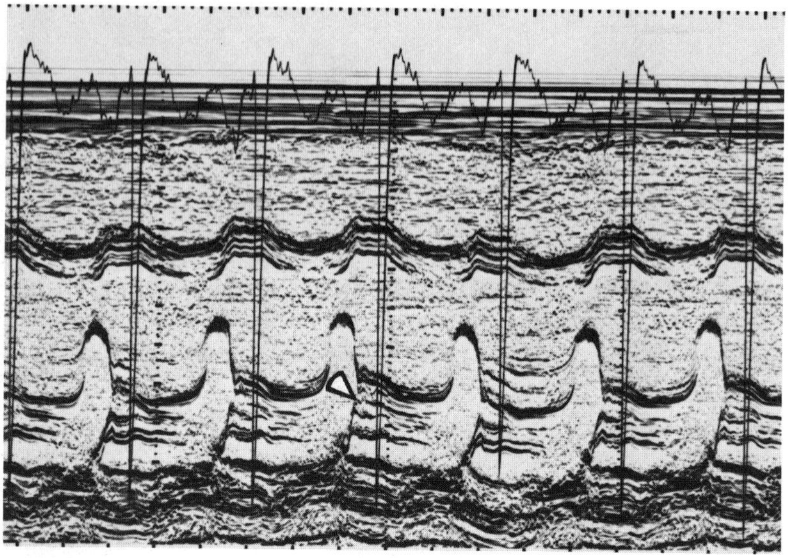

Figure 7.12
M-mode recording of the mitral valve from a patient with acute severe aortic regurgitation. Note the absence of any demonstrable diastolic fluttering of the anterior mitral leaflet. Moreover, due to significant elevation of left ventricular pressure in late diastole, premature closure of the mitral valve is clearly evident (open arrowhead). The ECG signal was amplified to show the time interval from premature mitral valve closure to the beginning of the next systolic cycle.

Valve Anatomy

The main abnormality in rheumatic mitral stenosis is fusion of the tips of the mitral leaflets. This results in restricted opening and obstruction of flow. The echocardiographic findings demonstrate thickened valve leaflets with diminished leaflet separation in diastole (Figure 7.13). The body of the leaflet is usually spared and distends under the influence of high left atrial pressure in diastole. This is reflected on the two-dimensional echocardiogram as a diastolic doming appearance. Because of persistently elevated left atrial pressures relative to left ventricular pressures in diastole, there is loss of the normal closure pattern of the mitral valve (Figure 7.14). The rate of leaflet closure in early diastole is diminished. This is reflected as a decreased E-F slope. Fusion of the tips of the anterior and posterior leaflets is very common. Hence, the leaflets demonstrate concordant motion, with the posterior leaflet moving forward together with the anterior leaflet in diastole (Figure 7.14).

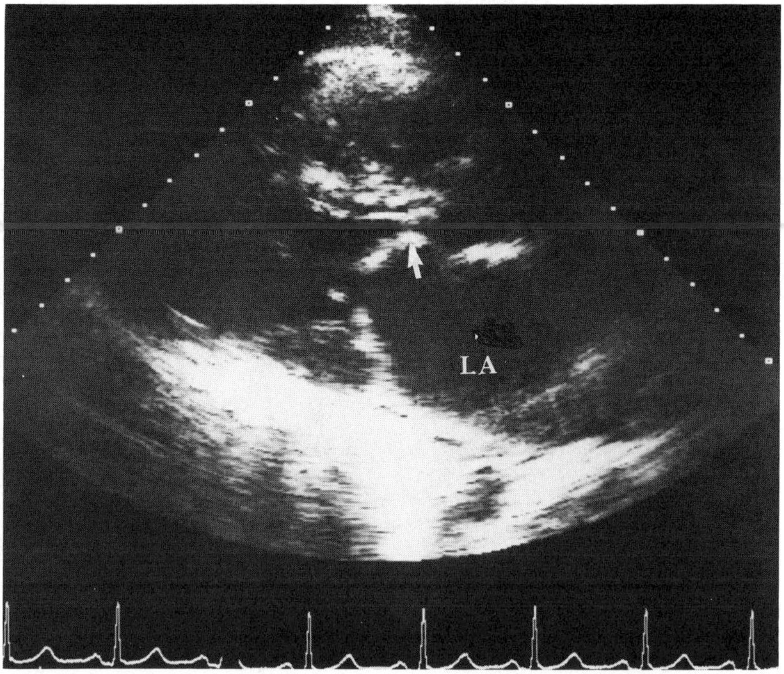

A

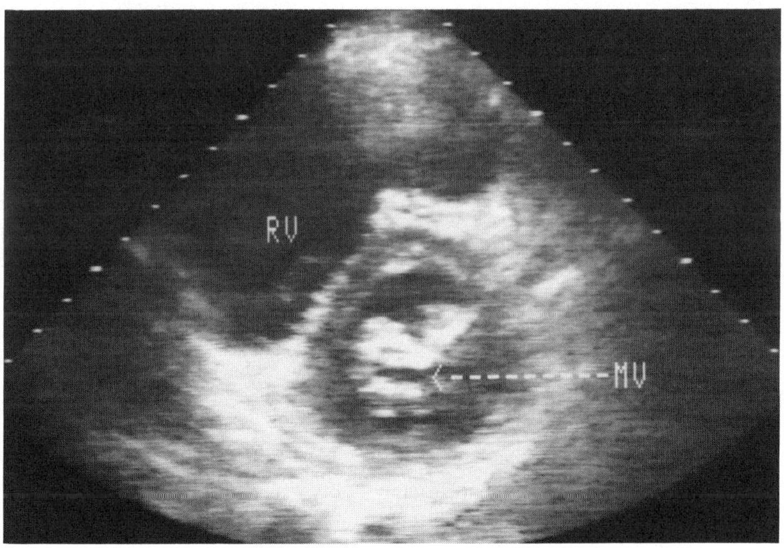

B

Figure 7.13
A. Diastolic frame of the mitral valve obtained from a parasternal long axis view, depicting the reduced valve opening and diastolic doming (arrow) of the anterior leaflet. B and C. Short axis and four-chamber apical views of the mitral valve, showing thickened leaflets with restricted diastolic excursion. Note the marked dilatation of the left atrium. LA = left atrium, LV = left ventricle, MV = mitral valve, RA = right atrium, RV = right ventricle.

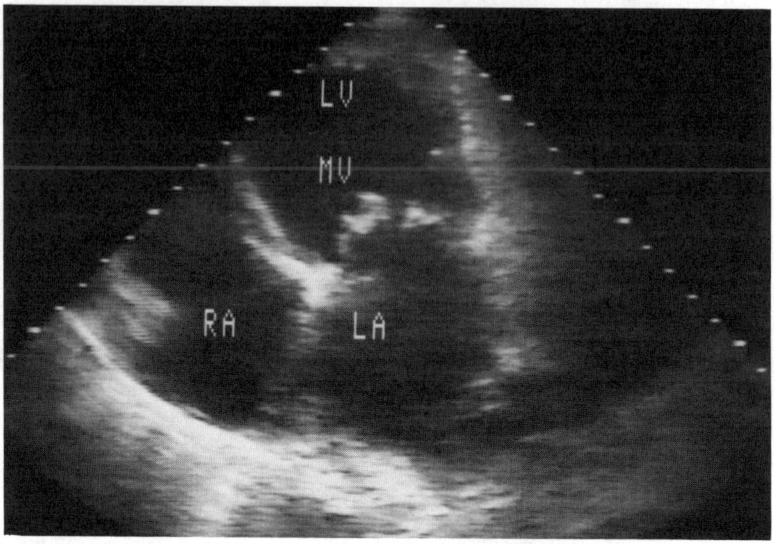

C
Figure 7.13 (continued)

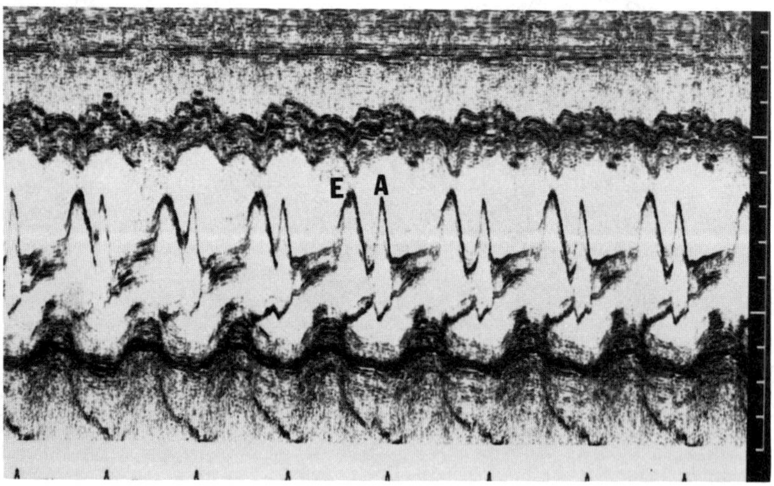

A
Figure 7.14
A. Normal mitral valve motion. B. Mild mitral stenosis. C. Moderate mitral stenosis. Compare the motion in A to the restricted and thickened leaflets in B and C. Note the loss of normal E and A waves despite the presence of sinus rhythm in all of these tracings.

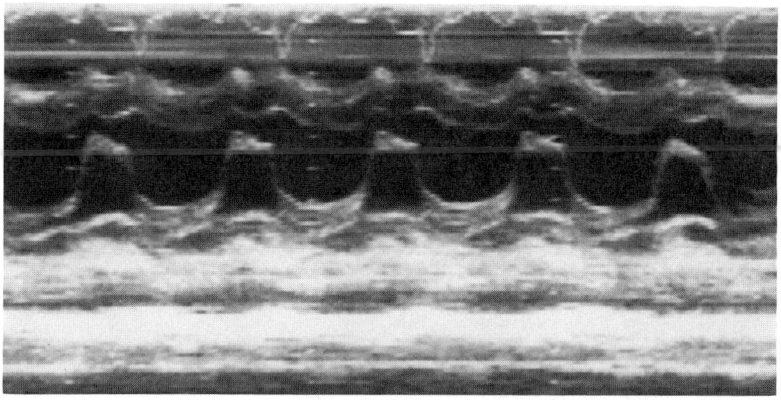

B

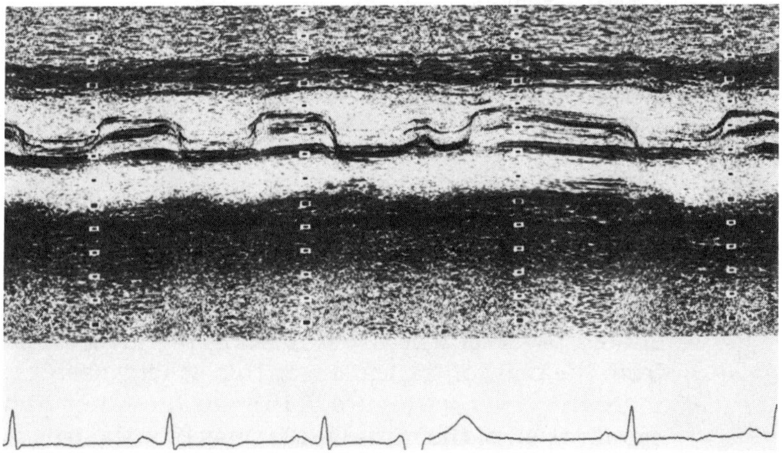

C

Figure 7.14 (continued)

Determining the Severity of Stenosis

The M-mode echocardiogram is highly sensitive in establishing the diagnosis of mitral stenosis, but not the severity. Leaflet separation and, subsequently, severity of obstruction may be measured on the M-mode recordings. However, if the ultrasound beam is inaccurately directed along the body of the leaflets rather than the tips, the degree of stenosis may be underestimated (Figure 7.15). As mentioned earlier, there is a decrease in the E-F slope in mitral stenosis, which reflects a significant pressure gradient across the mitral valve. Hence, the worse the stenosis is, the less the E-F slope is. A diminished E-F slope reflects impaired left ventricular filling, and this echocardiographic sign may be observed in patients with abnormal left ventricular diastolic relaxation in the absence of mitral stenosis.

The two-dimensional echocardiogram is more accurate

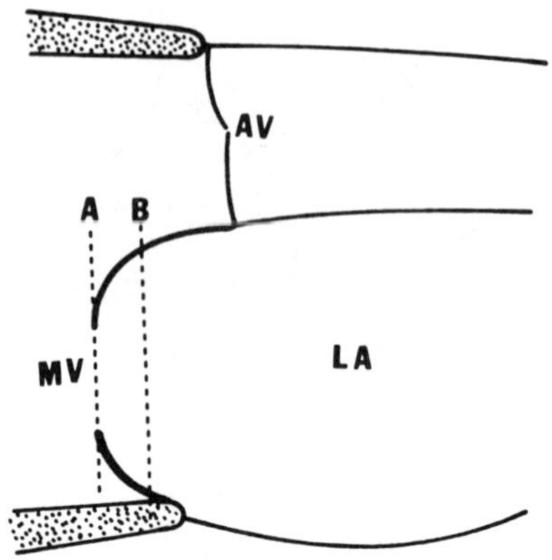

Figure 7.15
A parasternal long axis view in mitral stenosis. Leaflet separation measured from an M-mode ultrasound beam traversing the body of the mitral leaflets (B) will underestimate the severity of stenosis. A smaller valve excursion will be obtained if the beam is directed across the tips of the leaflets (A). MV = mitral valve, AV = aortic valve, LA = left atrium.

than the M-mode echocardiogram in determining the severity of the stenosis. Accurate measurements of the narrowed valve orifice can be made from the parasternal short axis view at the tips of the mitral leaflets (Figure 7.13). One should be careful to avoid making the area measurements from the body of the leaflets as this will invariably underestimate the severity (Figure 7.15). On the other hand, severe calcification of the mitral leaflet may blur the true margins of the valve orifice. If this occurs, measurements of the valve area may be less accurate.

Associated Findings

Persistently elevated left atrial pressure causes left atrial dilatation (Figure 7.13). Occasionally, thrombus formation in the left atrium may occur. Such thrombi are more commonly situated in the atrial appendage, which is difficult to visualize by echocardiography. Occasionally, a thrombus may detach from the atrial wall and embolize. However, a large thrombus may be trapped within the left atrium because of a relatively small mitral valve orifice (Figure 7.16).

The left ventricle is usually small with preserved overall contractility. The right ventricle may be dilated as a result of pulmonary hypertension, secondary to the persistently elevated left atrial pressure. Even though rheumatic heart disease commonly affects primarily the mitral valve, other valves may be involved. Associated aortic and, occasionally, tricuspid valve disease may be observed. Rheumatic involvement of the pulmonary valve is very rare.

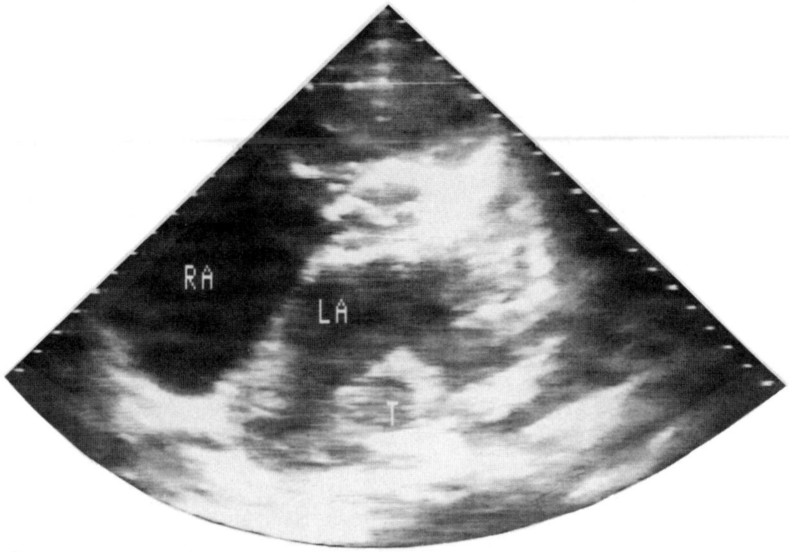

A

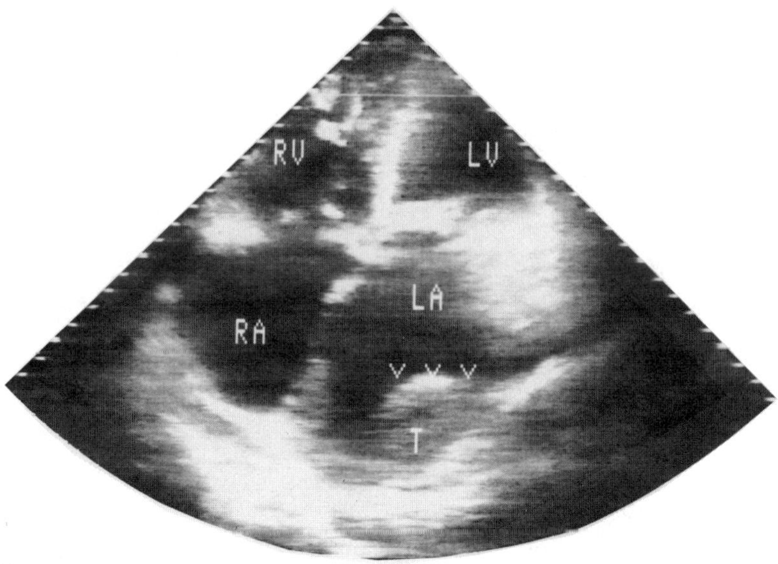

B

Figure 7.16
A. Short axis view, and B. Apical four-chamber view from a patient with mitral stenosis and thrombus (T) along the posterior aspect of the left atrium (LA). RA = right atrium, RV = right ventricle, LV = left ventricle.

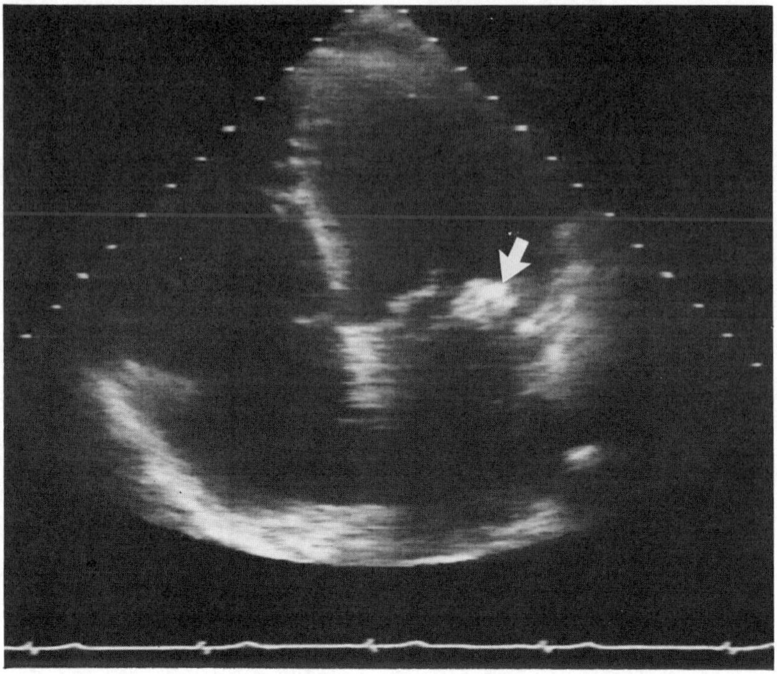

A

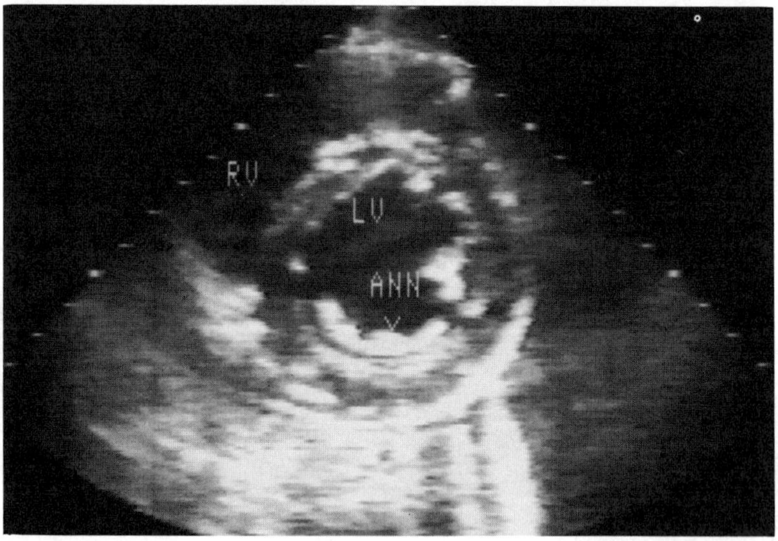

B

Figure 7.17
A. Apical four-chamber view from a patient with mitral annular calcification (arrow), depicting dense irregular echoes at the annulus. Note the normal appearance of the anterior mitral leaflet.
B. Short axis view showing extensive calcification along the annulus (ANN), which appears as a semicircle from this view.
C. M-mode recording across the mitral valve showing dense continuous echo densities of the calcified mitral annulus (MAC). Note the normal appearance of the anterior mitral leaflet (AML). RV = right ventricle, LV = left ventricle.

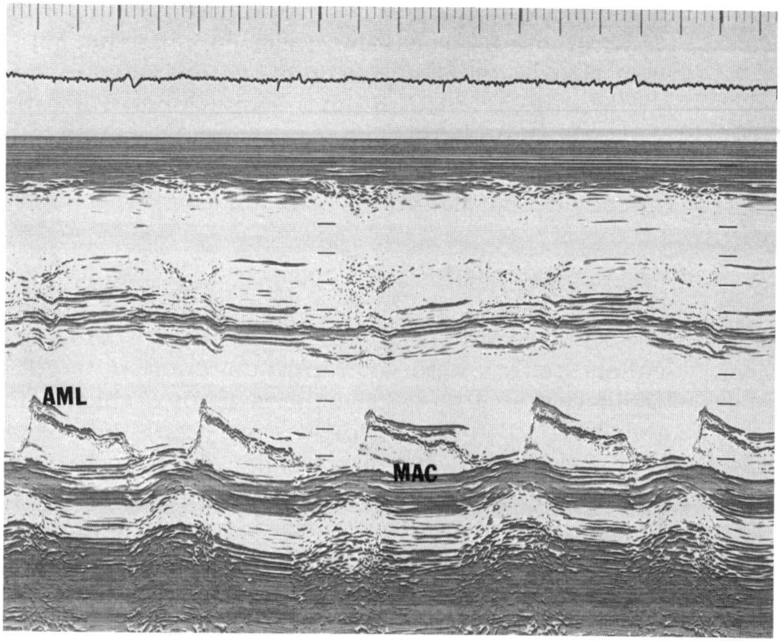

C
Figure 7.17 (continued)

Mitral Annular Calcification

The mitral annulus is continuously subjected to shearing forces related to ventricular contraction. With advancing age, fibrosis and calcification of the mitral annulus may occur, and are commonly observed by the sixth decade of life. Annular calcification may be observed in younger individuals with severe left ventricular pressure overload, such as with aortic stenosis, hypertrophic obstructive cardiomyopathy, or severe chronic hypertension. Moreover, abnormal calcium metabolism, as seen in patients with hyperparathyroidism or end-stage renal failure, may predispose for mitral annular calcification at a younger age.

Calcium deposition frequently extends into the posterior mitral leaflet, thereby restricting its mobility. Mitral regurgitation occurs in approximately one-half of patients with significant annular calcification. Extension of calcium deposition into the anterior mitral leaflet is less frequent, and rarely leads to any significant true obstruction to diastolic flow.

The calcified mitral annulus is highly echogenic and produces characteristic ultrasound appearance of enhanced echoes in the region of the annulus (Figure 7.17). On the M-mode echocardiogram, the calcified annulus appears as dense echoes adjacent to the posterior wall of the left ventricle throughout the cardiac cycle. This is to be distinguished from rheumatic calcification of the mitral valve, whereby in mitral annular calcification the anterior mitral leaflet is usually spared and exhibits normal unrestricted mobility. Occasionally, the calcification may extend into the chordae tendineae and papillary muscle head.

Chronic Mitral Regurgitation

The mitral valve is a complex structure composed of two leaflets, with supporting annulus, chordae tendineae, and papillary muscles. Abnormalities of any of these components may lead to mitral regurgitation. Common diseases that primarily involve the mitral leaflets include rheumatic heart disease and bacterial endocarditis. Mitral valve prolapse is a degenerative disease of the mitral leaflets, which become redundant relative to the size of the mitral annulus. The chordae tendineae may also be redundant, and at times may rupture and worsen the severity of mitral regurgitation.

Diseases that involve the supporting structure of the mitral valve leaflets leading to regurgitation include calcification of the mitral annulus, bacterial endocarditis with rupture of the chordae tendineae, and ischemia with or without infarction of the papillary muscles, which may rupture.

Mitral regurgitation may occur without any primary involvement of the mitral valve apparatus. This secondary cause of mitral regurgitation commonly occurs with any condition that causes severe dilatation of the left ventricle. Marked enlargement of the left ventricle causes passive dilatation of the mitral annulus with distension of the chordae tendineae; leaflet coaptation is incomplete, resulting in valve incompetence. Moreover, secondary causes of mitral regurgitation include extrinsic pressure from an extracardiac tumor mass, and occasionally from an intra-atrial myxoma.

Valve Anatomy

The echocardiographic examination of a patient suspected of having mitral regurgitation should be directed to confirm the presence of this hemodynamic abnormality as well as provide clues to the cause of the regurgitation and its severity.

Rheumatic heart disease will demonstrate thickening and abnormal mobility of the mitral leaflets. Vegetations may be seen in bacterial endocarditis (Figure 7.18). Flail mitral leaflets may cause coarse fluttering of the tip of the leaflets, best observed on the M-mode echocardiogram (Figure 7.10).

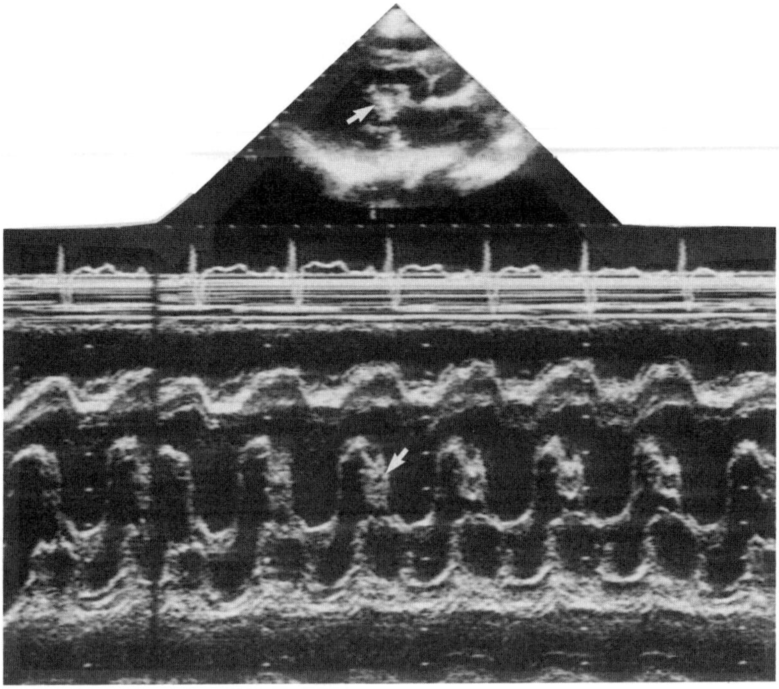

Figure 7.18
Vegetation (arrow) attached to the anterior mitral leaflet is clearly demonstrated on the two-dimensional parasternal long axis view and simultaneous M-mode recording across the mitral valve.

Prolapse of the mitral leaflets typically demonstrates ballooning of the affected leaflet into the left atrium during systole (Figure 7.19). The M-mode recording demonstrates posterior motion of the mitral leaflet in mid to late systole. However, the two-dimensional echocardiogram is more sensitive than M-mode echocardiography because mitral valve motion can be observed from multiple views. The parasternal long axis view and the apical four-chamber views are the best to demonstrate the prolapse. In this context, it is important to note that even though mitral valve prolapse is commonly associated with regurgitation, valve incompetency may not be present in every patient with echocardiographic evidence of prolapse. Since mitral valve prolapse is a dynamic process, variation of intracardiac pressures and volumes may affect the severity of the prolapse.

Determining the Severity

The presence of a flail mitral leaflet commonly suggests that the regurgitation is severe. However, in the absence of any gross pathologic evidence, evaluation of the severity of

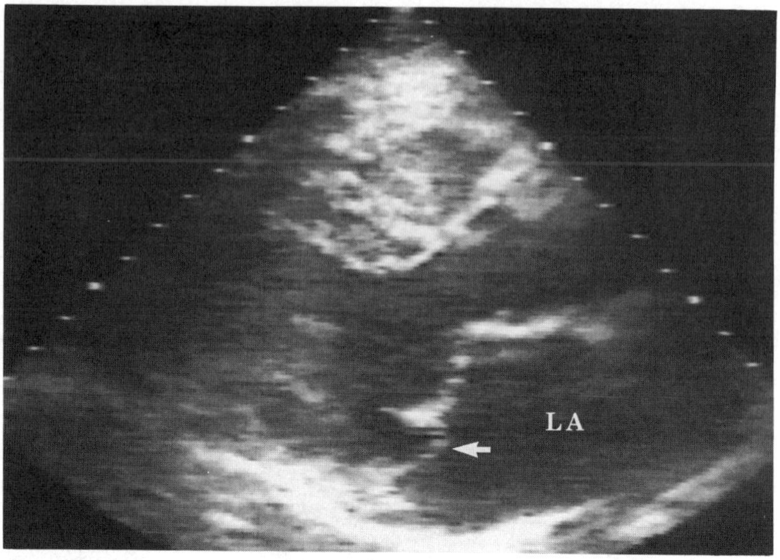

A

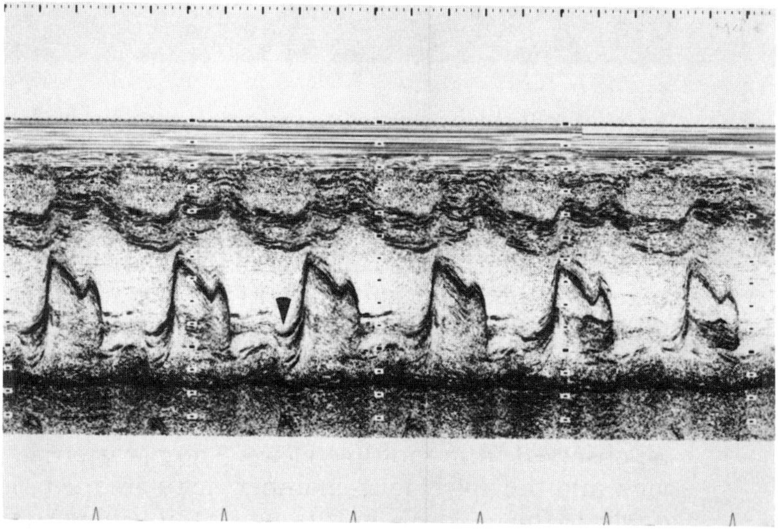

B

Figure 7.19
Mitral valve prolapse exhibits exaggerated posterior motion of one or both mitral leaflets in systole into the left atrium (LA). A. Note the buckling of the posterior mitral leaflet (arrow) in this parasternal long axis view. B. Note the posterior motion of both mitral leaflets at end systole (arrowhead), characteristic of mitral valve prolapse.

chronic mitral regurgitation is difficult. Indirect echocardiographic evidence of severe mitral regurgitation relies on demonstrating a dilated left atrium with left ventricular volume overload, in the absence of any other reason for left ventricular dilatation.

In severe regurgitation, progressive dilatation of the left ventricle occurs. This ultimately leads to various degrees of impaired contractility.

Associated Findings

Mitral regurgitation is commonly associated with a dilated left atrium. As the disease progresses, left atrial pressure becomes elevated. This can lead to pulmonary hypertension with right ventricular dilatation and hypertrophy.

If mitral regurgitation is secondary to coronary artery disease with papillary muscle dysfunction, the echocardiogram may demonstrate abnormal motion of the wall segments that are involved with ongoing ischemia or infarction.

Acute Mitral Regurgitation

This is commonly caused by a flail mitral leaflet secondary to bacterial endocarditis, mitral valve prolapse, or rupture of papillary muscles in a patient with acute myocardial infarction. The echocardiogram typically demonstrates the flail leaflet (Figures 7.10B, 6.8). The left ventricle is usually normal in size with preserved contractility unless severe acute myocardial infarction is present.

Tricuspid Valve

Tricuspid Stenosis

Isolated stenosis of the tricuspid valve is very rare. Tricuspid atresia is the congenital absence of this valve, with narrowing of the right ventricular inflow tract and a small right ventricular chamber. Acquired stenosis secondary to rheumatic heart disease is rare. The echocardiogram demonstrates changes similar to those observed in patients with mitral stenosis in regard to leaflet thickening and restricted mobility and reduced E-F slope. However, two-dimensional echocardiography is better suited to evaluate tricuspid valve stenosis. Carcinoid syndrome may cause tricuspid stenosis, but this is also rare. In this context, there is fibrosis and thickening of the body of the valve leaflet. In contrast to the fusion of leaflet tips in rheumatic stenosis, the tips of the tricuspid leaflets are usually spared in carcinoid disease.

The degree of associated right atrial dilatation is usually commensurate with the severity of obstruction.

Tricuspid Regurgitation

Bacterial endocarditis is the most common form of acquired tricuspid valve disease causing regurgitation (Figure 7.20). Two-dimensional echocardiography may demonstrate the vegetations and, occasionally, a ruptured leaflet. Rheumatic heart disease involving the tricuspid valve more commonly causes regurgitation than stenosis. The leaflets may be thickened with minimal restriction of mobility. Prolapse of the tricuspid valve leaflets may occur in association with mitral valve prolapse.

Right ventricular dysfunction is the most common cause of secondary tricuspid regurgitation. In this context, the valve leaflets are normal. Regurgitation occurs because of dilatation of the valve annulus and the right ventricle. The echocardiogram usually demonstrates right ventricular as well as right atrial dilatation (Figure 7.21). The inferior vena cava is often dilated as well.

Chronic severe tricuspid regurgitation leads to right ventricular volume overload. In the absence of significant left ventricular dysfunction, right ventricular overload may alter the motion of the interventricular septum. Normally, the interventricular septum is curved concave toward the left ventricular chamber. Moreover, left ventricular pressure in diastole is usually higher than right ventricular pressure, thus causing the interventricular septum to bulge into the right ventricle. When right ventricular dilatation occurs, there is stretching of the interventricular septum, which becomes flattened. Severe right ventricular dysfunction may lead to elevation of diastolic pressure. If this pressure exceeds left ventricular diastolic pressure, the interventricular septum tends to bulge into the left ventricle in diastole. However, during systole, left ventricular pressure exceeds right ventricular pressure, thus leading to paradoxical motion of the interventricular septum into the right ventricle in systole. This alteration of septal motion during systole and diastole is reflected on the echocardiogram (Figure 7.22) and is consistent with right ventricular volume overload.

Contrast echocardiography may be used for the echocardiographic diagnosis of tricuspid regurgitation. The microbubbles, injected in a peripheral vein in the arm, travel through the superior vena cava to the right atrium. These microbubbles then traverse the right ventricle into the pulmonary artery (Figure 7.23). In the normal heart, these microbubbles are not seen within the inferior vena cava. How-

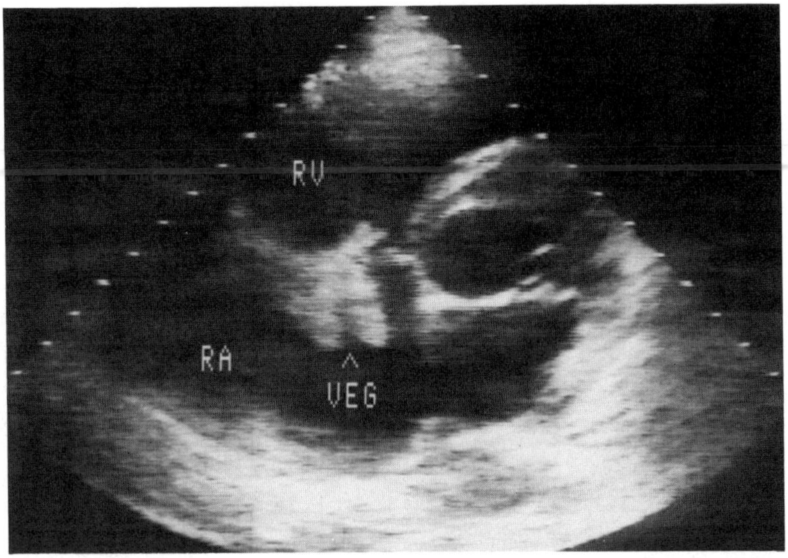

A

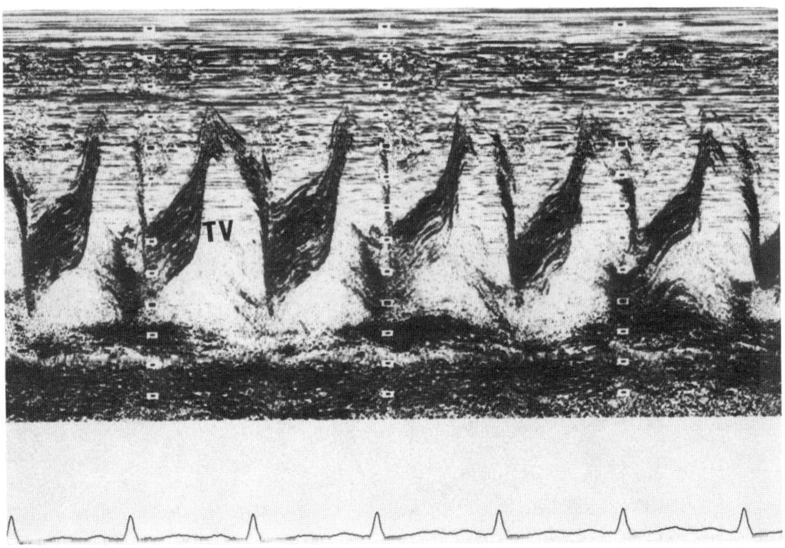

B

Figure 7.20
A. Short axis view showing large vegetation (VEG) on the tricuspid valve, prolapsing into the right atrium (RA) in systole.
B. M-mode recording across the tricuspid valve (TV), showing markedly thickened leaflet with multiple linear echo densities consistent with vegetation. RV = right ventricle.

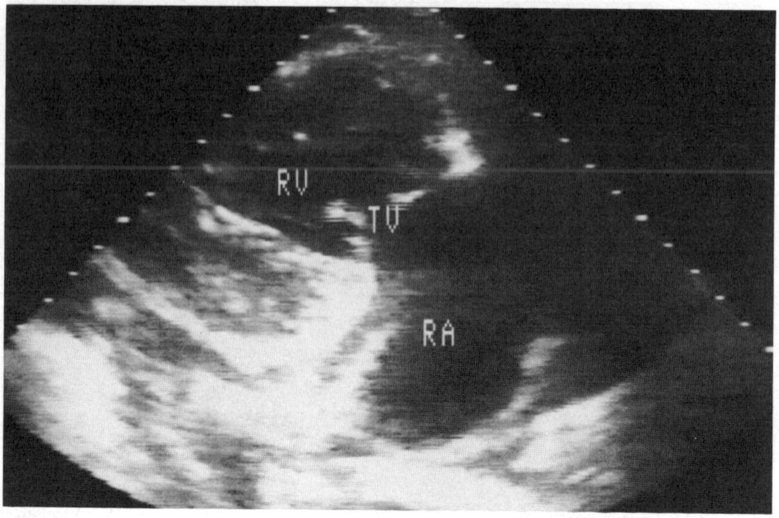

A

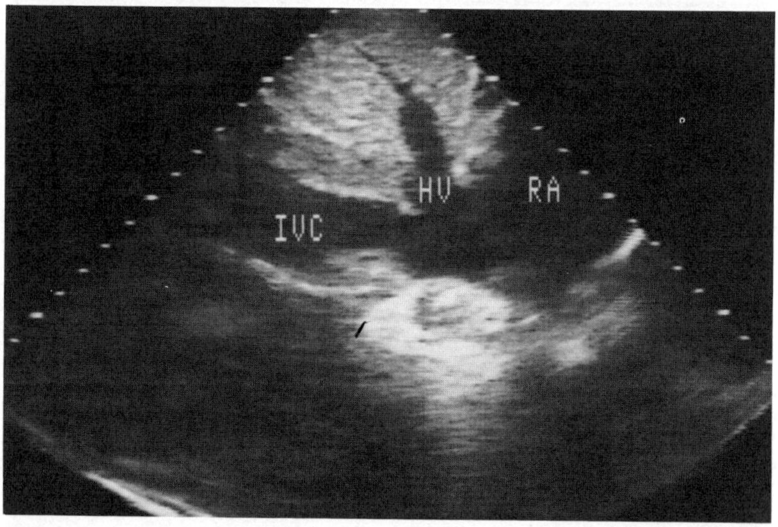

B

Figure 7.21
A. Right ventricular inflow tract view demonstrating dilated right atrium (RA) and ventricle (RV). B. Subcostal view of a patient with significant tricuspid regurgitation, demonstrating dilated inferior vena cava (IVC) and hepatic vein (HV). TV = tricuspid valve.

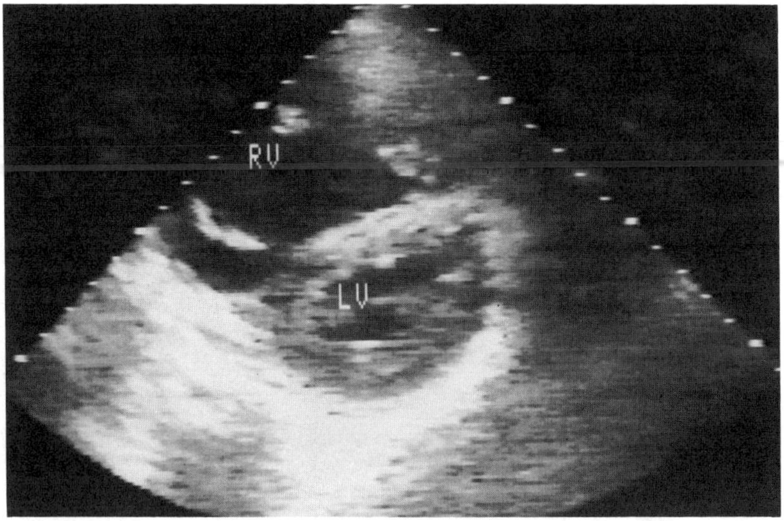

A

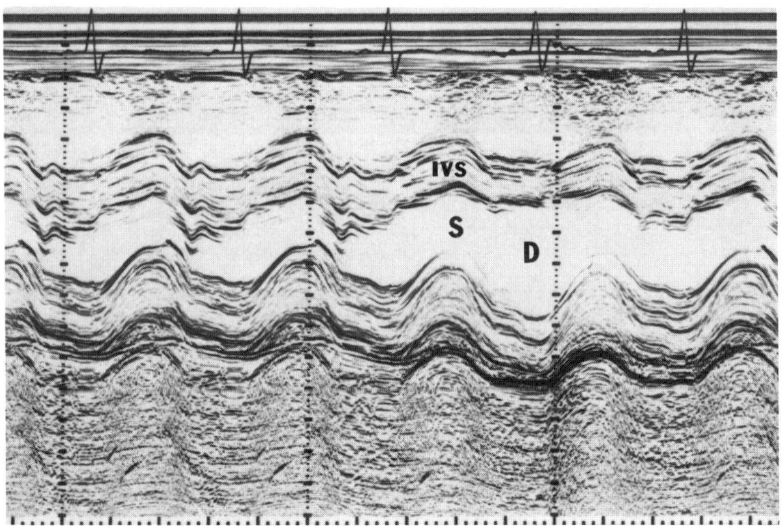

B

Figure 7.22

A. Short axis view from a patient with tricuspid regurgitation and markedly dilated right ventricle (RV). Note the flattened interventricular septum with loss of normal diastolic curvature.

B. M-mode recording of the interventricular septum (IVS) clearly demonstrates the paradoxical motion, whereby the septum moves anteriorly in systole (S) and posteriorly in diastole (D). LV = left ventricle.

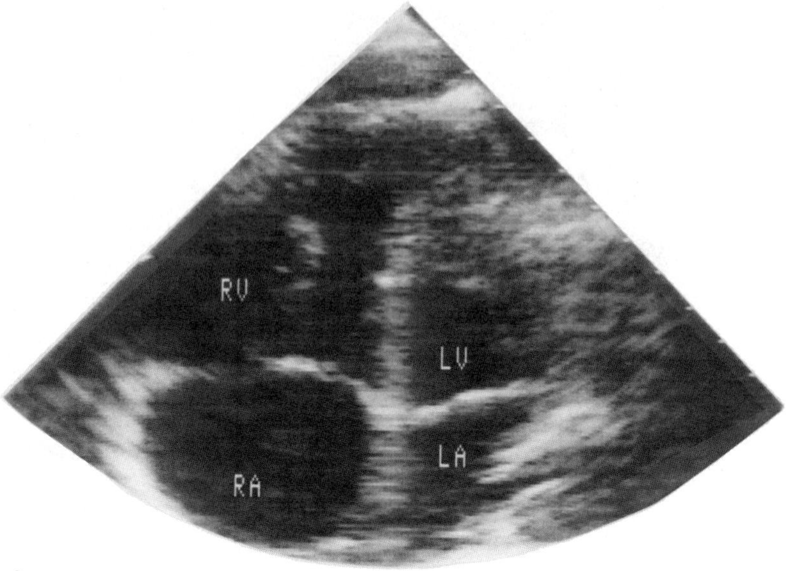

A

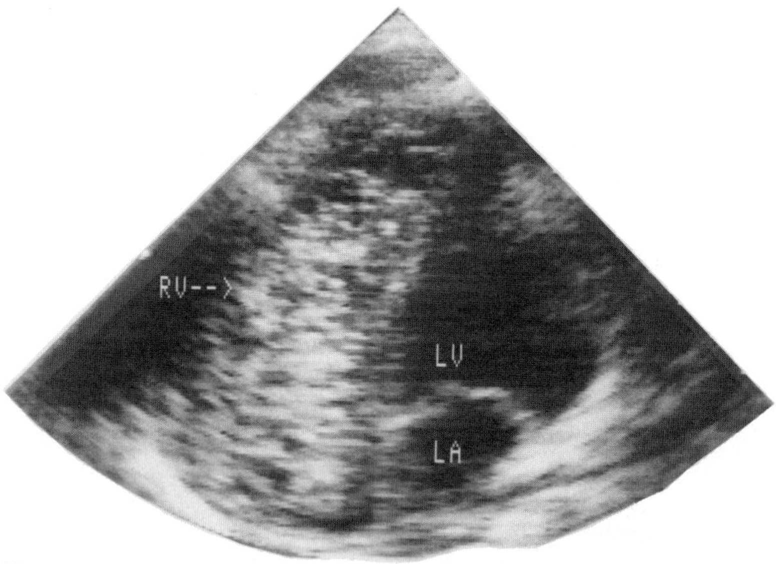

B

Figure 7.23
Rapid infusion of sonicated saline solution into a peripheral vein generates microbubbles, creating an interface that reflects ultrasound and that can be traced on the two-dimensional recording as the microbubbles travel through the cardiac chambers. A. Four-chamber apical view before injection of the sonicated saline solution. B. The right chambers are opacified with the microbubbles as they traverse the right atrium and right ventricle (RV). LA = left atrium, LV = left ventricle, RA = right atrium.

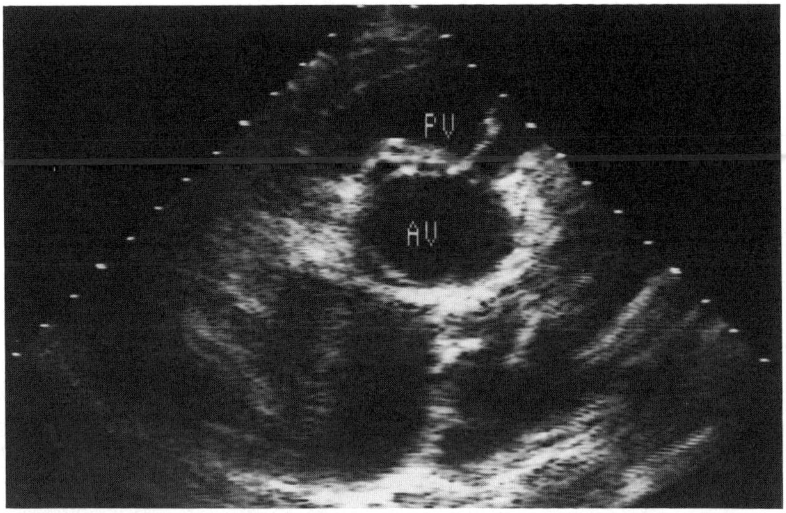

Figure 7.24
Systolic frame from the short axis parasternal window, showing restricted motion of the posterior pulmonary valve leaflet (PV). Note the wide-open aortic valve leaflets (AV), for comparison.

ever, when tricuspid regurgitation is present, regurgitant blood concentrated with microbubbles is seen within the inferior vena cava, indicating retrograde blood flow. Moreover, there is usually a delayed clearance of these microbubbles, which may be seen traveling back and forth across the tricuspid valve for many cardiac cycles before they finally dissolve and disappear.

Pulmonary Valve

Pulmonary Stenosis

Stenosis of the pulmonary valve is not often seen in the adult population. This is usually congenital. Acquired stenosis is rarely seen in patients with carcinoid syndrome. Echocardiography demonstrates thickened leaflets with restricted opening and doming of the body of the leaflets during systole (Figure 7.24). The M-mode echocardiogram usually depicts an exaggerated A wave on the pulmonary valve tracing, consistent with increased right atrial and ventricular pressures during late diastole relative to the pulmonary artery diastolic pressure. Because of obstruction to right ventricular emptying, hypertrophy of this chamber occurs.

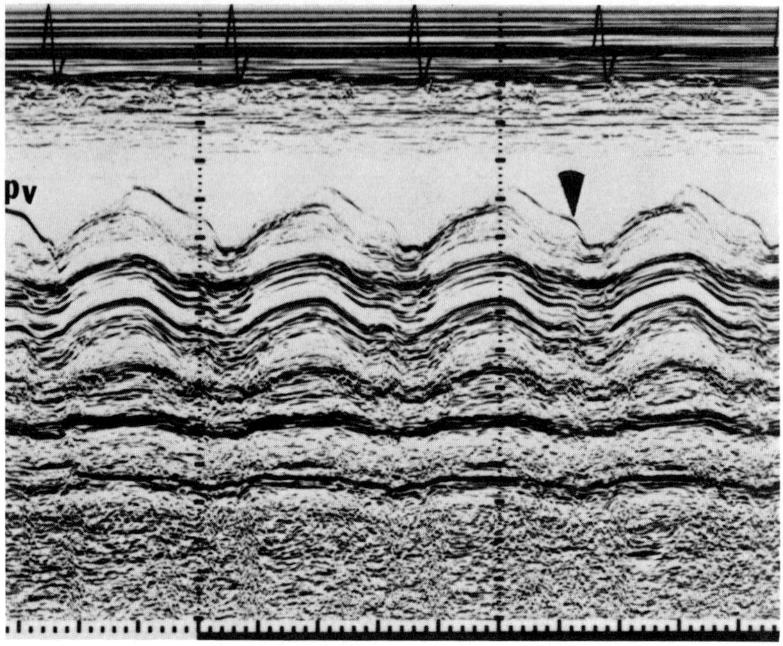

Figure 7.25
M-mode recording of the pulmonary valve (pv) from a patient with right ventricular volume overload without pulmonary hypertension. Note the premature opening of the pulmonary valve (arrowhead) before the onset of systole, consistent with significant elevation of diastolic pressure in the right side of the heart.

Pulmonary Regurgitation

Bacterial endocarditis of the pulmonary valve is rare. Pulmonary regurgitation most commonly occurs secondary to pulmonary hypertension with no structural abnormality of this valve. Various degrees of right ventricular dilatation and hypertrophy may occur, depending on the severity of the volume and pressure overload. Right atrial dilatation is frequently encountered as well. Premature opening of the pulmonary valve, prior to onset of ventricular systole, may occasionally be noted on the echocardiogram in patients with right ventricular volume overload without pulmonary hypertension. In this context, right ventricular diastolic pressure exceeds pulmonary artery pressure, forcing premature opening of the valve (Figure 7.25).

8 Doppler Ultrasonography in Valvular Heart Disease

Cardiac valvular pathologic conditions cause abnormalities of the velocity and direction of blood flow across the diseased cardiac valve. These abnormalities may be divided into three categories:

1. Stenotic valvular lesions in which flow is in a normal direction relative to the cardiac cycle and cardiac valve being examined; however, the velocity of flow is abnormally higher than expected.
2. Regurgitant valvular lesions in which flow is abnormal relative to the cardiac cycle and valve being insonated.
3. Complex flow patterns comprising mixed valvular lesions (e.g., stenosis and regurgitation of one or more cardiac valves).

Stenotic Valvular Lesions

A stenotic cardiac valve causes blood flow disturbances simi lar to water flow disturbances observed with a narrow nozzle at the end of a water hose. When the nozzle is wide open, water flows smoothly out of the nozzle. The flow is almost laminar, and the velocity is of normal magnitude and is mainly dependent on the amount of flow controlled by the water faucet at the other end of the hose. If the nozzle is adjusted to a smaller opening, maintaining the same amount of flow, then the velocity of water coming out of the nozzle is higher and the flow becomes turbulent. The magnitude of increase in the velocity is dependent on the degree

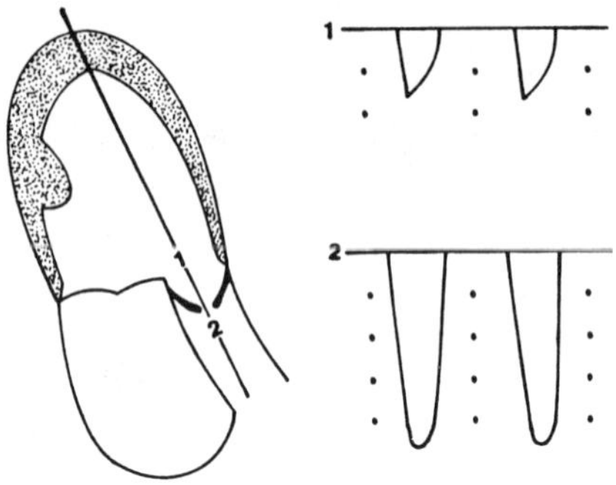

Figure 8.1
An apical two-dimensional image in aortic stenosis. PW mode Doppler recording in the left ventricular outflow tract (sample volume location 1) depicts relatively normal velocity of flow in that region. PW mode Doppler recording at the level of the aortic valve leaflets (sample volume location 2) depicts high-velocity jet consistent with relative obstruction of flow in that region.

of narrowing of the nozzle head. In general, the narrower the orifice is, the higher the velocity is. A stenotic cardiac valve will cause blood flow abnormalities similar to that observed for a narrow nozzle on a water hose. The cardiac chamber that is pumping the blood across the stenotic valve acts as the faucet that regulates the amount of flow.

It is very important to realize that the increase in the velocity occurs mainly downstream to the site of the obstruction to flow (Figure 3.5). For example, velocity of blood flow across a stenotic aortic valve is near normal in the left ventricular outflow tract; this velocity increases significantly at the level of the aortic valve itself or in the aortic root (Figure 8.1). Also, in mitral valve stenosis, an increase in velocity is expected only at the level of the valve or within the left ventricular inflow tract and not within the left atrium (Figure 8.2). With increasing severity of obstruction, a small stream of blood flow is detected, referred to as the jet of flow. Eddy currents may occur at the boundaries of this jet with a high proportion of blood elements moving in various directions (parajet). This type of flow is turbulent (Figure 3.5).

The typical Doppler recording of this abnormal flow pattern shows a high velocity or frequency shift in the normal direction of flow, depending on the valve being insonated and location of the transducer on the chest wall. However, in the presence of turbulence, some frequency shifts or velocities may be recorded in the other direction as well. If PW mode Doppler is used, aliasing may occur if the frequency shifts caused by these high velocities exceed the Nyquist limit as discussed earlier. Shifting the zero baseline up or

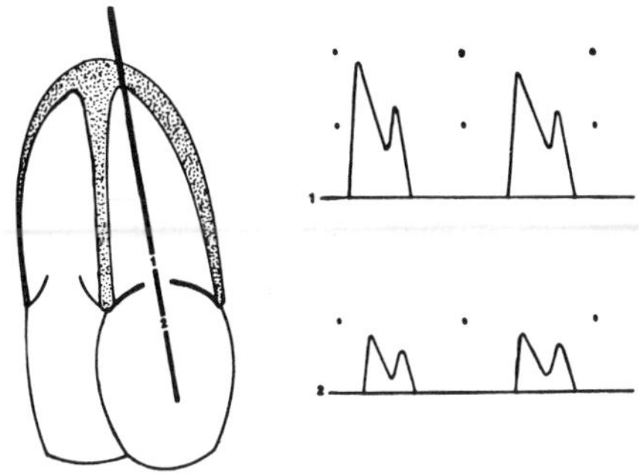

Figure 8.2
An apical two-dimensional image in mitral stenosis. PW mode Doppler recording in the left atrium proximal to the mitral annulus (sample volume location 2) depicts normal velocity of flow in that region. PW mode recording at the tips of the mitral leaflets (sample volume location 1) depicts high-velocity jet consistent with relative obstruction of flow in that region.

down on the Doppler recording may help eliminate this problem if the frequency shift is less than the PRF employed. Unfortunately, this maneuver may not be sufficient in many situations where the velocities are sufficiently high to cause severe aliasing. This problem underscores the value of combining PW mode with CW mode in examinations of valvular stenosis. CW mode is used to record the highest velocities along the ultrasound beam; then the PW mode is applied to determine the anatomic location within the heart at which these high-velocity jets are occurring. Conversely, the PW mode may be used first to locate the anatomic location of high-velocity jet, followed by the CW mode to determine the true velocity at that particular location. When examining patients with a single valvular abnormality, it may be obvious that the highest velocities recorded by CW mode are coming from a location downstream to the diseased valve; thus, a PW mode recording may not be needed. However, multiple valvular lesions or complex congenital heart diseases may produce high velocities at anatomic locations that may not be accurately determined without the use of the PW mode as well.

Aortic Valve Stenosis

The average normal aortic valve area in adults is approximately 3 cm^2. As aortic valvular stenosis develops, there is gradual narrowing of the orifice area. If the stroke volume (i.e., the amount of blood ejected through the valve per beat) remains constant, then an increase in the velocity of blood will be observed in systole. If the valve is competent, then

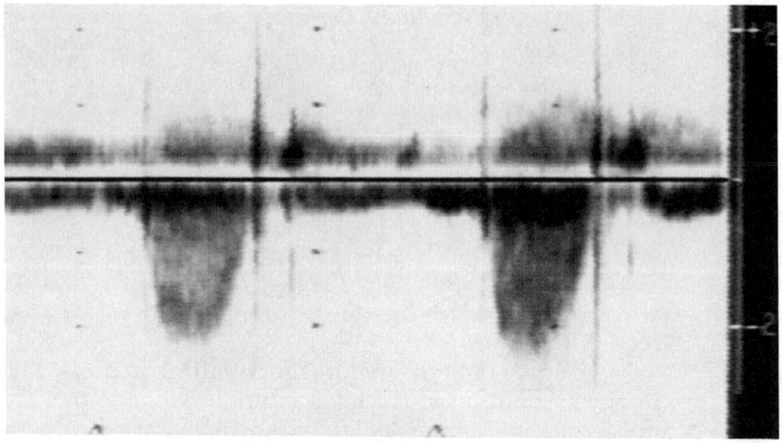

A

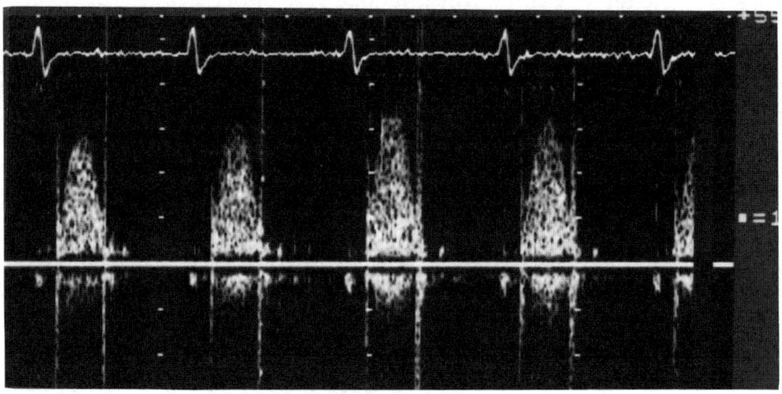

B

Figure 8.3
A. CW mode recording with the transducer in an apical location, depicting systolic high velocity of flow across a stenotic aortic valve. B. Systolic aortic flow recorded from a right parasternal location.

aortic flow is only in systole and occurs in the normal direction (i.e., from the left ventricle to the aorta). There is no retrograde flow in diastole.

Aortic flow may be recorded from transducer locations similar to those in normal situations, i.e., apical, suprasternal, or substernal (Figure 8.3). It is common to have an eccentric jet of flow across the diseased aortic valve, which is commonly oriented anteriorly and toward the right. Therefore, keeping in mind the effect of the incidence angle (θ) and the azimuthal plane, a good two-dimensional image showing the Doppler ultrasound beam in the center of the aortic root may not necessarily produce adequate Doppler recordings of the highest true velocity of flow. Hence, it is not uncommon to record the highest velocities across the aortic valve from

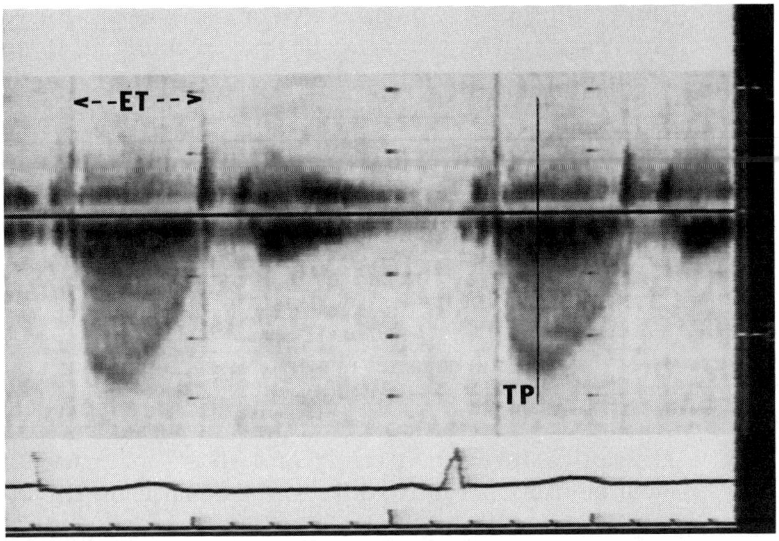

Figure 8.4
CW mode recording of aortic stenosis jet at 50 mm/sec paper speed. The amplitude signals delineate the duration of the ejection time (ET). Time to peak flow (TP) is measured from the beginning of flow to the time of highest velocity. The TP/ET ratio of less than 0.5 in this patient suggests that the aortic stenosis is not very severe.

transducer locations in the left lower parasternal area or even on the right side of the sternum in the second or third intercostal spaces. Such unusual locations to record aortic flow may show Doppler velocity recordings above or below the zero baseline, depending on the direction of flow relative to angulation of the transducer (Figure 8.3). It is also important to remember that the highest velocities occur downstream from the aortic valve within the aortic root and not in the left ventricular outflow tract. The quality of the two-dimensional image may need to be sacrificed in order to obtain the best Doppler signals.

Quantitative evaluation of the severity of obstruction will be discussed later. Semiquantitative analysis may be performed by measuring the duration of flow (ejection time [ET]) and the time from onset of flow to the time of occurrence of peak velocity (TP). The ratio of these two intervals may be used as a rough indication of the severity of obstruction (Figure 8.4). A TP/ET ratio of less than or equal to 0.5 indicates mild obstruction. A ratio of greater than 0.5 indicates high-grade obstruction.

Mitral Valve Stenosis

The average normal area of the mitral valve in adults is approximately 5 cm^2. Similar to aortic valve stenosis, gradual narrowing of the mitral valve orifice will produce a gradual increase in the velocities of flow in diastole. If the valve is competent, then mitral flow occurs only in diastole and in the normal direction (i.e., from the left atrium to the left ventricle). There is no retrograde flow in systole.

Transmitral flow is best recorded with the transducer in an apical position, with the ultrasound beam directed in the same manner for recording normal mitral flow (superiorly and posteriorly). The highest velocities are recorded within the left ventricular inflow tract, just at the tips of the fused mitral valve leaflet (Figure 8.2).

If the cardiac rhythm is still sinus rhythm with a preserved atrial kick, the velocity recording will be of similar configuration to that of normal mitral flow; however, the peak velocities in early diastole and those following atrial kick will be higher (Figure 8.5). The E-F slope on the M-mode recording is diminished. This has been shown to reflect a reduced rate of emptying of the left atrium (Figure 7.14). A hemodynamic correlate of this M-mode finding is the diminished deceleration rate of the Doppler velocity recordings in early diastole (Figure 8.5). This is consistent with the fact that in mitral stenosis, left atrial emptying is impaired and a pressure gradient persists between the left atrium and the left ventricle in diastole. This concept may be applied to estimate the anatomic valve area, as will be discussed in Chapter 21.

Most patients with a high degree of mitral stenosis develop atrial fibrillation. With this cardiac rhythm, there is no effective atrial contraction. The atrial kick is lost, resulting in the loss of the A wave on the M-mode echocardiogram, as well as the loss of the second peak velocity on the Doppler recording (Figure 8.5).

The peak velocities attained in mitral stenosis cannot be as high as those velocities encountered across the aortic valve in aortic stenosis. This is because the left atrium is a so-called low-pressure chamber and cannot generate high pressures like the left ventricle (high-pressure chamber). Moreover, the velocities primarily reflect the pressure gradient across the valve, i.e., the difference in pressure between the left atrium and the left ventricle in diastole. This pressure gradient is much less than the pressure gradient across the aortic valve in aortic stenosis (difference in pressure between the left ventricle and the aorta in systole).

Color Doppler imaging demonstrates a wide jet of flow originating from the mitral valve orifice. Because of high velocity of flow, the Nyquist limit is frequently exceeded. The usual orange color is mixed with blue. Turbulence causes mosaic color appearance as well (Plate 4).

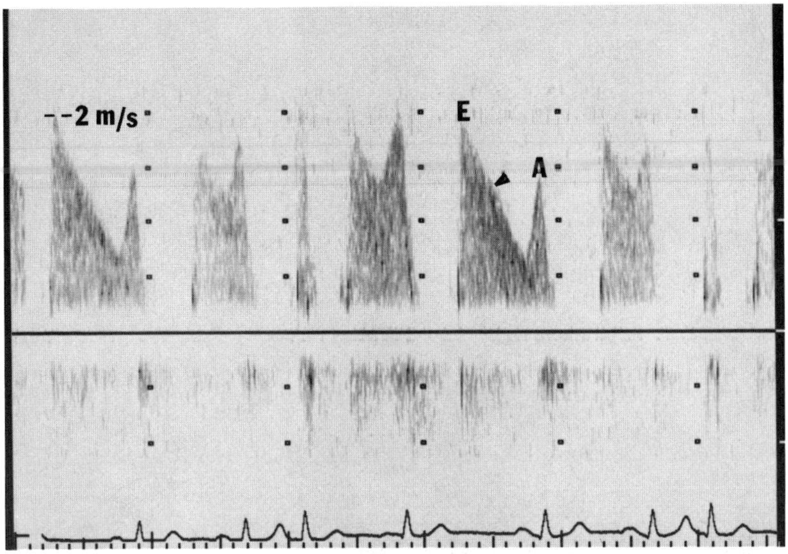

A

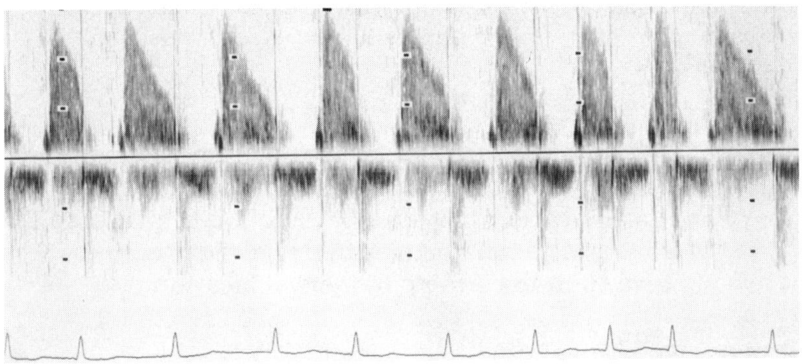

B

Figure 8.5
A. CW mode Doppler recording from a patient with mitral stenosis and sinus rhythm and premature atrial contractions. Note the preserved E and A velocities, which are higher than normal. Also note the slow rate of deceleration of flow after the E velocity (arrowhead) as compared to normal (see Figure 5.1). B. CW mode recording of mitral stenosis from a patient in atrial fibrillation. Note the absence of A velocity.

Tricuspid Valve Stenosis

Since the average anatomic area of the tricuspid valve is normally approximately 7 cm^2, a severely narrowed tricuspid orifice is rarely encountered. Doppler recordings across a stenosed tricuspid valve demonstrate similar patterns as those seen in mitral stenosis. Transducer locations to record

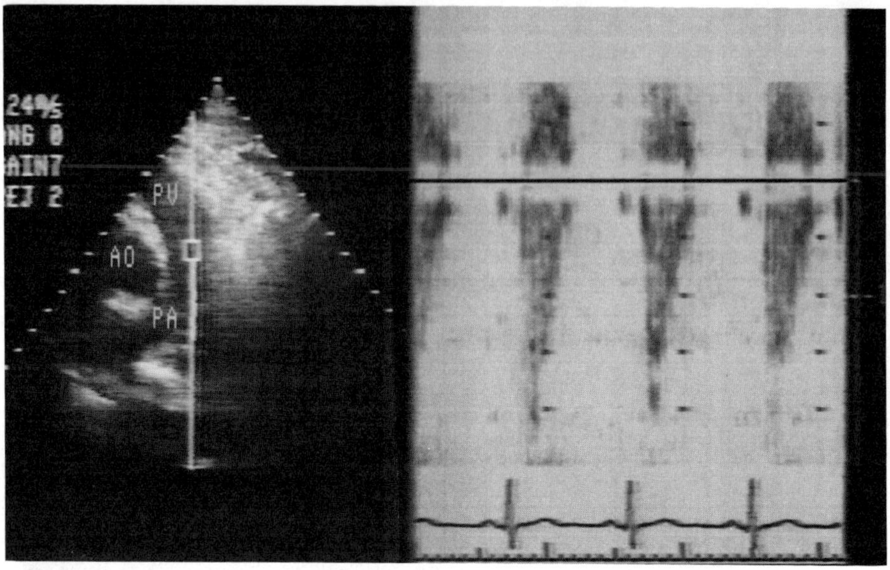

Figure 8.6
Mild pulmonary stenosis with increased velocity of flow recorded from a parasternal location. PA = pulmonary artery, AO = aorta, PV = pulmonary valve.

tricuspid flow are similar to those employed to visualize this valve by two-dimensional echocardiography. In general, the apical location provides better alignment of the Doppler ultrasound beam to the abnormal flow across the tricuspid valve than does the parasternal location.

Pulmonary Valve Stenosis

Pulmonary valve stenosis is more commonly seen in children than in adults. The Doppler recordings demonstrate higher than normal velocities across the pulmonary valve (Figure 8.6). At times, the subcostal locations may allow better access to examine pulmonic flow than the standard left parasternal location.

Regurgitant Valvular Lesions

Incompetent cardiac valves will allow blood to flow in a retrograde manner at a time in the cardiac cycle when there is normally no flow across the valve in question. The anatomic area through which the retrograde flow occurs is usually very small, thus behaving as a stenotic lesion producing high velocities with turbulence. However, such flow occurs at the wrong time in the cardiac cycle and in the opposite direction to that which is expected for normal flow (Figures 8.7, 8.8).

Again using the analogy of the water hose with a wide open nozzle, increasing the volume of water flow from the faucet causes a higher velocity of flow at the nozzle even if it is wide open. Therefore, the velocity of flow is directly proportionate to the volume of flow in the absence of obstruction. This phenomenon can be observed across regurgitant cardiac valves as well. In the case of aortic regurgitation, the left ventricle fills in diastole with blood coming from two sources (Figure 7.9): blood coming from the left atrium and regurgitant blood from the aorta. Hence, during systole, this ventricle ejects a higher volume of blood across the aortic valve. This results in a slightly higher velocity of flow in systole even though there is no obstruction.

Aortic Regurgitation

Normal flow across the aortic valve occurs in systole from the left ventricle to the aorta (forward flow). An incompetent aortic valve will allow blood to go backward (from the aorta to the left ventricle) in diastole (regurgitant flow) (Figure 7.9). Aortic regurgitation starts immediately after the closure of the aortic valve at end systole and persists throughout diastole until the next systolic starts (Figure 8.7).

Knowledge of the pressure changes in the aorta and the left ventricle throughout the cardiac cycle helps to explain why aortic regurgitant flow occurs in the manner just described (Figure 8.9). Normally, the direction of flow is from a high-pressure chamber to a low-pressure chamber. At end systole, the pressure within the ascending aorta is higher than that in the left ventricle; therefore, an incompetent aortic valve will allow blood to flow backward into the left ventricle. When the next systolic cycle starts, the left ventricle begins to contract with an abrupt increase in its internal pressure. As soon as left ventricular pressure exceeds aortic pressure, regurgitant flow stops, the aortic valve opens, and blood flows in the normal direction from the left ventricle into the aorta. Therefore, one may realize that there are no isovolumic relaxation (IRP) or isovolumic contraction periods (ICP) for the left ventricle since it starts filling with aortic regurgitant flow as soon as diastole starts, and it is still filling in early systole during the pre-ejection period. One should also note that aortic regurgitant flow starts before the mitral valve opens and continues until shortly after it closes (Figure 8.9). This is simply because left atrial pressure is usually less than aortic diastolic pressure. Therefore, the crossover time between aortic and left ventricular pressures

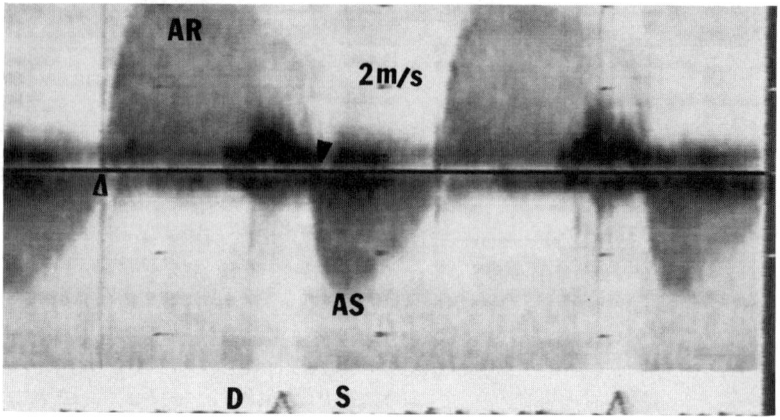

A

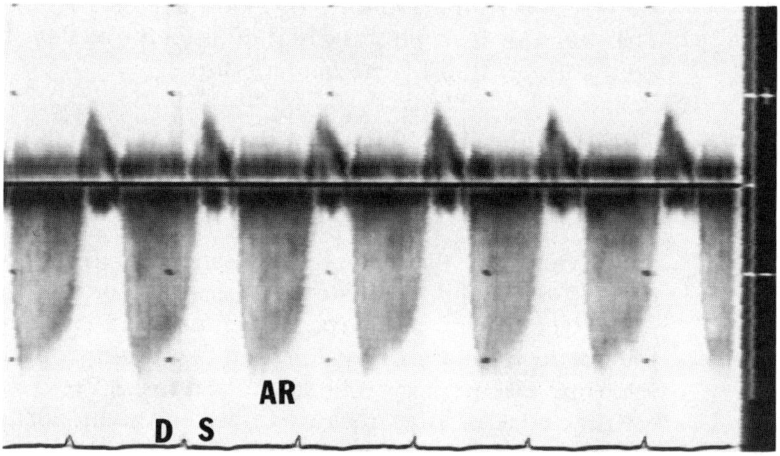

B

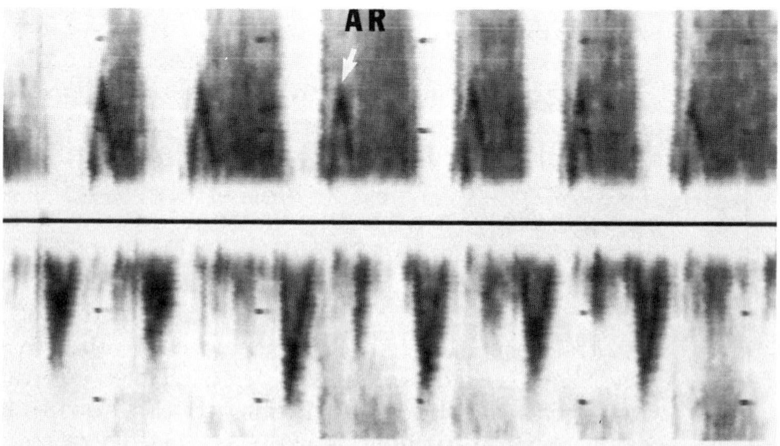

C

Figure 8.7

A. CW mode recording, with the transducer in an apical location, across the aortic valve in a patient with mild aortic stenosis (AS) and significant regurgitation (AR). Note the increased forward ve-

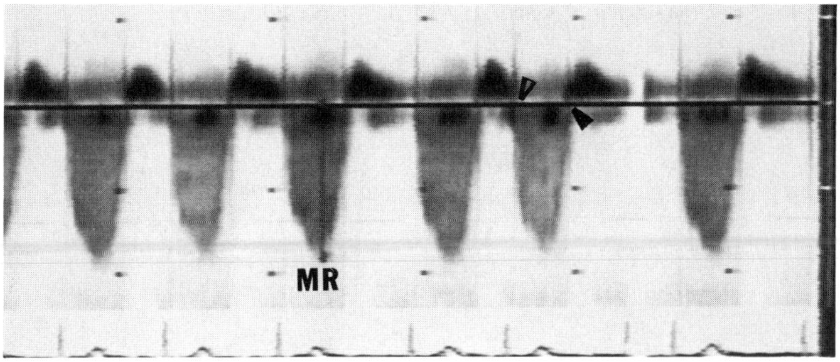

A

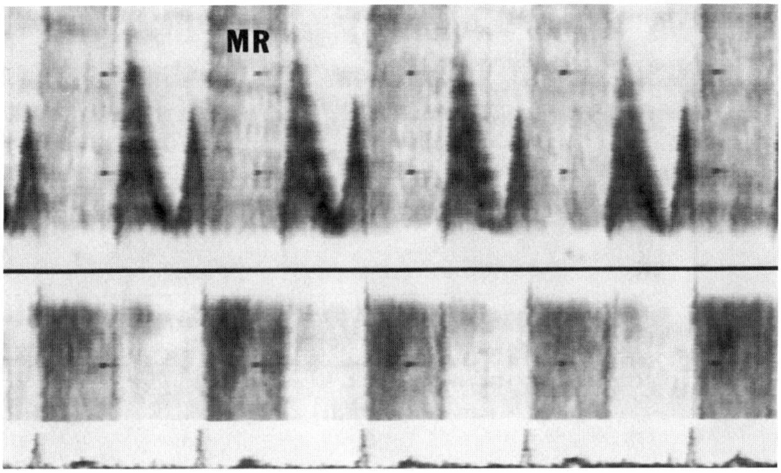

B

Figure 8.8
A. CW mode recording of high-velocity jet of mitral regurgitation (MR) in systole. Note that mitral regurgitant flow starts immediately after the end of forward flow (open arrowhead) in early systole and terminates immediately before the onset of forward flow of the next diastolic cycle (closed arrowhead). B. PW mode recording of mitral regurgitation (MR) with severe aliasing.

Figure 8.7 (continued)
locity in systole, away from the transducer, and high-velocity regurgitation in diastole. Also, note the aortic regurgitant flow starts immediately after the end of forward flow (open arrowhead) and terminates immediately before the onset of forward flow of the next systolic cycle (closed arrowhead). B. Aortic regurgitation recorded from the suprasternal notch from a patient with Marfan's syndrome and markedly dilated aortic root. From this transducer location, systolic aortic flow is toward the transducer and regurgitant flow (AR) is away from the transducer. D = diastole, S = systole. C. PW mode recording from an apical location in the left ventricular outflow tract in aortic insufficiency. Note the high velocity, with aliasing in diastole. Also note that this regurgitant jet (AR) starts before the onset of forward diastolic mitral flow (arrow).

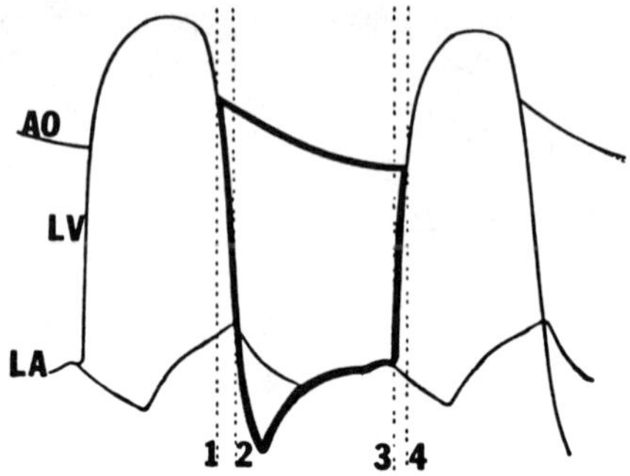

A

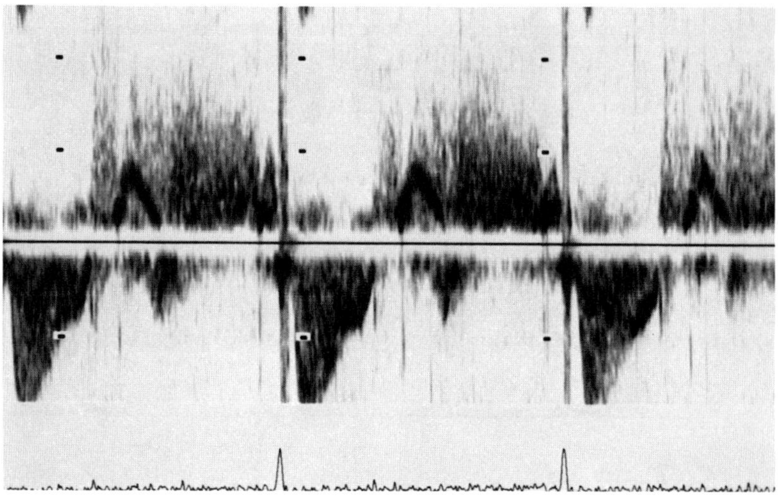

B

Figure 8.9
A. Simultaneous aortic (AO), left ventricular (LV), and left atrial (LA) pressures in hemodynamically significant chronic aortic regurgitation. Regurgitant aortic flow starts immediately at the crossover between aortic and left ventricular pressures in early diastole (time interval 1) and is abruptly terminated when left ventricular pressure exceeds aortic pressure early during the subsequent systolic cycle (time interval 4) (see Figure 8.7). Note that onset of mitral flow (at left ventricular–left atrial pressure crossover in early diastole, time interval 2) occurs after aortic regurgitation had already started. Also, mitral flow terminates (at left ventricular–left atrial pressure crossover in early systole, time interval 3) prior to the termination of aortic regurgitation. Hence, duration of mitral flow is shorter than the duration of aortic regurgitation. B. CW mode recording of aortic regurgitation with mitral flow in early diastole, superimposed on aortic regurgitant flow. Note that the onset of aortic regurgitant flow precedes the onset of mitral flow in diastole.

is different than the crossover time between left ventricular and left atrial pressures.

The Doppler recordings will demonstrate high initial velocities due to a high-pressure gradient between the aortic root and the left ventricle in early diastole. As this initial pressure gradient decreases throughout diastole, so does the velocity of regurgitant flow. With the onset of the next systolic cycle, the velocity recording will show a sudden drop to zero and a quick reversal of flow back to the aorta during ventricular ejection (Figures 8.7, 8.9). Aortic regurgitant flow is best recorded with the transducer in an apical location and may also be recorded from a suprasternal position, with the ultrasound beam directed within the ascending aorta. However, in this latter location, peak regurgitant velocities may not be accurately determined because the highest velocities occur in the left ventricular outflow tract, which is difficult to insonate from the suprasternal location.

Although forward aortic flow is obviously in the opposite direction of the regurgitant flow, the directions of these two opposing flows may not necessarily be parallel. Thus, adequate Doppler recordings of forward flow may fail to show the highest regurgitant velocities and vice versa. One has to realize that the regurgitant orifice is small and may have an eccentric location in the aortic valve leaflets. It is not unusual to encounter difficulties in locating the regurgitant jet in conditions of mild aortic regurgitation. Another fact to be remembered is that forward flow and regurgitant flow occur at different periods in the cardiac cycle. A small angle (θ) in systole may significantly increase in diastole because the heart is constantly moving, while the transducer and, subsequently, the direction of the ultrasound beam are relatively stable on the chest wall.

Finally, recordings of forward aortic flow may demonstrate a slightly higher peak velocity with a longer ejection time. These are mainly related to the increase in flow seen with aortic regurgitation and not due to obstruction of the aortic valve in systole.

Semiquantitative analysis of the severity of aortic regurgitation may be performed by mapping the anatomic area within the left ventricular cavity where any regurgitant flow may be recorded. PW mode is used for this purpose. Mild regurgitation can be demonstrated only when the sample volume is located within the left ventricular outflow tract, just behind the aortic valve. Severe regurgitation may be recorded deep within the left ventricular chamber all the way to the apex (Figure 8.10). Mapping of flow can be performed from an apical or parasternal location. Unfortunately, this technique is not very reliable for adequate evaluation of the

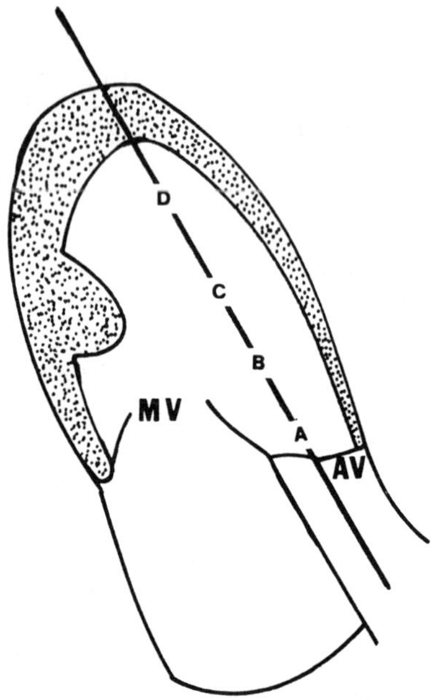

Figure 8.10
Two-dimensional apical view in aortic regurgitation. Regurgitant jet that can only be detected in the left ventricular outflow tract (sample volume location A) suggests mild regurgitation, whereas a regurgitant jet detected within the left ventricular apex (sample volume location D) suggests severe regurgitation. MV = mitral valve, AV = aortic valve.

severity of regurgitation. In this context, one has to consider the size of the left ventricle and direction of the regurgitant jet. Mild to moderate regurgitation into a relatively small left ventricle may allow Doppler recordings of the regurgitant flow within the left ventricular apex. If this occurs, the severity of the regurgitation will be overestimated. On the other hand, a large eccentric regurgitant jet directed toward the mitral valve may not be recorded if the sample volume is positioned close to the left ventricular apex, hence underestimating the severity of regurgitation.

Another technique for the semiquantitative estimation of the severity of regurgitation is based on the abnormal hemodynamics of mild versus severe aortic regurgitation. In mild regurgitation, the aortic–left ventricular pressure gradient remains significantly elevated throughout diastole. The resulting Doppler regurgitant velocity is accordingly elevated throughout diastole. In contrast, the aortic–left ventricular pressure gradient in severe regurgitation rapidly diminishes toward late diastole, reflecting the abnormally elevated left

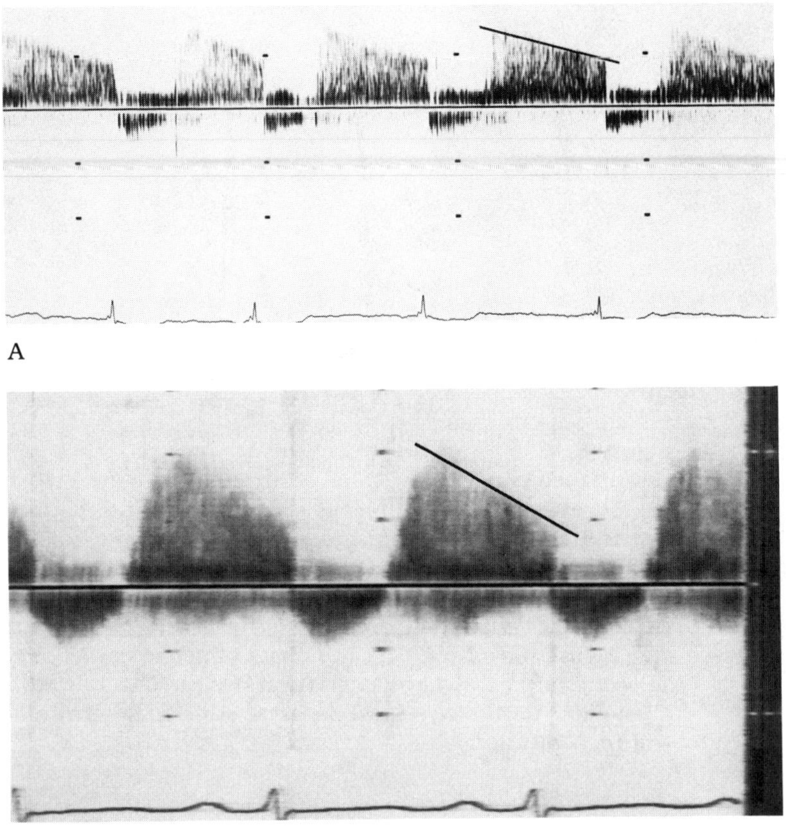

A

B

Figure 8.11
A. Mild aortic regurgitation. Note the gradual deceleration of the velocity of aortic regurgitation throughout diastole. B. Severe aortic regurgitation. Note the relatively rapid deceleration of aortic regurgitant velocity in diastole.

ventricular diastolic pressure. The resulting Doppler diastolic velocity exhibits a rapid deceleration rate. The time interval needed for the initial pressure gradient in early diastole to drop to one-half its value is referred to as the pressure half-time. Mild regurgitation causes very long intervals, whereas the pressure half-time in severe regurgitation is significantly reduced (Figure 8.11).

Color Doppler imaging demonstrates the aortic regurgitant jet originating in the left ventricular outflow tract, just proximal to the aortic valve. More severe regurgitation causes wider jets that extend deeper within the left ventricle. Aliasing and turbulence produce an orange jet with superimposed blue and mosaic colors as well (Plate 5A).

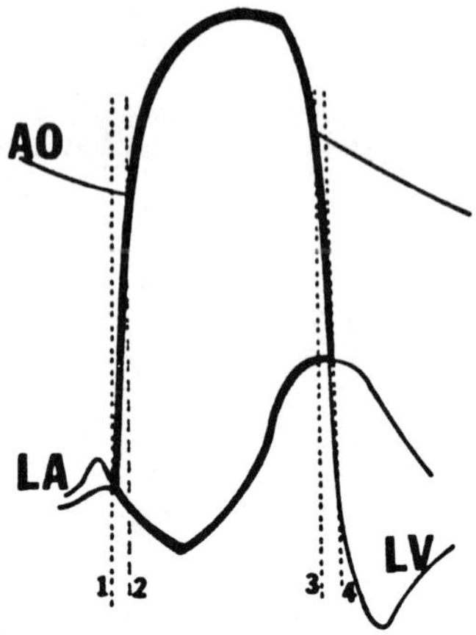

Figure 8.12
Simultaneous aortic (AO), left ventricular (LV), and left atrial (LA) pressures in hemodynamically significant mitral regurgitation. Regurgitant mitral flow starts immediately at the crossover between left ventricular and atrial pressures in early systole (time interval 1) and is abruptly terminated when left atrial pressure exceeds left ventricular pressure early in diastole (time interval 4) (see Figure 8.8). Note that the onset of aortic flow (time interval 2) occurs after mitral regurgitation has already started. Also, aortic flow terminates (time interval 3) prior to termination of mitral regurgitation.

Mitral Regurgitation

Normal mitral flow occurs in diastole from the left atrium to the left ventricle. An incompetent mitral valve will allow blood to go backward from the left ventricle to the left atrium in systole. Mitral regurgitant flow starts immediately after the crossover of left ventricular and left atrial pressure in early systole and persists until the onset of the second pressure crossover in early diastole (Figure 8.12). Similar to what was previously discussed for aortic regurgitation, there is no ICP or IRP for the left ventricle. Doppler recordings of mitral regurgitant flow are best obtained from an apical position, with the ultrasound beam directed across the mitral valve annulus. Eccentric regurgitant jets are not unusual. These are more commonly encountered when regurgitation is caused by papillary muscle dysfunction or mitral valve prolapse.

The highest regurgitant velocity occurs downstream to flow just behind the mitral valve within the left atrium. The velocity of the regurgitant flow closely follows the changes in the pressure gradient between the left ventricle and left atrium in systole. A rapid rise in velocity is seen. Peak velocity is rounded and not sharp, followed by a rapid deceleration toward the end of systole. In conditions associated with a noncompliant left atrial wall, the regurgitant volume may not be accommodated without a simultaneous significant increase in left atrial pressure. Thus, the pressure gradient drops markedly in mid and late systole (as left atrial pressure increases with a high V wave). The resulting velocity recordings will be altered accordingly.

In the absence of atrial fibrillation, forward mitral flow (from the left atrium to the left ventricle) in diastole may show a normal pattern with early and late velocity peaks. However, depending on the severity of regurgitation, these forward velocities may be slightly higher than normal. Moreover, the rate of deceleration of velocity in early diastole may be slower than normal. This does not mean stenosis; rather, it is a reflection of increased flow, when more time is needed to empty the large volume of blood within the atrium, leading to a longer duration of flow in early diastole. Despite the decrease in this rate of deceleration, it is still faster than what would be expected in mitral stenosis. In addition, abnormalities in left ventricular relaxation may also reduce these deceleration rates.

Similar to what was discussed in the previous section, forward mitral flow may not be parallel to regurgitant flow. The former occurs in diastole and the latter occurs in systole. Adjustments in the direction of the ultrasound beam may be needed to record the highest velocities in either direction. Similar to aortic regurgitation, mapping of the extent of the regurgitant jet within the left atrium provides a semiquantitative estimate of the severity of mitral regurgitation. However, this approach is also limited by the size of the left atrium and the presence of eccentric jets of flow (Figure 8.13).

Color Doppler imaging demonstrates the mitral regurgitant jet in the left atrium as blue. Aliasing and turbulence may cause superimposed orange and mosaic colors as well. More severe regurgitation causes wider jets that extend deeper into the left atrial cavity. Eccentric jets can be easily localized with color flow imaging (Plates 6, 7).

Pulmonic Regurgitation

Similar to aortic regurgitation, regurgitant pulmonic flow occurs in diastole from the pulmonary artery to the right ventricle. There are no right ventricular isovolumic contraction and relaxation periods (Figure 8.14).

Pulmonic regurgitant flow is best recorded from a parasternal transducer location, with the ultrasound beam di-

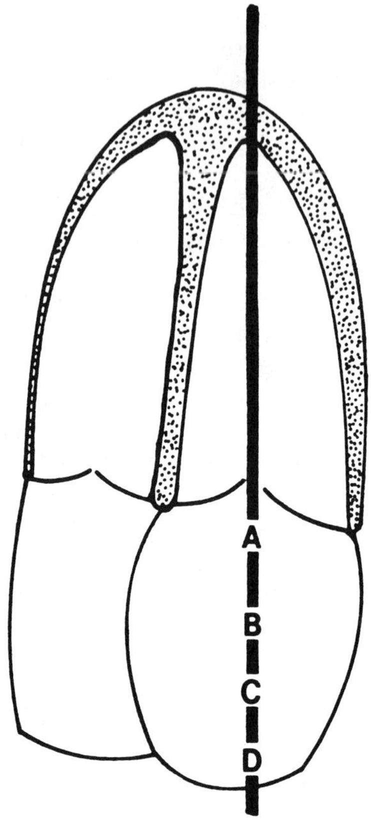

Figure 8.13
Two-dimensional apical view in mitral regurgitation. Regurgitant jet that can only be detected at the mitral annulus (sample volume location A) suggests mild regurgitation, whereas a regurgitant jet detected close to the left atrial posterior wall (sample volume location D) suggests severe regurgitation.

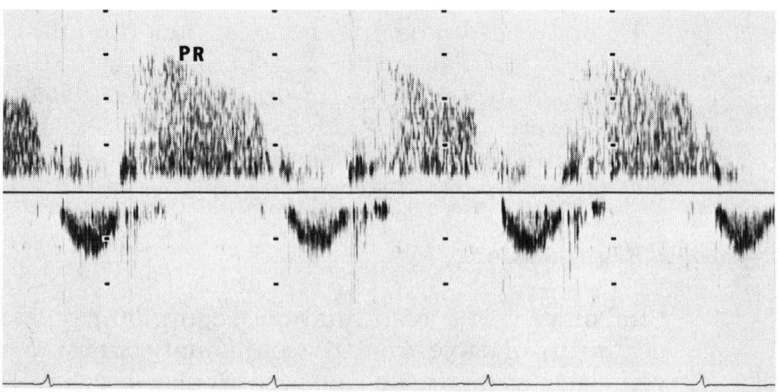

Figure 8.14
CW mode recording of pulmonary regurgitation (PR) obtained from a left parasternal location.

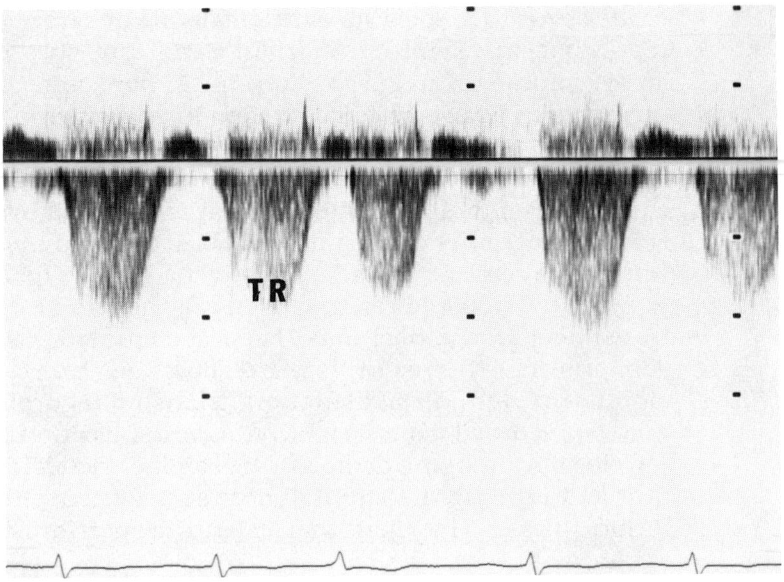

Figure 8.15
CW mode recording of tricuspid regurgitation (TR) obtained from an apical location. The velocity varies in this recording because the rhythm is atrial fibrillation with variable ventricular rate.

rected along the right ventricular outflow tract. Occasionally, the subcostal approach may be helpful. In general, pulmonary arterial and right ventricular pressures are usually much less than aortic and left ventricular pressures; thus, right-sided pressure gradients in diastole are less than the left-sided gradients seen in aortic regurgitation. Therefore, the peak regurgitant velocities are expected to be smaller than those observed in aortic regurgitation. Also similar to aortic regurgitation, the direction of forward and regurgitant pulmonic flow may not be parallel, and peak forward pulmonic velocities may be slightly increased. The highest velocities of the regurgitant flow occur downstream from the pulmonary valve in diastole, i.e., within the right ventricular outflow tract.

Color flow imaging demonstrates orange jet of pulmonic regurgitation in the right ventricular outflow tract. Wider jets suggest more severe regurgitation (Plate 8).

Tricuspid Regurgitation

Similar to mitral regurgitation, tricuspid regurgitation occurs in systole. There is no ICP and IRP for the right ventricle. Peak velocity of the regurgitant flow occurs within the right atrium just behind the tricuspid valve (Figure 8.15).

Abnormalities of flow in the superior and inferior venae

cavae occur in association with moderate or severe tricuspid regurgitation. Elevation of right atrial pressure due to a large volume of regurgitation in a noncompliant right atrium may cause reversal of flow in the superior and inferior venae cavae. At times this reversal of flow may even be observed within the hepatic vein. These findings represent the hemodynamic correlates of what is observed by contrast echocardiography where microbubbles are seen moving in a retrograde manner in the inferior vena cava or hepatic vein in systole. Tricuspid regurgitation may be recorded with the transducer in the positions that are commonly used to record normal tricuspid forward flow. At times, due to significant right atrial dilatation, tricuspid regurgitant flow may be recorded from a right parasternal location as well.

Color flow imaging demonstrates a blue tricuspid regurgitant jet in the right atrium. A more severe tricuspid regurgitation causes wider jets that extend deeper into the right atrial cavity (Plate 9).

Valvular Regurgitation: Overview

Doppler ultrasound has been shown to be highly sensitive in detecting regurgitant flow patterns. At times, mild valvular regurgitation can be recorded only by Doppler ultrasound when there have not been any audible murmurs on clinical examination or any other abnormality on the echocardiogram. Frequently, minimal tricuspid or pulmonary regurgitation may be detected by Doppler in the absence of any demonstrable pathology on the echocardiogram. Such minimal regurgitant flows are probably physiologic and are of no significant hemodynamic consequence.

Complex Flow Patterns

Multiple valvular pathologic conditions may coexist. A particular cardiac valve may be stenotic and incompetent at the same time. Thus, the resulting Doppler recordings will reflect the hemodynamic abnormalities of stenosis and regurgitation as described earlier in this chapter (Figure 8.16).

Problems arise when two different cardiac valves are diseased, giving rise to abnormal flow patterns that occur at the same time in the cardiac cycle. These abnormal flow patterns may cause confusion unless simultaneous two-dimensional imaging is performed with the judicious interplay of PW and CW mode Doppler ultrasound. The following discussion will focus on certain multiple valvular pathologic states that are commonly encountered, and point out certain features that may distinguish the differences and, subsequently, the origin of these abnormal flow patterns.

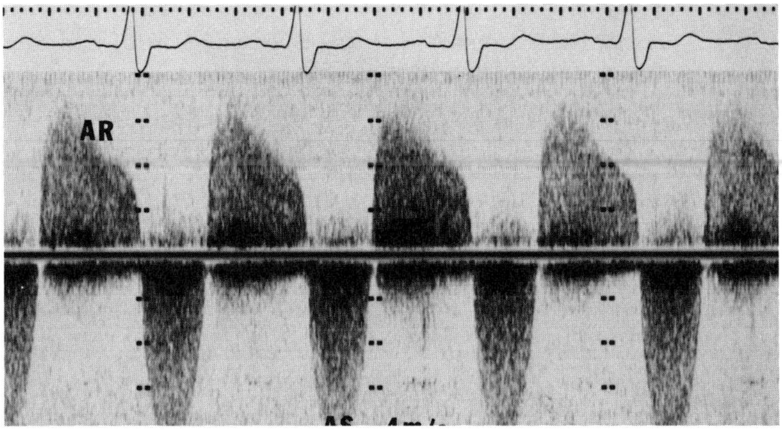

A

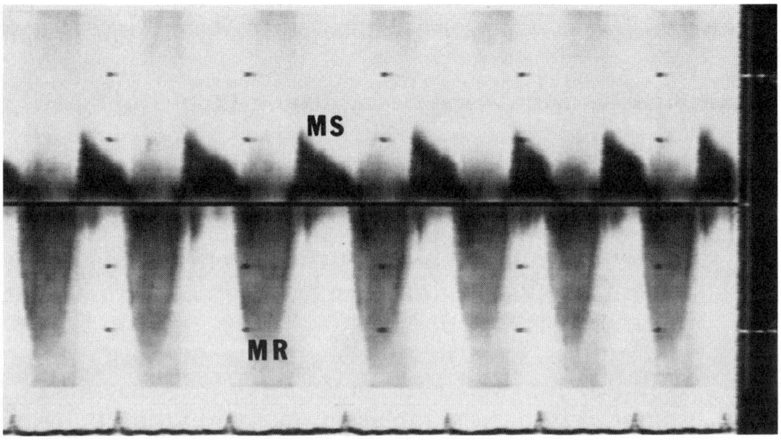

B

Figure 8.16
A. CW mode recording from a patient with significant aortic stenosis (AS) and regurgitation (AR). Note the markedly increased forward velocity in systole (approximately 4 m/sec) as well as the aortic regurgitation in diastole with relatively rapid deceleration rate, suggesting hemodynamically significant regurgitation.
B. CW mode recording from a patient with significant mitral stenosis (MS) and regurgitation (MR) in atrial fibrillation. Note the markedly increased forward velocity (approximately 2 m/sec). Mitral regurgitant jet was easily recorded in this patient, and was mapped close to the left atrial posterior wall, suggesting significant regurgitation.

Table 8.1
Features that distinguish the Doppler recordings of mitral regurgitation from those of aortic stenosis

	Mitral regurgitation	Aortic stenosis
Flow in systole	+	+
High velocity of flow	+	+
Transducer location		
Apical	+	+
Suprasternal	−	+
Audio signal	Softer	Harsher
Duration of flow	Longer	Shorter
Forward mitral flow (in diastole)	+	±

Key: + = present; − = absent; ± = present or absent.

Aortic Stenosis with Mitral Regurgitation (Table 8.1)

Aortic stenosis and mitral regurgitation demonstrate high-velocity patterns in systole. With the transducer in an apical position, both flow patterns occur away from the transducer and are displayed below the baseline. Therefore, independent Doppler recordings may show similar flow patterns that can be easily confused.

At the start of the Doppler examination, the operator should first verify the presence of these lesions by using PW mode, with the sample volume within the left atrium to demonstrate mitral regurgitation and then within the aortic root to demonstrate aortic stenosis. If the velocities are high, then frequency aliasing may occur and the CW mode must then be used to record the highest possible velocities. If adequate Doppler recordings are obtained in conjunction with a good two-dimensional image, then the direction of the Doppler ultrasound cursor will help identify the origin of the high velocities being recorded. However, as mentioned earlier, it is not uncommon to encounter situations where the quality of the two-dimensional image is sacrificed in order to obtain adequate Doppler recordings. Therefore, one should rely on other factors to determine the origin of the high velocities being recorded. The audio signal is a very helpful differentiator. Aortic stenotic flow produces Doppler frequency shifts with harsh sounds, while the audio signal of mitral regurgitant flow is softer in quality. The duration of the systolic flow is also important. Recall that there are no ICPs and IRPs for the left ventricle in conditions of mitral

Table 8.2
Features that distinguish the Doppler recordings of mitral stenosis from those of aortic regurgitation

	Mitral stenosis	Aortic regurgitation
Flow in diastole	+	+
High velocity of flow is usually	< 2 m/sec	> 2 m/sec
Transducer location		
Apical	+	+
Suprasternal	−	+
Audio signal	Harsher	Softer
Duration of flow	Shorter	Longer
Forward aortic flow (in systole)	±	+
Atrial kick		
Sinus rhythm	+	−
Atrial fibrillation	−	−

Key: + = present; − = absent; ± = present or absent.

regurgitation, while these intervals are preserved in aortic stenosis. Hence, when two patterns with high velocities are recorded with minimal angulation of the transducer, the pattern with the longer duration of flow is most probably caused by mitral regurgitation (Figure 8.12). Aortic stenotic flow can be recorded with the transducer in a suprasternal location. The pattern obtained from this location can be compared to the other two patterns recorded from the apical locations (with respect to peak velocities and duration of flow) and thus help eliminate confusion. An important point to keep in mind is that angulation of the transducer may produce recordings of different peak velocities depending on the angle (θ); however, irrespective of this angulation, the duration of a particular flow pattern is not expected to differ significantly. Finally, forward mitral flow in diastole may be easier to recognize when the true mitral regurgitant flow is being recorded; however, in the CW mode, this diastolic mitral flow may still be seen if one is recording aortic systolic flow from a more lateral apical location.

Aortic Regurgitation with Mitral Stenosis (Table 8.2)

Aortic regurgitation with mitral stenosis is a common finding in patients with rheumatic heart disease. Both patterns of flow occur in diastole and are recorded within the left ventricle. If the cardiac rhythm is still sinus, then there should be no confusion in resolving this issue since mitral flow will demonstrate two peak velocities—one during early diastole and the second after the atrial kick. Aortic regurgitant flow will demonstrate a single peak velocity with gradual deceleration throughout diastole. With the transducer in an apical location, both flow patterns may be superimposed and minimal angulation of the transducer may be necessary to show the two different flow patterns. Problems may arise if the cardiac rhythm is that of atrial fibrillation, because the loss of the atrial kick renders the mitral diastolic flow indistinguishable from aortic regurgitant flow except for some subtle features.

The most obvious distinguishing feature between these two patterns of flow is the peak velocity in early diastole. The gradients across the mitral valve rarely cause velocities greater than 2 m/sec, while aortic regurgitant flow velocities are usually much higher. Also, there is no IRP and ICP for the left ventricle in conditions of aortic regurgitation; thus, the duration of aortic regurgitant flow is longer than the duration of forward mitral flow in diastole (Figure 8.9). The audio signal from mitral stenosis is harsher than that from aortic regurgitation. Forward systolic flow in the left ventricular outflow tract may be easier to record when sampling aortic regurgitant flow, although if the left ventricle is not dilated, forward systolic flow can be recorded simultaneously with mitral flow. Finally, aortic regurgitant flow may be recorded from a suprasternal location, although peak velocities may be underestimated with the transducer in this position. Color flow Doppler imaging is the best noninvasive method to resolve this issue. With color flow imaging, one can easily observe two distinct jets of flow within the left ventricular cavity and can also determine the time of onset of these two different jets (Plate 10).

9 Prosthetic Cardiac Valves

Progressive worsening of valvular disease will ultimately affect cardiac function. Open heart surgery for replacement of a defective cardiac valve may help improve cardiac function and alleviate symptoms of heart failure. In general, there are three types of cardiac valve prostheses: ball valves, disc valves, and bioprosthetic valves. Each valve is designed to simulate normal valve function by providing minimal resistance to flow and also preventing regurgitation. Each of these prosthetic cardiac valves has its advantages and disadvantages.

The echocardiographic examination of any prosthetic valve should be directed to the evaluation of the structure of the prosthesis, opening and closing motion of its movable parts, stability of the prosthesis within the heart, and its functional capacity as a replacement of a native cardiac valve. In addition, the echocardiogram should provide information regarding the response of the heart to the hemodynamic alterations induced by the prosthesis.

Normal Echocardiographic Patterns

Ball Valve Prosthesis

The Starr-Edwards valve is a prototype of the ball valve prosthesis (Figure 9.1). A ball made of titanium metal or Silastic material is housed within a metallic cage. Flow across the valve forces the ball into the open position, touching the inner edges of the cage. Temporary reversal of the flow forces

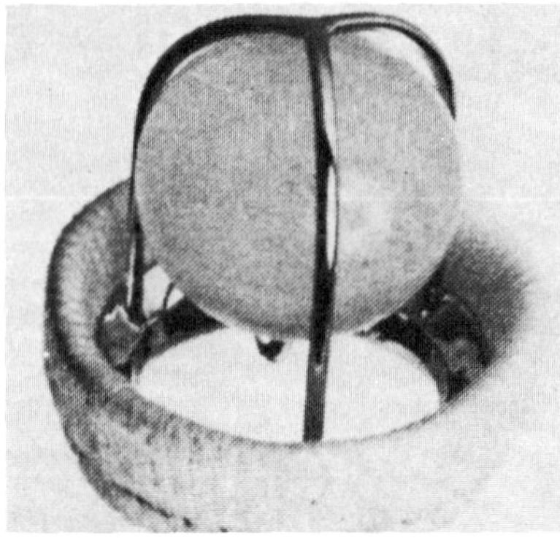

Figure 9.1
Starr-Edwards ball valve prosthesis. Note the ball within the metallic cage in the open position. (From A. D. Hagan and A. N. DeMaria, *Clinical Applications of Two-Dimensional Echocardiography and Cardiac Doppler* [2nd ed.]. Boston: Little, Brown, 1989. P. 426.)

the ball into the closed position, whereby it rests on the sewing ring and occludes the prosthetic valve opening, thus preventing regurgitation.

The metallic elements of such prostheses are highly echogenic and cause bright echoes on the two-dimensional echocardiogram. Typically, normal M-mode recordings of the ball valve prosthesis will demonstrate two dense linear echoes that represent the cage and sewing ring. These prosthetic elements exhibit motion similar to the valve annulus to which they are sutured. Echoes from the ball valve will reflect its motion throughout the cardiac cycle (Figure 9.2).

A linear echo, reflected from the anterior surface of the ball valve, will approximate the echoes from the cage of the prosthesis when the valve is in the open position. However, when the valve is in the closed position, this linear echo rapidly moves to a central location, midway between the echoes from the cage and sewing ring. There are no echoes reflected from the posterior surface of the metallic ball valve. Instead, dense linear echoes representing reverberations commonly extend along the length of the echocardiographic field, posterior to the prosthesis. On the other hand, echoes reflected from the posterior surface of a Silastic ball valve cause typical patterns on the M-mode recording (Figure 9.2). These echoes will be parallel to the echoes reflected from the anterior surface of the ball valve; however, they will be displayed behind the echoes from the sewing ring as if originating from a location outside the prosthetic valve. This artifactual appearance of the echoes reflected from the posterior surface of the Silastic ball valve is related to the fact that the velocity of

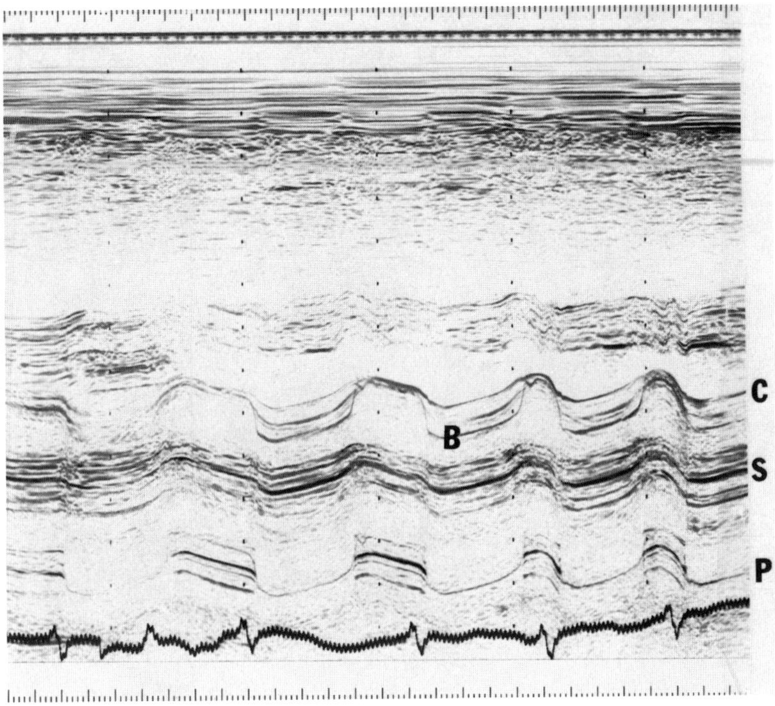

Figure 9.2
M-mode recording of a ball valve prosthesis in the mitral position. The anterior surface of this Silastic ball (B) exhibits anterior and posterior motion throughout the cardiac cycle. Note the echoes (B) are contained within the cage (C). In systole, the ball rests on the sewing ring (S). Echoes reflected from the posterior surface of the ball (P) exhibit similar motion to those reflected from B; however, they appear outside the cage, posterior to the heart. See text for detail.

ultrasound is slower in Silastic material than in human tissue. Subsequently, it takes longer for the ultrasound beam to travel within the Silastic ball. Since depth or distance perception by the ultrasound equipment is derived from time measurements based on normal velocity of ultrasound in tissue, the delayed travel time of the ultrasound pulse is falsely attributed to farther depth location of the posterior surface of the Silastic ball.

Disc Valve Prosthesis

As the name implies, a disc (Figure 9.3), instead of a ball, is used to occlude the sewing ring. There are three general types of disc valve prostheses: floating disc, monocuspid tilting disc, and bicuspid tilting disc.

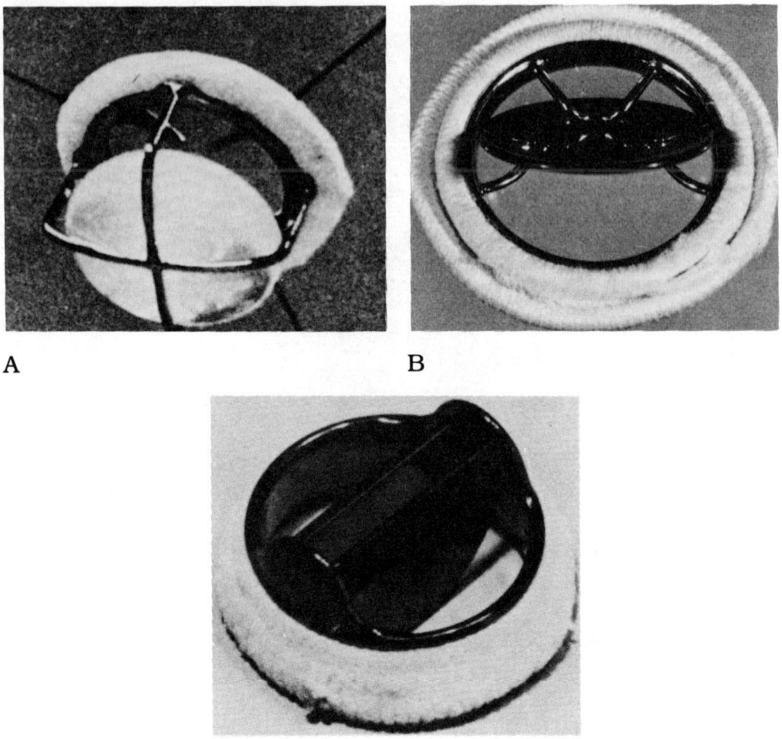

A B

C

Figure 9.3
A. Beall valve floating disc prosthesis. B. Bjork-Shiley tilting disc valve prosthesis. C. St. Jude bicuspid tilting valve prosthesis. All valves are shown in the open position. (From A. D. Hagan and A. N. DeMaria, *Clinical Applications of Two-Dimensional Echocardiography and Cardiac Doppler* [2nd ed.]. Boston: Little, Brown, 1989. Pp. 426–427.)

Floating Disc

The Beall-Surgitool valve is a prototype of such prostheses. The disc is housed within two metallic struts. The M-mode echocardiogram demonstrates two parallel lines representing the sewing ring and one of the metallic struts. In between these two parallel lines, a third linear echo represents the floating disc. When in the open position, the disc touches the struts, and when closed, it rests on the sewing ring. Similar to the ball valve prosthesis, the apical view is better suited than the parasternal view for adequate evaluation of disc excursions.

Monocuspid Tilting Disc

The Bjork-Shiley tilting disc prosthesis is the most common type of disc valve prostheses. The disc is anchored to the sewing ring so that it tilts to open (Figures 9.4, 9.5). Depending on its orientation during surgical insertion, the echocardiographic appearance and degree of excursion of the disc are largely dependent on transducer location and imaging plane. M-mode recordings are usually recorded from the usual parasternal location with minor angulation. An implant in the mitral position will demonstrate dense linear echoes originating from the sewing ring. When the disc tilts to open, it generates multiple dense linear echoes. On the M-mode recording, there is rapid anterior motion into the left ventricular cavity followed by gradual posterior motion that parallels the posterior motion of the sewing ring and mitral annulus in diastole. Ventricular contraction causes sudden closure of the disc valve prosthesis (Figure 9.6).

When the prosthesis is positioned in the aortic valve region, M-mode recordings from the parasternal view demonstrate dense linear echoes in close approximation and parallel to the anterior and posterior walls of the aorta (Figure 9.7). Echoes from the disc will only appear during systole when the valve is opened.

Biscupid Tilting Disc

The St. Jude valve is made of two tilting discs (Figure 9.3). When in the open position, both discs tilt together and become parallel to each other, producing two parallel linear echoes. When closed, the discs rest within the sewing ring and disappear from the ultrasound image (Figure 9.8). The parasternal views are best suited to evaluate this type of prosthesis. However, depending on the orientation of the prosthesis during surgical implantation, adequate visualization on echocardiography may be difficult, necessitating angulated parasternal views.

Bioprosthetic Valves

Unlike mechanical ball or disc valve prostheses, the leaflets of bioprosthetic valves (Figure 9.9) are made of natural biologic material that is chemically treated, then mounted on the metallic sewing ring, and supported by three stents that project from the sewing ring.

The aortic valve of the pig is used for porcine bioprostheses, whereas the pericardium excised from sheep is used for leaflets in a bovine bioprosthesis. Both types of such prosthetic valves are tricuspid and are used to replace any cardiac valve.

Visualization of bioprosthetic valves is usually employed by the routine echocardiographic windows. The metallic ele-

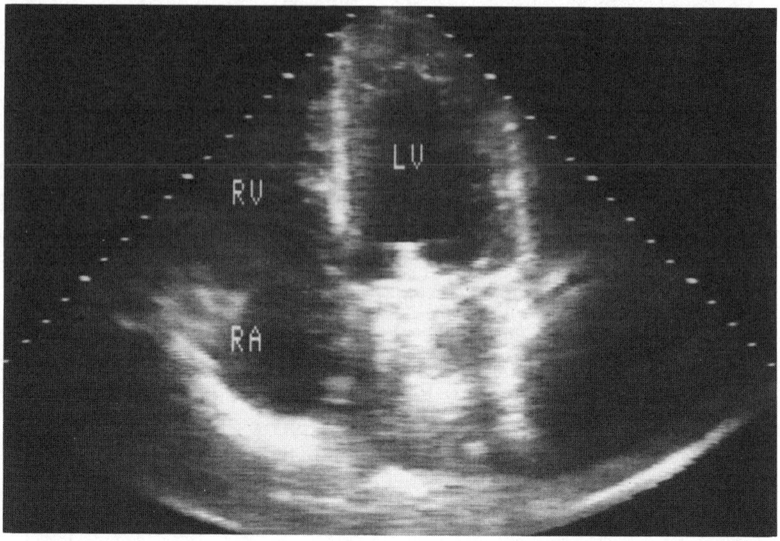

A

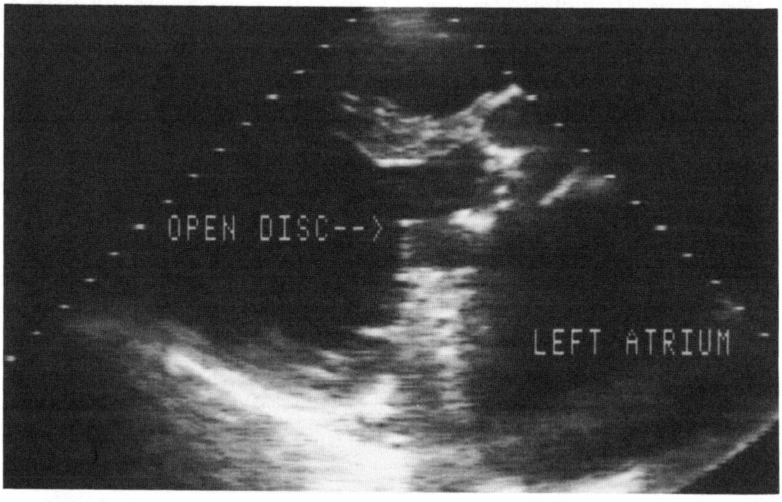

B

Figure 9.4
A. Apical four-chamber view, and B. Parasternal long axis view, showing a tilting disc prosthesis in the mitral position. Both frames are during diastole, with the disc in the open position. Note the prominent ill-defined reverberations and acoustic shadowing caused by the metallic elements of the sewing ring. LV = left ventricle, RV = right ventricle, RA = right atrium.

ment of a bioprosthesis is highly echogenic. Only two stents are visualized at any one time on an M-mode echocardiogram (Figures 9.10, 9.11). This is because the three stents are positioned at 120-degree angles from each other, and the third stent will always be out of the plane of the ultrasound beam. These stents and the sewing ring will produce two

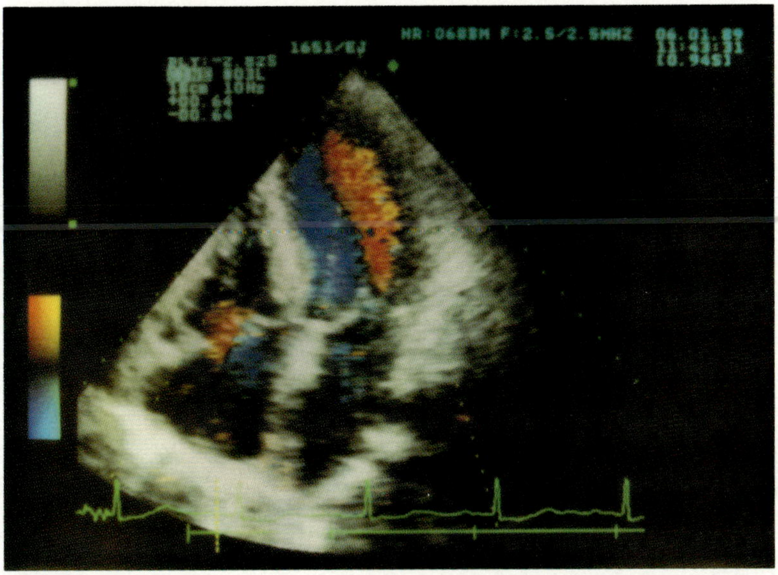

Plate 1
Apical four-chamber view showing normal flow pattern across the mitral valve in diastole. Flow is toward the transducer and is displayed in orange. As the blood is reflected at the apex toward the left ventricular outflow tract (vortices), its color changes into blue because it is going away from the transducer. See text for details.

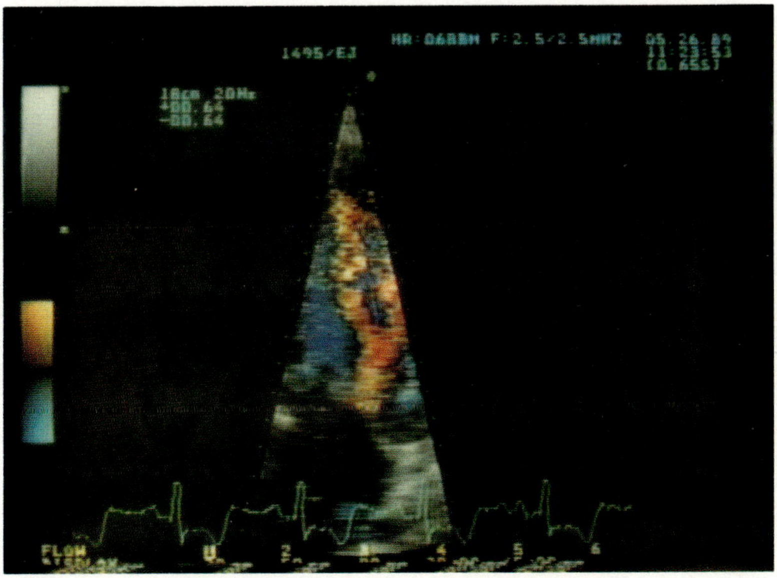

Plate 2
Apical view showing transmitral flow in diastole, in orange. The velocity of flow at the center of the jet is depicted in blue due to aliasing of color.

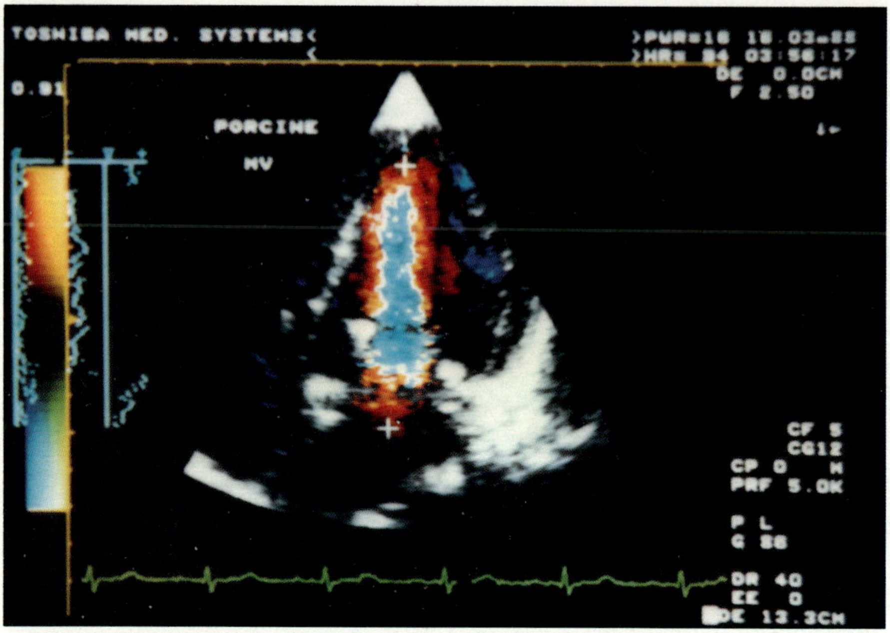

Plate 3
Apical four-chamber view from a patient with porcine mitral valve (MV) bioprosthesis. Severe aliasing with mosaic color patterns is due to significantly high velocity of flow. Note the orange color with central white and blue.

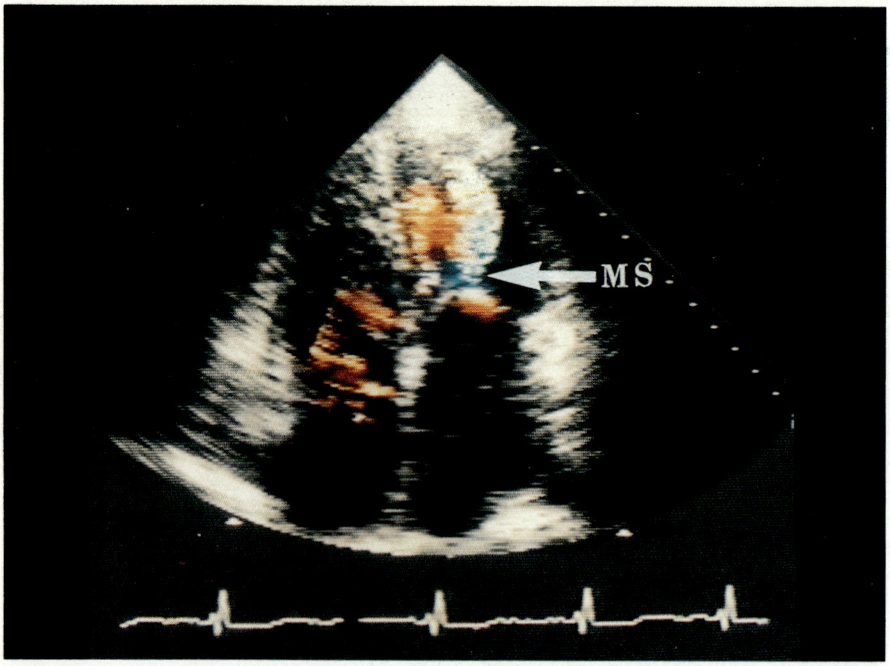

Plate 4
Apical four-chamber view from a patient with mitral stenosis (MS), with severe aliasing and turbulence. Note the prominent white color with shades of orange and blue.

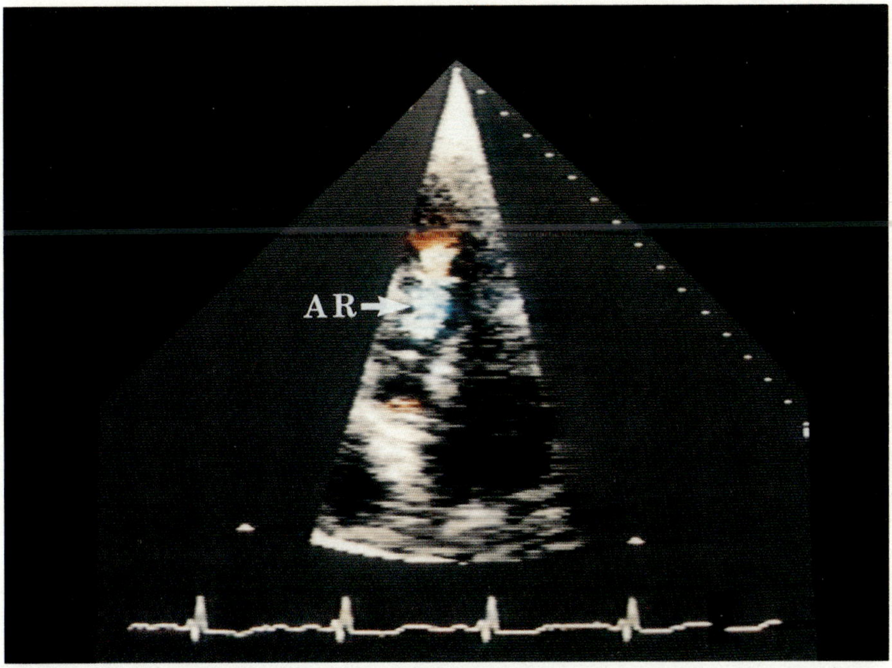

A

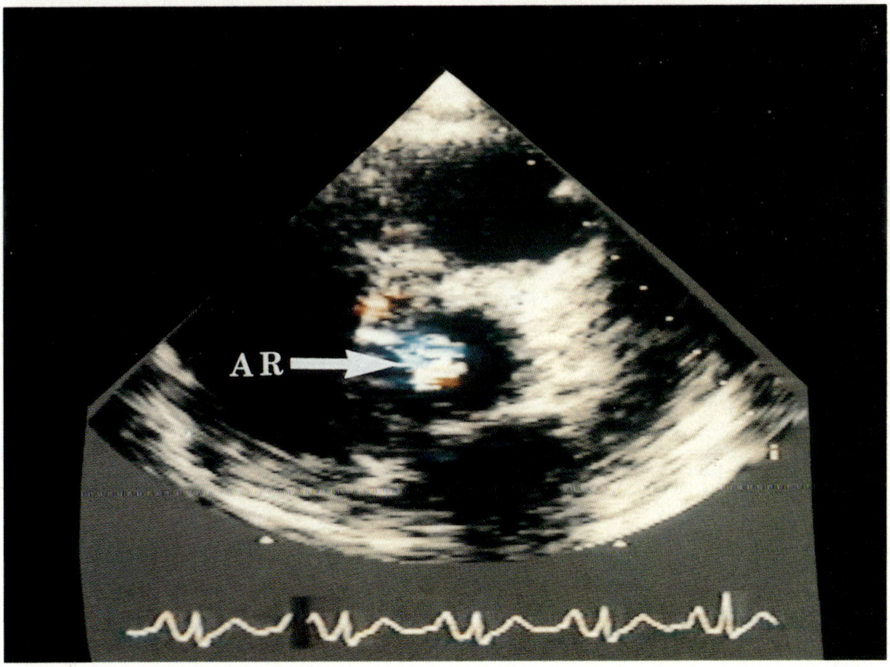

B

Plate 5
A. Apical view showing the left ventricular outflow tract from a patient with aortic regurgitation (AR). The high-velocity turbulent jet in diastole causes mosaic color pattern. B. Short axis view showing the aortic regurgitant jet (AR) at the center of the aortic valve.

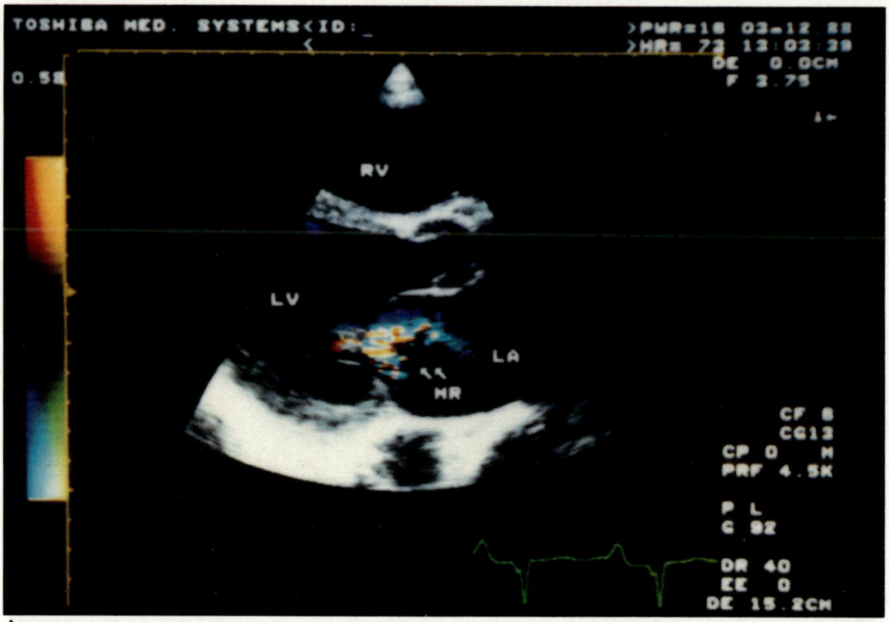

A

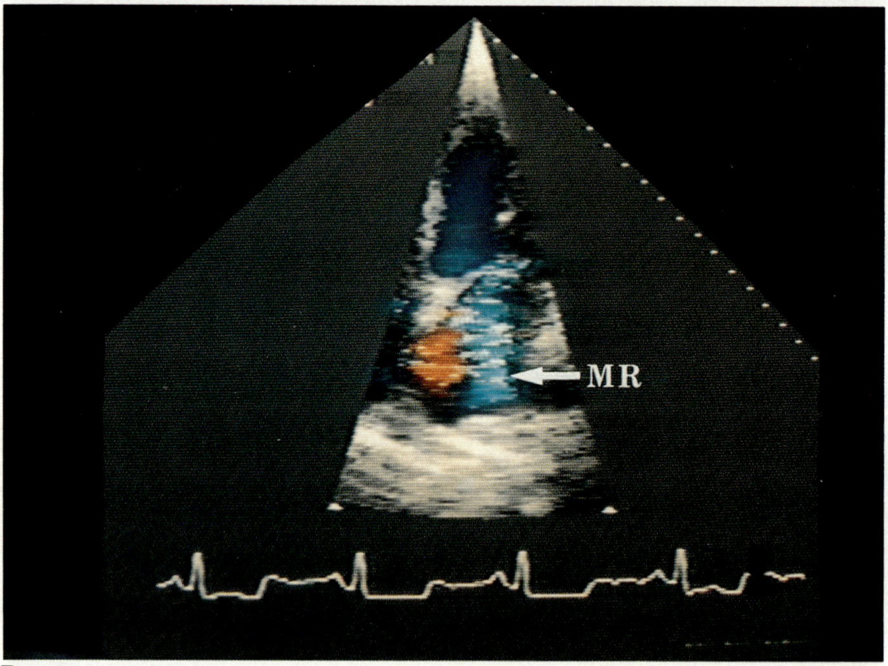

B

Plate 6

Parasternal long axis view (A) and apical four-chamber view (B) showing high-velocity jets in mitral regurgitation (MR). LA = left atrium, LV = left ventricle, RV = right ventricle.

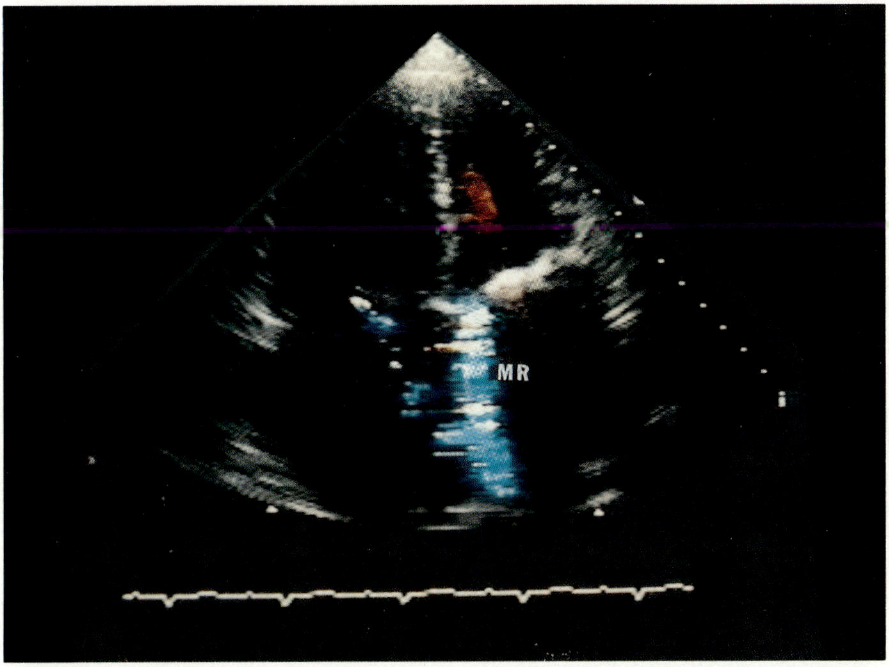

Plate 7
Apical four-chamber view showing an eccentric mitral regurgitant jet (MR). Such eccentric jets may be missed on conventional Doppler recordings.

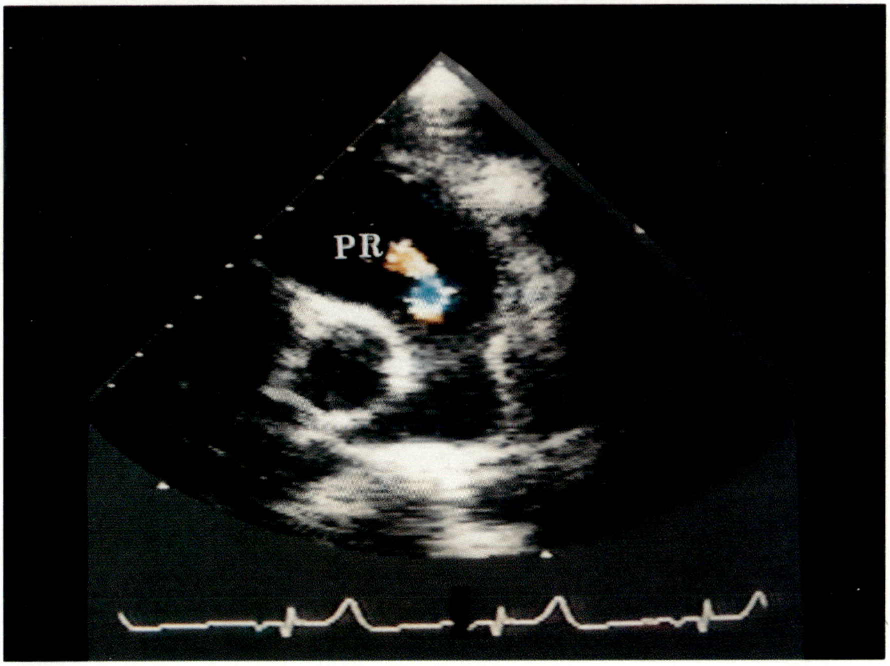

Plate 8
Parasternal short axis view showing a dilated right ventricular outflow tract and pulmonary artery with high-velocity pulmonic regurgitant jet (PR).

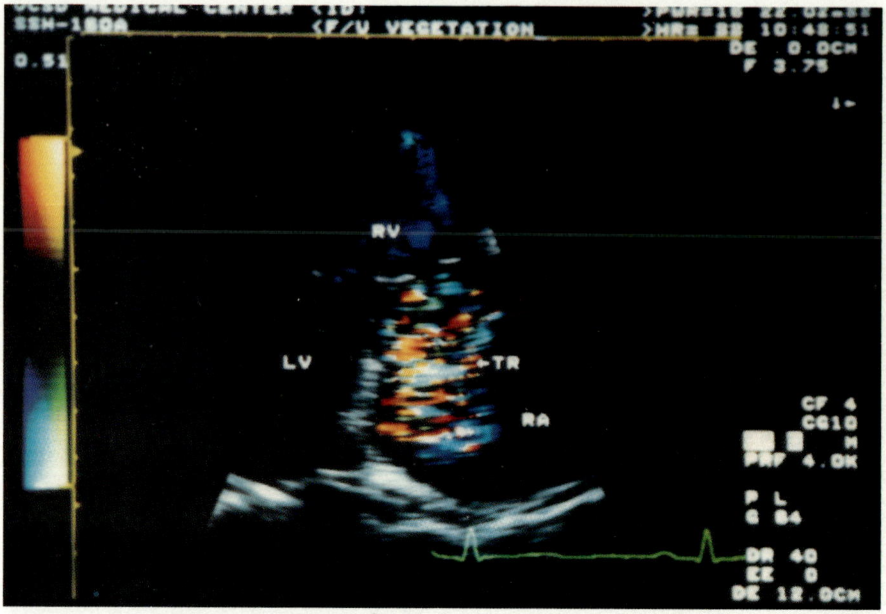

Plate 9
Parasternal, right-ventricular, inflow tract view showing tricuspid regurgitation jet (TR) in the right atrium (RA). LV = left ventricle, RV = right ventricle.

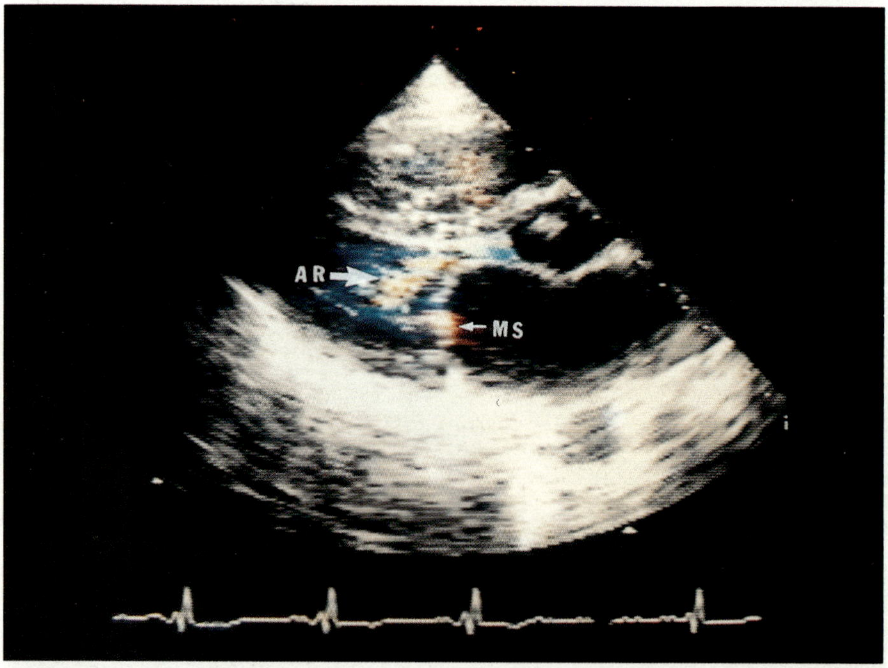

Plate 10
Parasternal long axis view showing combined mitral stenosis jet (MS) and aortic regurgitation jet (AR) can be distinguished in this diastolic frame.

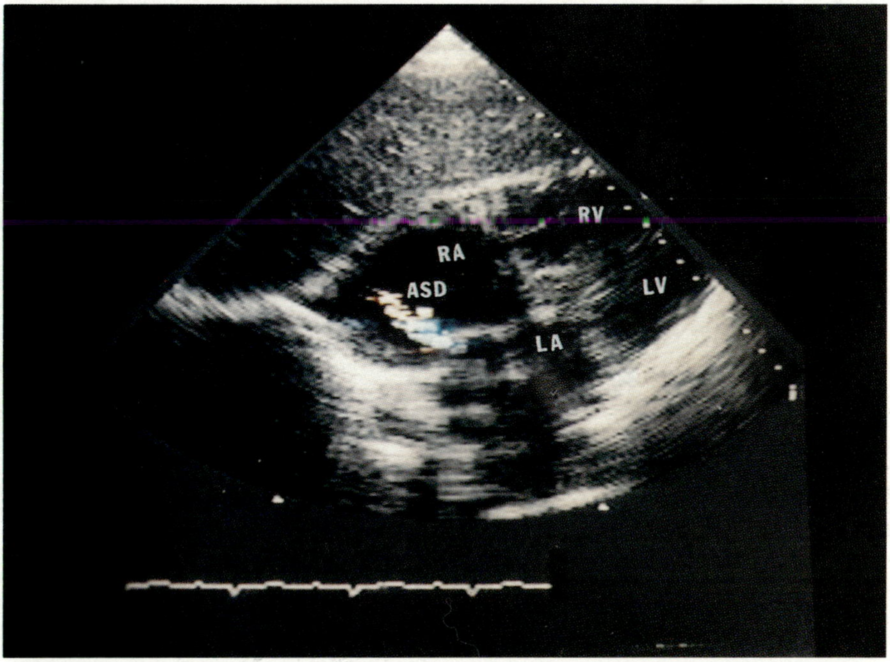

Plate 11
Subcostal four-chamber view showing left-to-right shunt jet into the right atrium (RA) in atrial septal defect (ASD). LA = left atrium, RV = right ventricle, LV = left ventricle.

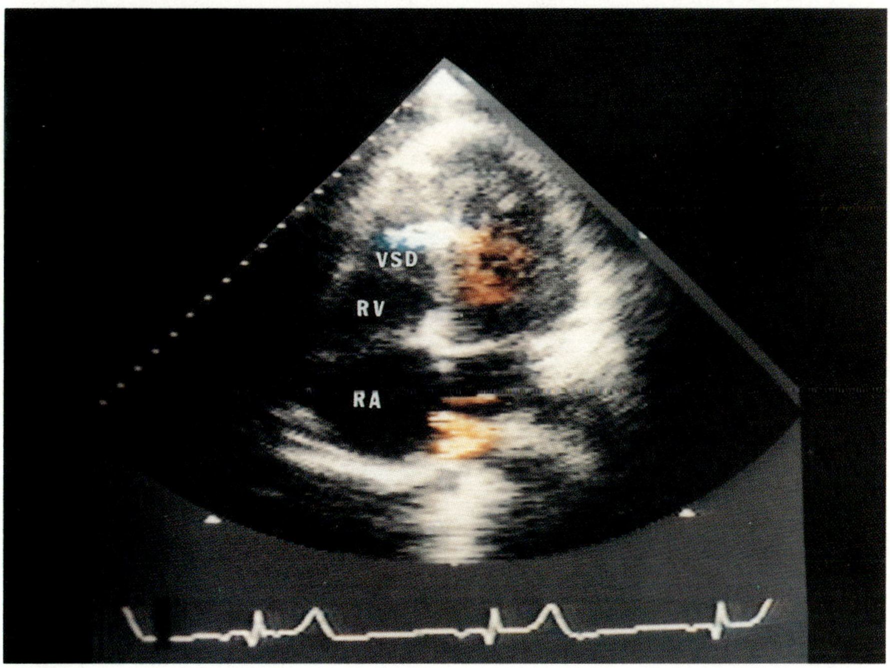

Plate 12
Apical four-chamber view showing left-to-right shunt jet across a muscular ventricular septal defect (VSD). RV = right ventricle, RA = right atrium.

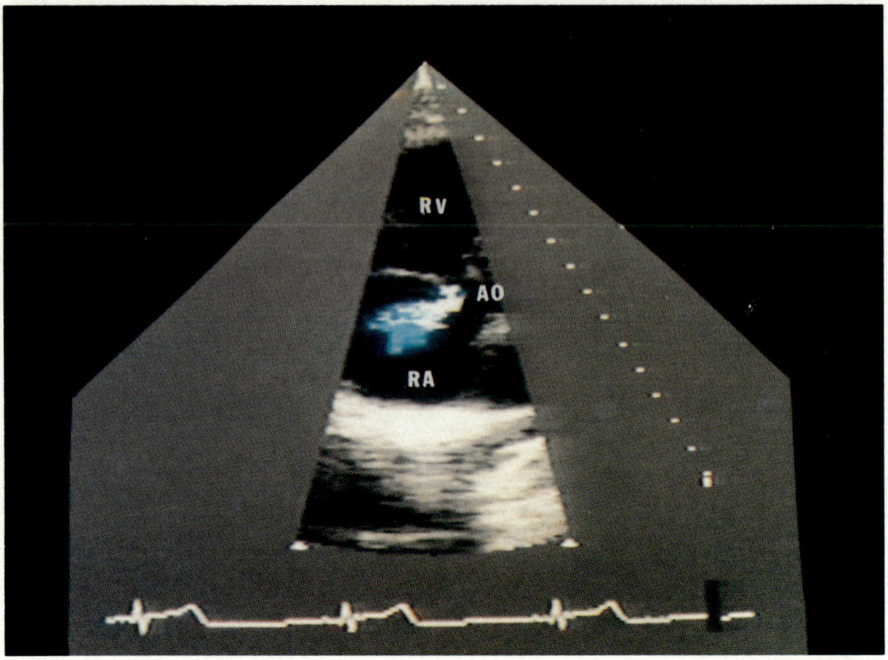

Plate 13
Parasternal short axis view showing high-velocity jet from a ruptured sinus of Valsalva with aortic-to-right atrial shunt. AO = aortic root, RA = right atrium, RV = right ventricle.

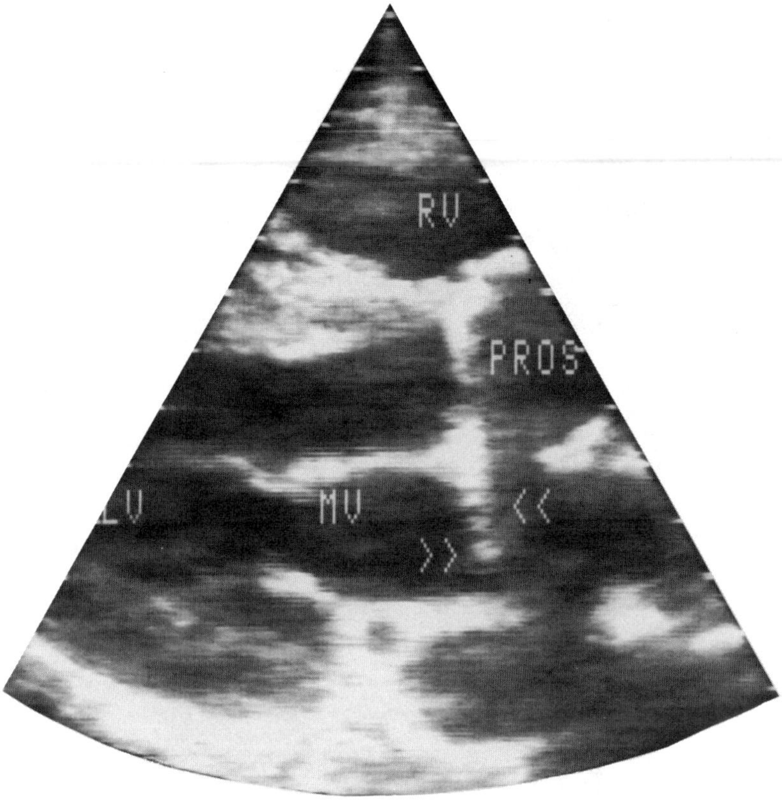

Figure 9.5
Parasternal long axis view of a tilting disc prosthesis (PROS) in the aortic position. The disc rests in the sewing ring in this diastolic frame. Note the prominent reverberations (arrowheads). LV = left ventricle, RV = right ventricle, MV = mitral valve.

parallel linear echo densities that exhibit motion coherent with the valve annulus. Normal tissue leaflets of the bioprosthesis are usually faintly visualized and exhibit motion similar to that of a normal aortic valve with the typical box-shape appearance when the valve is in the open position (Figure 9.11). A similar echocardiographic appearance is noted even for prosthetic implants in the mitral position.

Cardiac Response to the Prosthetic Implant

A new prosthetic implant alleviates the hemodynamic overload caused by the diseased cardiac valve that was replaced. This allows regression of most of the adaptive changes undergone by the heart as a response to the previous hemodynamic abnormalities. The degree of improvement is largely dependent on the status of the cardiac function prior to valve replacement. The most dramatic change is usually

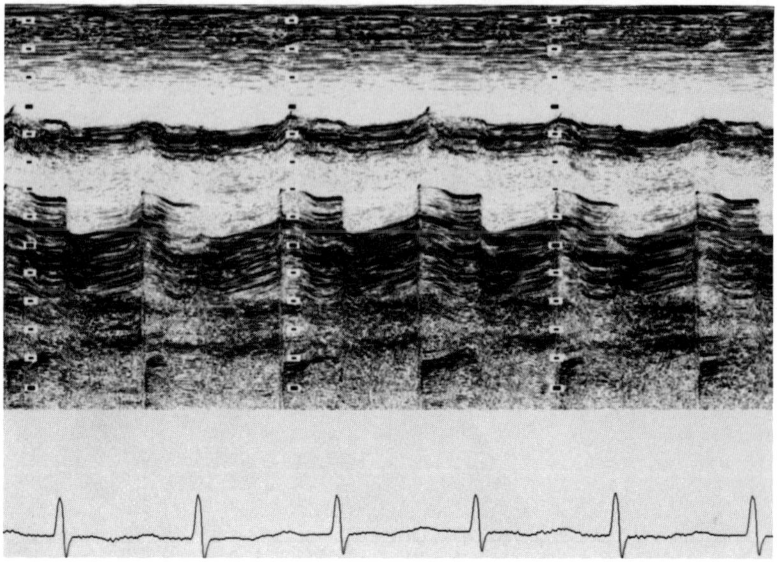

Figure 9.6
M-mode recording of a Bjork-Shiley disc valve prosthesis in the mitral position. Note the rapid opening and closing motion of the disc. Multiple linear echoes are generated by reverberations from the sewing ring.

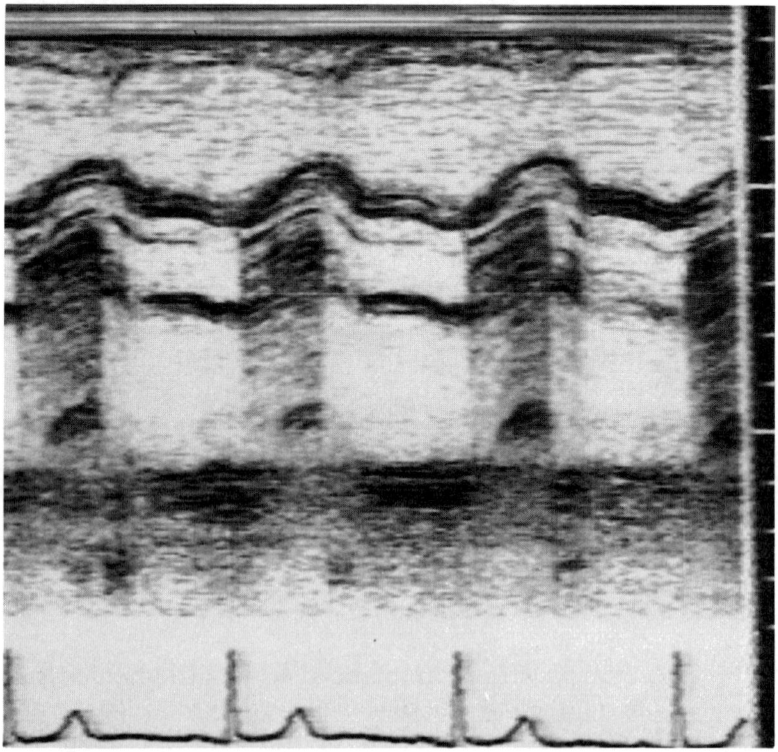

Figure 9.7
M-mode recording of a Bjork-Shiley disc valve prosthesis in the aortic position. Note the dense linear echoes generated only in systole, with reverberations extending into the left atrial cavity.

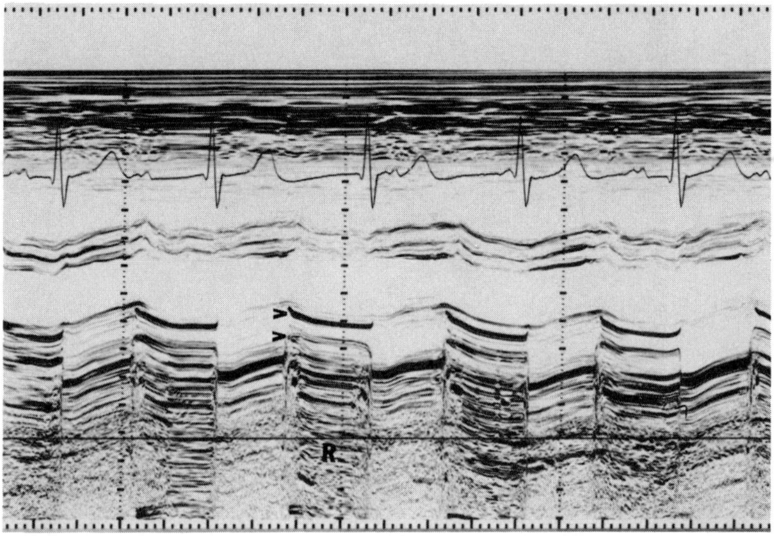

Figure 9.8
M-mode recording of a St. Jude metallic prosthesis in the mitral position. Note the prominent two parallel linear echoes originating from both discs in diastole, in the open position (open arrowheads). The discs are not visible in systole. Reverberations (R) from the sewing ring are also prominent.

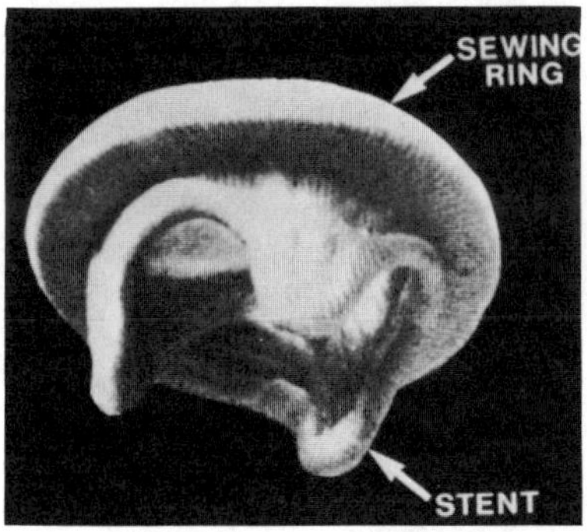

Figure 9.9
Hancock porcine bioprosthesis. Note the large stents that support the valve leaflets. (From A. D. Hagan and A. N. DeMaria, *Clinical Applications of Two-Dimensional Echocardiography and Cardiac Doppler* [2nd ed.]. Boston: Little, Brown, 1989. Pp. 426–427.)

observed in patients following aortic valve replacement for severe aortic stenosis. This abnormality causes pressure overload with significant left ventricular hypertrophy. Following valve replacement, the left ventricle is relieved from this pressure overload. Serial echocardiograms following aortic valve replacement will invariably demonstrate variable degrees of regression of left ventricular hypertrophy, with

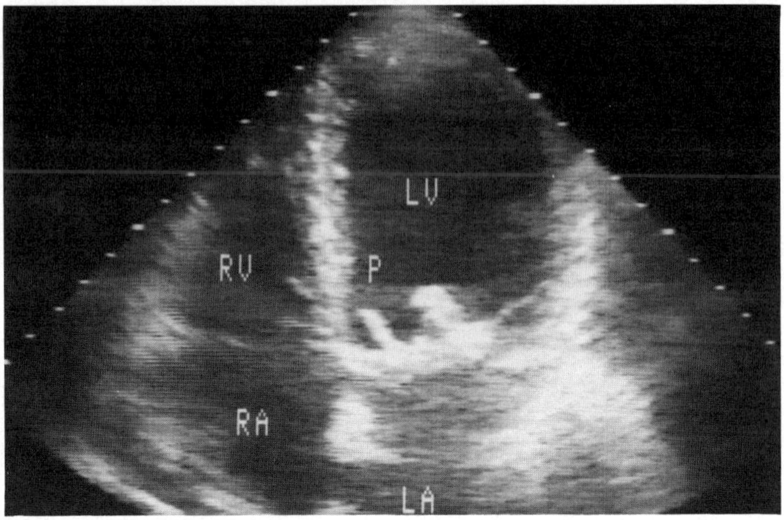

A

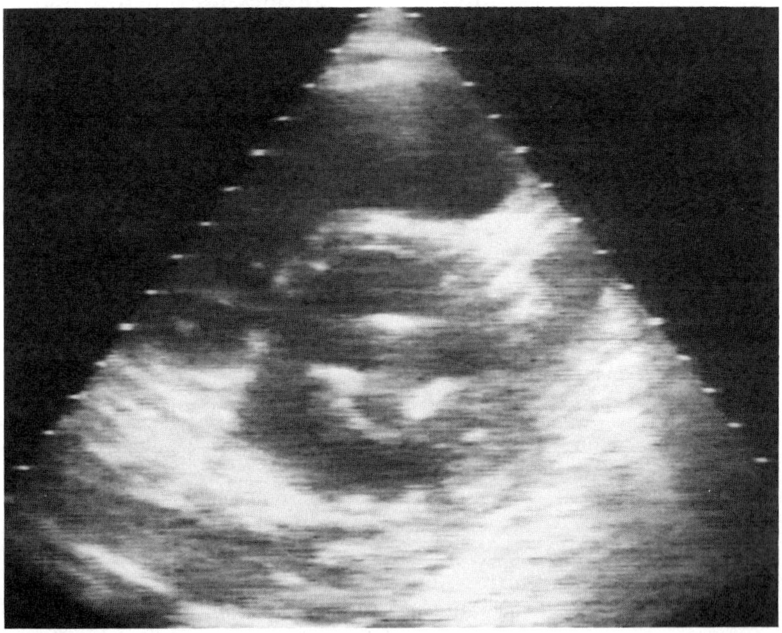

B

Figure 9.10
A. Apical four-chamber view depicting two stents of a bioprosthesis in the mitral position (P). B. Short axis view of the same bioprosthesis showing a cross-sectional image of the three stents of the bioprosthesis. LV = left ventricle, RV = right ventricle, RA = right atrium, LA = left atrium.

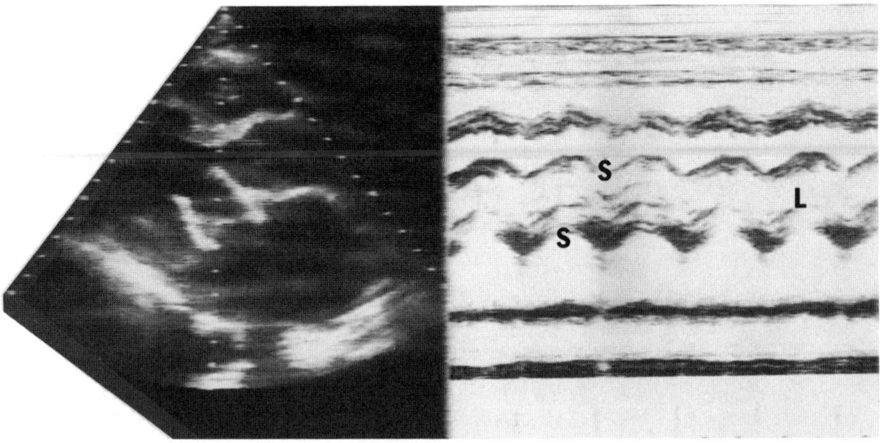

Figure 9.11
Parasternal two-dimensional view of the bioprosthesis in the mitral position. The leaflets (L) of a newly implanted bioprosthesis are only faintly visualized. Only the stents (S) are visualized. Note the parallel wavy lines generated on the M-mode recording.

improvement of overall contractile performance over a period of several months.

In mitral valve stenosis, replacement of the mitral valve causes a decrease in the previously elevated left atrial pressure. This may be associated with a gradual decrease in left atrial size. However, the left atrium will always remain larger than normal.

With respect to regurgitant valvular lesions, replacement of diseased aortic or mitral valves alleviates the volume overload on the left ventricle. Ventricular size may decrease slightly, but will always remain enlarged to some degree. Unfortunately, improvement of contractility is more subtle and is less dramatic. In fact, temporary worsening of left ventricular function may be noted immediately after valve replacement.

The interventricular septum commonly exhibits atypical or paradoxical motion during the first 6 months after open heart surgery. The true reason for this atypical septal motion is not well understood. It is thought to be secondary to postoperative adhesions along the anterior border of the heart and the chest wall, and does not necessarily reflect any damage to the interventricular septum, which thickens normally during systole (Figure 9.12).

Mechanical Prosthetic Valve Malfunction

All prosthetic valves have been designed to attempt to simulate normal function of the native valve being replaced. How-

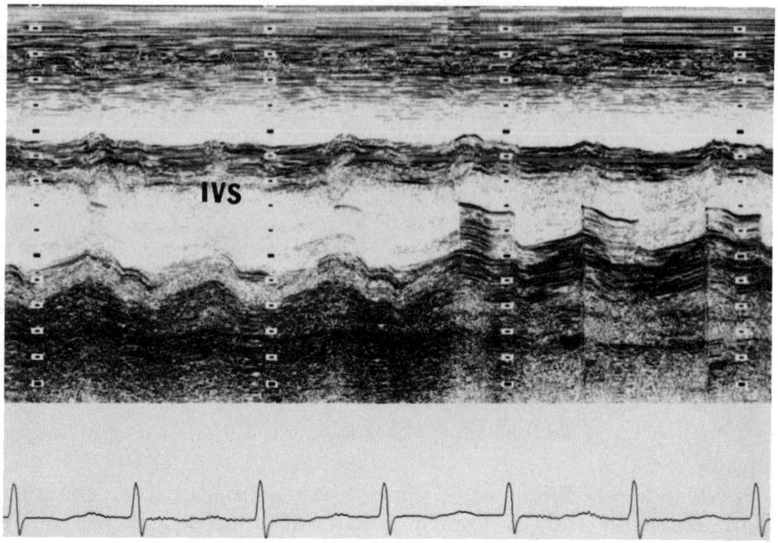

Figure 9.12
Paradoxical motion of the interventricular septum (IVS) is readily apparent in this M-mode recording from a patient with a mitral valve disc prosthesis.

ever, acting as foreign objects in the body, prosthetic valves may be involved in, or may even induce, multiple abnormalities that are potentially life threatening.

Thombus Formation

Deposition of platelets on various elements of a mechanical prosthesis predisposes for thrombus formation. This is the most common abnormality leading to malfunction of a mechanical valve prosthesis (Figure 9.13). A relatively large thrombus typically prevents normal closure of the ball valve or disc, resulting in regurgitation. Less frequently, a relatively large thrombus adherent to the cage or struts of the mechanical prosthesis may restrict adequate valve opening. This could lead to functional obstruction with consequences similar to stenosis of the natural cardiac valve, but occurs at a relatively fast rate and does not allow enough time for normal cardiac adaptive mechanisms to respond to this new overload.

Because of the highly echogenic elements of mechanical prosthetic valves, it is difficult at times to reliably identify small thrombi on the prosthesis. Occasionally, abnormal excursion or closure of the ball or disc valve may be the only clue to the thrombus formation.

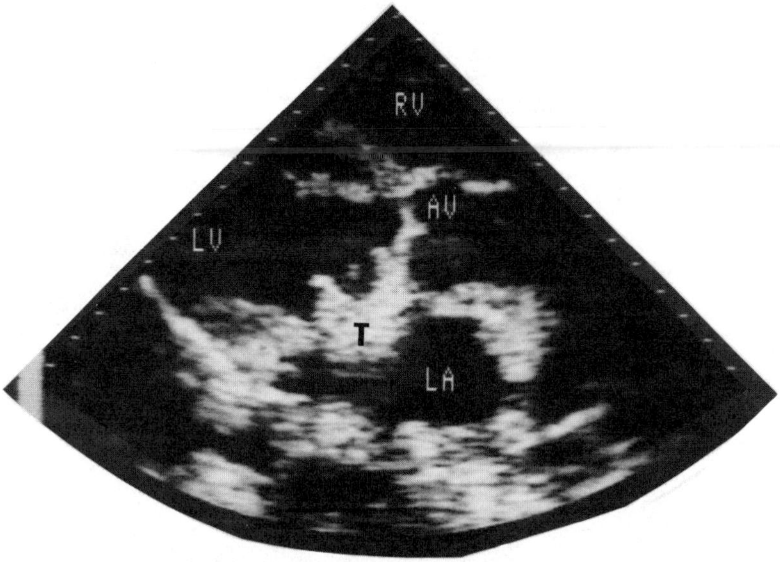

Figure 9.13
Parasternal long axis view of a prosthesis in the mitral position with unusually prominent echoes on the sewing ring, highly suspicious for thrombus formation (T). RV = right ventricle, LV = left ventricle, AV = aortic valve, LA = left atrium.

At times, M-mode echocardiography may provide a better assessment of the mobile elements of a prosthetic valve than two-dimensional echocardiography. A normal disc frequently produces echoes with sharp edges during the rapid opening and closing movements. This is in contrast to the rounded contour of the echoes produced by a slowly moving disc restricted by thrombus formation (Figure 9.14).

Bacterial Endocarditis

Acting as foreign bodies, prosthetic valves are easy targets for bacterial endocarditis and development of vegetations. Relatively large vegetations, acting similar to thrombus formation, may restrict normal valve closure and allow for regurgitation. Moreover, in the setting of bacterial endocarditis involving a prosthesis, the incidence of abscess formation is higher than that of vegetation on native valves. Antibiotics alone may not be adequate to control the infection. Progressive valvular regurgitation is very common, at times necessitating surgical replacement of the infected prosthesis.

Similar to thrombus formation, vegetative growths on the mechanical prosthesis are also difficult to identify. However,

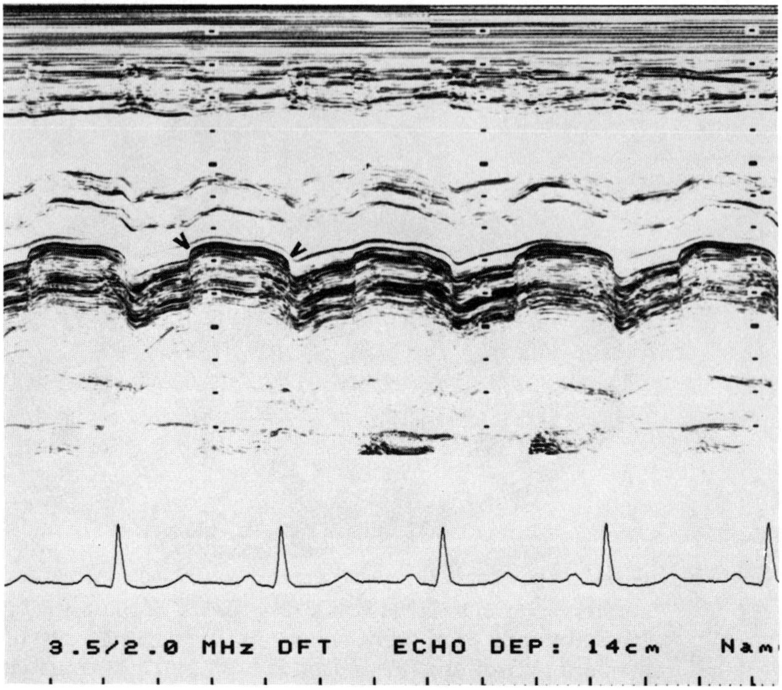

Figure 9.14
A thrombus on this tilting disc prosthesis in the mitral position caused substantial slow opening and closure movements of the disc, with diminished diastolic excursion. Note the rounded contour (open arrowheads) during opening and closure motion. This is in contrast to the sharp contours commonly seen with a normally functioning prosthesis (see Figure 9.6).

large mobile vegetations may be seen prolapsing back and forth across the sewing ring (Figure 9.15). Abscess formation along the sewing ring may be identified as a localized area of ultrasound density, different from the surrounding tissues. Dehiscence of the prosthetic implant is not uncommon in such conditions (discussion follows).

Dehiscence

This refers to the rupture of one or more sutures that anchor the sewing ring of the prosthesis to the annulus of the excised cardiac valve. Dehiscence of the prosthesis is frequently a complication that occurs early after surgery, and may occur because of abscess formation at the valve annulus in patients with bacterial endocarditis. Irrespective of the

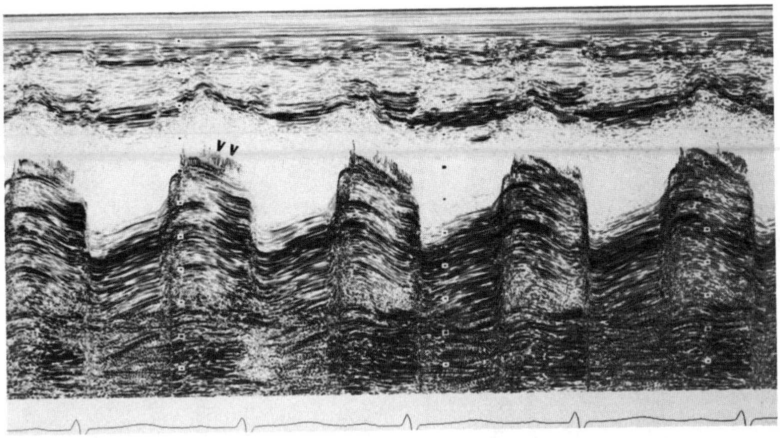

Figure 9.15
Note the irregular shaggy echoes of a vegetation on this disc valve prosthesis in the mitral position (open arrowheads). Also note the rounded contour of the opening and closure motion of the disc, suggesting relative restriction of disc mobility due to the vegetation.

cause of dehiscence of the prosthesis, paravalvular regurgitation is very common, and may necessitate surgical intervention.

Dehiscence allows exaggerated motion of the prosthetic valve apparatus relative to the valve annulus. In extreme situations, the sewing ring may be seen prolapsing outside the plane of the valve annulus throughout the cardiac cycle. Such hypermobility is commonly referred to as rocking motion of the prosthetic implant and frequently suggests significant dehiscence.

Variance

Ball or disc valves made of Silastic material may absorb lipids from the blood and may actually change in size or shape. Mechanical wear and tear of the poppet or disc causes loss of smooth contour, and at times, leads to cracking or chipping. This may cause the poppet or disc to malfunction, and at times, to stick to the cage or struts. A decrease in the size of the poppet or disc may allow it to break loose from the cage or struts, thus causing acute severe regurgitation. On the other hand, a swollen poppet may stick on the cage in the open position, and will also cause regurgitation. These complications are less frequently encountered with the newer models of mechanical prosthesis.

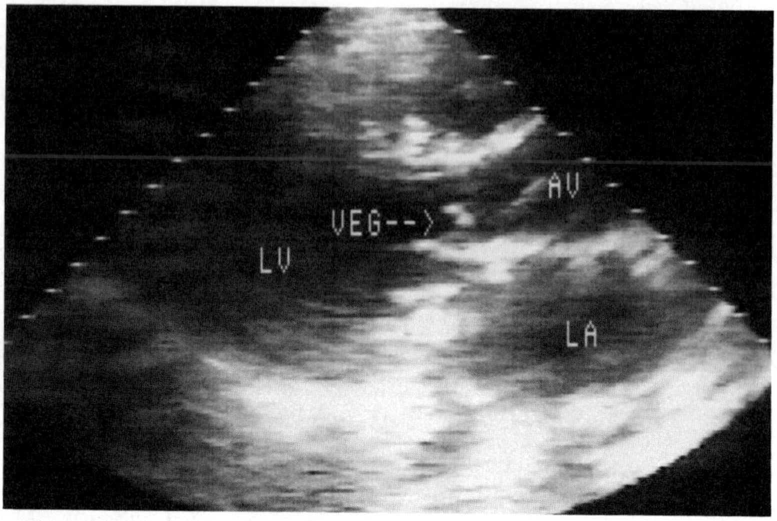

Figure 9.16
Parasternal long axis view of a bioprosthesis in the mitral position, depicting hypermobile mass, consistent with vegetation (VEG). AV = aortic valve, LV = left ventricle, RV = right ventricle.

Bioprosthetic Valve Malfunction

Bioprosthetic valves were primarily designed to avoid complications encountered with mechanical prosthesis in regards to thrombus formation. Hence, the incidence of thrombosis is much lower with tissue prostheses, drastically reducing the need for anticoagulant therapy after valve replacement.

Bacterial Endocarditis

Similar to mechanical prostheses, vegetations localized to the stents of the bioprosthesis may be difficult to identify. However, vegetations on the tissue leaflets may cause echocardiographic findings similar to vegetations on native cardiac valves (Figure 9.16).

Dehiscence

Dehiscence causes findings similar to those for mechanical prosthetic valves.

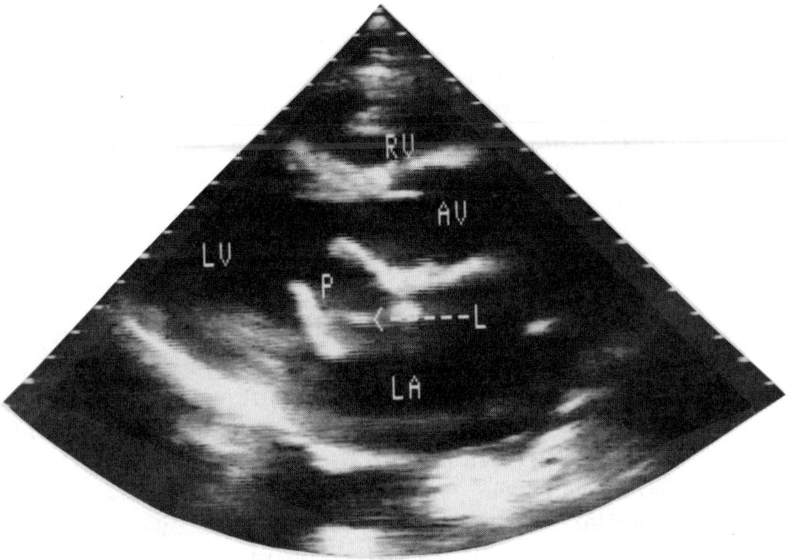

Figure 9.17
Parasternal long axis view of a bioprosthesis (P) in the mitral position, with prominent echoes originating from calcified bioprosthetic leaflets (L). LV = left ventricle, RV = right ventricle, LA = left atrium, AV = aortic valve.

Degeneration and Calcification

The chemical treatment of the bioprosthesis provides relative protection to the tissue material, which ultimately degenerates. Thus, fenestration and occasional rupture of a bioprosthetic leaflet are not unusual within approximately 5 to 10 years after its implantation. This may lead to significant regurgitation. On the other hand, deposition of calcium on the bioprosthetic leaflets leads to progressive thickening and restriction of leaflet mobility (Figure 9.17). This may ultimately lead to stenosis of the bioprosthesis with relative obstruction to blood flow.

Fenestration of a bioprosthetic leaflet is difficult to visualize on echocardiography. Normal bioprosthetic leaflets are usually faintly visualized on routine echocardiography, whereas progressive deposition of calcium makes the leaflets more echogenic.

Pseudo Valve Malfunction

Certain clinical situations arise when cardiac dysfunction after valve replacement may be attributed to the prosthetic implant despite normal function of the prosthetic valve.

Valve-Heart Mismatch

Prosthetic valves, whether mechanical or bioprosthetic, are available in different sizes depending on the location (mitral prosthesis is usually bigger than an aortic one) and also depending on the size of the heart itself. Valve-heart mismatch may occur when the size of the prosthetic implant is not adequate for a particular patient. This may create hemodynamic compromise despite the fact that the prosthesis is functioning normally. For example, a normally functioning aortic prosthesis may be relatively too small in regards to the volume of blood flow across it. This may actually simulate aortic valvular stenosis with similar hemodynamic sequelae. A relatively large ball valve prosthesis implanted in the mitral position protrudes into the left ventricular outflow tract of a small ventricle, causing relative obstruction to the left ventricular outflow tract. Either of these two examples may contribute to low cardiac output despite normal function of the prosthetic valve. Newer surgical techniques have significantly reduced the incidence of valve-heart mismatch.

Low Cardiac Output

In general, surgical replacement of the diseased cardiac valve results in progressive improvement of overall cardiac function. Sometimes, cardiac function continues to deteriorate following valve replacement and occasionally may be erroneously attributed to prosthetic valve malfunction. Improved surgical techniques allow successful valve replacement in patients with significant left ventricular dysfunction. Hence, alleviation of the hemodynamic overload caused by the diseased valve may not necessarily reverse the course of events. In such patients, low cardiac output with reduced rate of flow across the prosthesis may cause diminished opening of the prosthetic valve. This may superficially simulate valve malfunction with restricted valve opening. However, left ventricular contractile performance will always be significantly impaired and will help distinguish the cause of the low cardiac output.

Cardiac Rhythm and Conduction Abnormalities

Irregular cardiac rhythm, such as in atrial fibrillation, allows variable intervals of blood flow across the prosthetic valve. Therefore, motion of the prosthetic valve will be chaotic with variable excursions, similar to what would be expected for the native cardiac valve in the same position.

Flow across a prosthetic valve is primarily dependent on the transvalvular pressure gradient. Hence, any abnormality that alters this pressure difference may be associated with unusual motion of the prosthetic implant and may falsely simulate malfunction. This is best demonstrated in patients with mitral disc prosthesis and a prolonged PR interval, whereby, following atrial contraction, left atrial and ventricular pressures equilibrate. Transprosthetic flow stops and the prosthetic disc slowly drifts into the closed position. This slow motion will generate echocardiographic images with rounded contour during valve closure and may falsely suggest thrombus formation.

Doppler Evaluation of Prosthetic Cardiac Valves

Prosthetic cardiac valves always cause some obstruction to forward flow irrespective of the anatomic location. Therefore, a normally functioning prosthetic valve causes forward velocities slightly higher than expected for a corresponding normally functioning native valve. Moreover, normally functioning prosthetic valves may allow trivial regurgitation.

Normal Flow Patterns across Prosthetic Valves

The opening and closing motions of prosthetic valves are easy to record with Doppler ultrasound. Metallic valves produce much higher signals than tissue valves (Figure 9.18).

The transducer locations to record flow across prosthetic valves are similar to those used for native valves. However, the operator must be aware that the direction of flow across a prosthetic valve may not be central to the valve ring. Moreover, tilting disc valves, except for the St. Jude with double discs, may produce two streams of flow, on both sides of the disc. The ball on a ball valve prosthesis will not allow central flow across the valve.

Doppler Recordings of Prosthetic Valve Malfunction

Prosthetic valve stenosis (e.g., calcification of a tissue prosthetic valve or thrombus on a metallic valve) will cause an increase in obstruction with an associated increase in the velocity of transprosthetic flow. This may be regarded in the same way as native valvular stenosis. The direction of the jet of flow may be eccentric and the flow may be of higher velocities than the normal baseline recordings (Figure 9.19).

Regurgitant flow across a prosthetic valve may produce

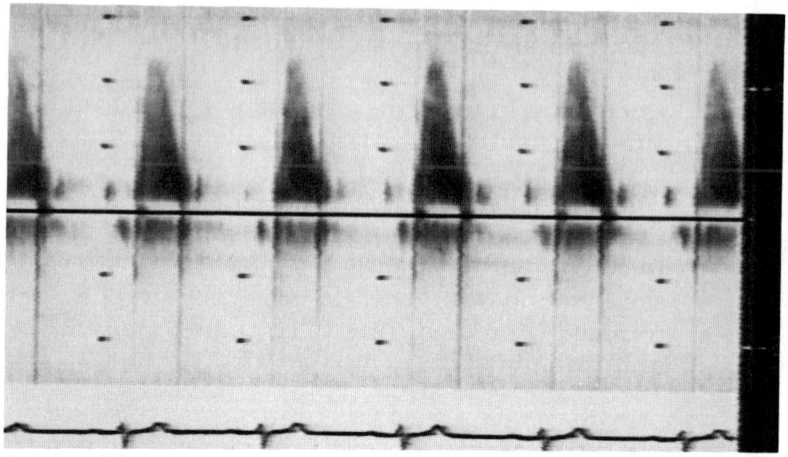

A

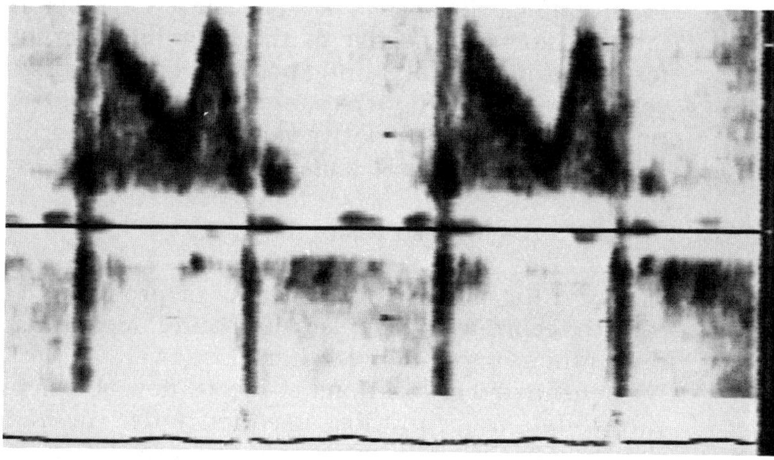

B

Figure 9.18
Slightly increased velocities of flow across normally functioning prosthetic valves are very commonly encountered by Doppler ultrasound. The opening and closure amplitude signals are also frequently recorded. A. Superstemal recording of aortic mechanical prosthesis. B. Apical recording of mitral mechanical prosthesis in sinus rhythm.

Doppler recordings of regurgitation similar to the native incompetent valve. However, one should realize that ultrasound does not pass through metallic valves. The apical position for the transducer is adequate to examine regurgitant flow across a metallic aortic valve prosthesis, since the valve itself lies anatomically distal to the area of interest, i.e., the left ventricular outflow tract. However, the apical position is not adequate for examining regurgitant flow across a

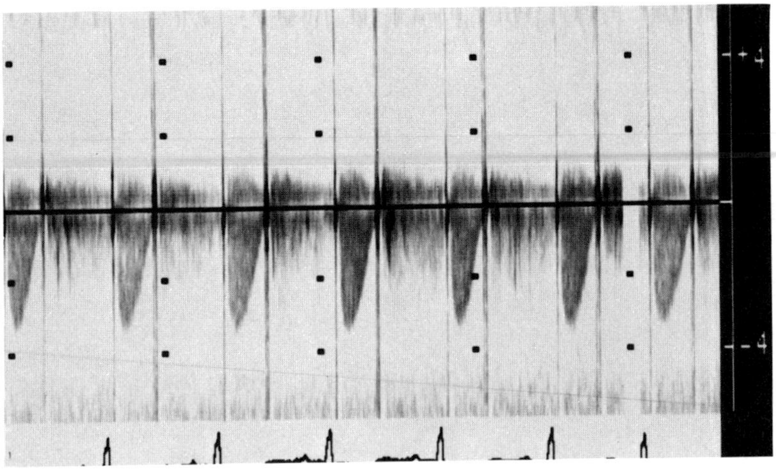

Figure 9.19
Abnormal increased Doppler velocities, noted across this prosthesis in the aortic position. Note the similarity of such recordings to those obtained from patients with stenosis of native aortic valves. The opening and closure amplitude signals are prominent on this recording.

metallic mitral valve prosthesis because the area of interest (i.e., the left atrium) lies distal to the prosthetic valve. The Doppler ultrasound beam cannot traverse the closed metallic valve in systole and the resulting signals are inadequate for interpretation. If this occurs, one may adopt a low parasternal location for the transducer whereby the left atrium is insonated by a Doppler ultrasound beam that does not pass across the metallic prosthesis. Two-dimensional echocardiography may be very helpful in this situation as a guide for the Doppler cursor. This maneuvering may allow adequate Doppler recordings to confirm the presence of regurgitation across the prosthetic valve and semiquantitative estimation of severity. However, it is not possible to clearly differentiate valvular from paravalvular leaks. Color Doppler imaging is particularly useful in the detection of abnormal prosthetic regurgitation since such regurgitant jets are commonly eccentric and may be difficult to detect with conventional Doppler ultrasound.

10 Cardiomyopathies and Myocarditis

Cardiomyopathy is a general term used to refer to cardiac muscle diseases of unknown cause. This group of cardiac diseases is divided into three general categories: (1) hypertrophic cardiomyopathy; (2) dilated cardiomyopathy; and (3) restricted cardiomyopathy.

Hypertrophic Cardiomyopathy

Wall Thickness

The hallmark of this cardiac muscle disease is cell hypertrophy, with disarray of the myocardial fibers as seen on microscopic examinations of the diseased myocardium. The abnormal myocardial structure may be localized to only one segment of the cardiac muscle wall, but at times, generalized involvement does occur. Most commonly, the interventricular septum is involved. Recent reports have identified localized involvement in the left ventricular apex, but rarely in the posterior wall or right ventricle only.

Contractility

Typically, there is hyperdynamic contractile performance of the left ventricle, with super normal ejection fraction. Left ventricular volume in diastole is normal or usually decreased. The hyperdynamic contraction in systole leads to a very small, and at times, obliterated, cavity at the end of systolic contraction.

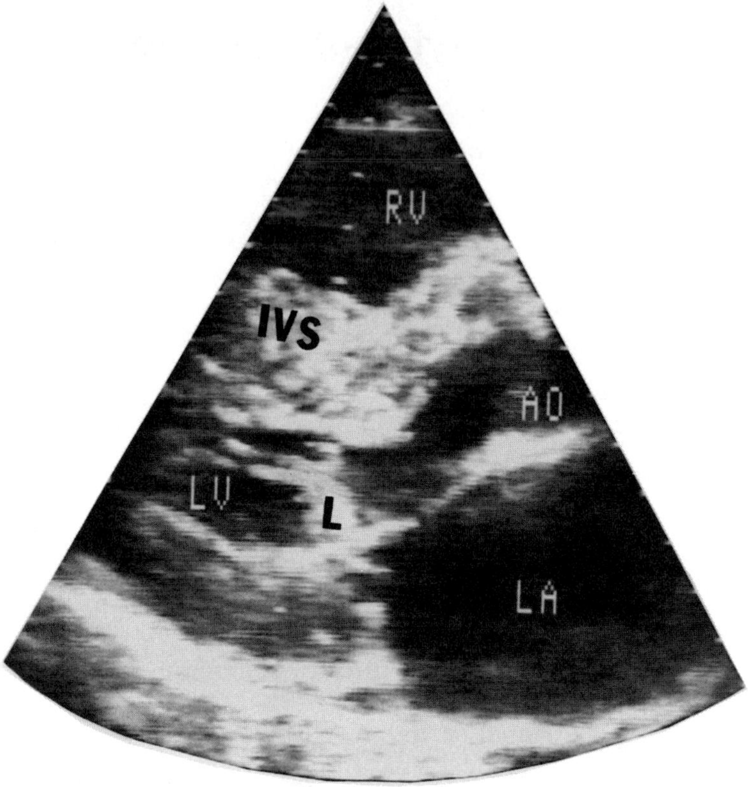

A

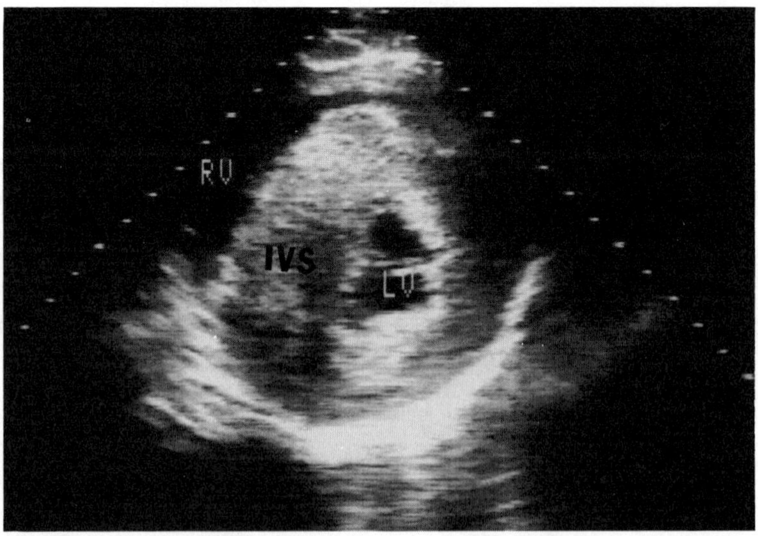

B

Echocardiographic Findings

The echocardiogram is an excellent noninvasive method for the diagnosis of hypertrophic cardiomyopathy. The markedly thickened myocardial wall is readily identifiable on the echocardiogram (Figure 10.1). A characteristic finding is the sparkling appearance of the diseased muscle, which is more echogenic than the normal myocardium. Despite the small chamber size and hyperdynamic contractile performance, it is not unusual to observe diminished wall motion in the affected segments. This is usually seen in the interventricular septum, which exhibits marked hypertrophy but minimal excursions in systole.

Idiopathic hypertrophic subaortic stenosis (IHSS) is an old term used to refer to one form of hypertrophic cardiomyopathy, whereby the interventricular septum is markedly hypertrophied in relation to other myocardial segments. Typically, the ratio of wall thickness of the interventricular septum to the left ventricular posterior wall is 1:1 in normal subjects. In patients with left ventricular hypertrophy secondary to systemic hypertension or aortic valve stenosis, this ratio remains normal. However, in IHSS, this ratio becomes 1.4 : 1 or even greater, depending on the severity of the disease. This finding is not diagnostic of this condition; however, it is strongly suggestive of it.

Outflow Tract Obstruction

When the markedly hypertrophied interventricular septum contracts in systole, it encroaches on the narrow left ventricular outflow tract, which becomes even narrower. This frequently leads to relative obstruction of left ventricular emptying in mid to late systole, thus, the term obstructive cardiomyopathy.

The anterior mitral leaflet also plays a role in the genesis of obstruction of the left ventricular outflow tract. It is not un-

---

Figure 10.1
A. Parasternal long axis view of hypertrophic cardiomyopathy. Note the marked increased thickness of the interventricular septum (IVS) and narrow left ventricular (LV) cavity. The left atrium (LA) is frequently dilated. Also note the systolic anterior motion of the anterior mitral leaflet (L), protruding into the left ventricular outflow tract, suggestive of outflow obstruction (see text and Figure 10.2). B. Parasternal short axis view also showing marked increased thickness of the interventricular septum with a small left ventricular cavity in this systolic frame. RV = right ventricle; AO = aorta

usual to observe the anterior mitral leaflet protruding into the already narrowed outflow tract in systole. It is not clear whether this is a contributory cause of the obstruction, or just a passive phenomenon of the suction effect imposed by the rapidly accelerating blood flow in the left ventricular outflow tract. This abnormal motion of the anterior mitral leaflet can be readily seen on the echocardiogram. This was first described on the M-mode echocardiogram as an anterior motion (toward the chest wall) in systole, thus, the term systolic anterior motion. It is not unusual to observe the anterior mitral leaflet touching the interventricular septum in systole (Figure 10.2). When systolic anterior motion is recorded on the echocardiogram, obstruction to the left ventricular outflow tract is very likely present. Increasing severity of obstruction may lead to an earlier occurrence of anterior motion in systole, with a longer duration of contact of the anterior mitral leaflet to the interventricular septum.

The presence of systolic anterior motion is not diagnostic of obstructive cardiomyopathy. Systolic anterior motion may be observed in hyperdynamic ventricles other than hypertrophic cardiomyopathy. It has been noted to occur also in mitral valve prolapse due to the redundant leaflets.

Another echocardiographic sign of obstruction of the left ventricular outflow tract is the abnormal motion of the aortic valve. Commonly, the aortic valve remains open throughout the ejection phase in systole. In the presence of obstruction of the left ventricular outflow tract, the hyperdynamic ventricle ejects most of its stroke volume rapidly in early systole. Moreover, increasing obstruction in mid to late systole markedly decreases blood flow. The resulting effect is a tendency for the aortic valve to start to close in mid to late systole. This is commonly referred to as midsystolic closure of the aortic valve (Figure 10.3). Since this phenomenon is simply a reflection of diminished transaortic blood flow in mid to late systole, it may occur in conditions other than obstructive cardiomyopathy that also cause a decrease in blood flow across the aortic valve. Systolic closure of the aortic valve may be observed in the presence of fixed membranous subaortic stenosis and, occasionally, in patients with severe mitral regurgitation in the absence of associated aortic valve disease.

The obstruction of left ventricular outflow is dynamic and variable. The onset and severity of this obstruction are not fixed, in contrast to the fixed obstruction in aortic valvular stenosis. The degree of obstruction in hypertrophic cardiomyopathy is dependent on several hemodynamic parameters. Various hemodynamic maneuvers may alter these parameters and subsequently alter the severity of obstruction.

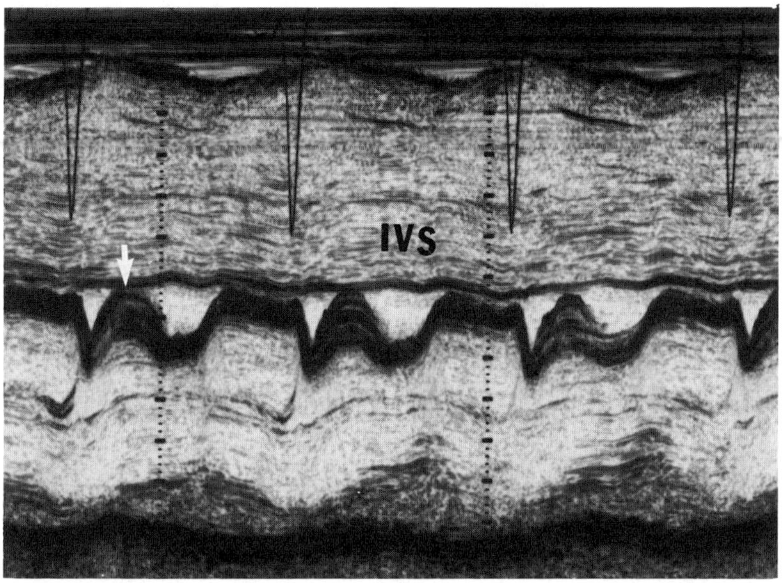

A

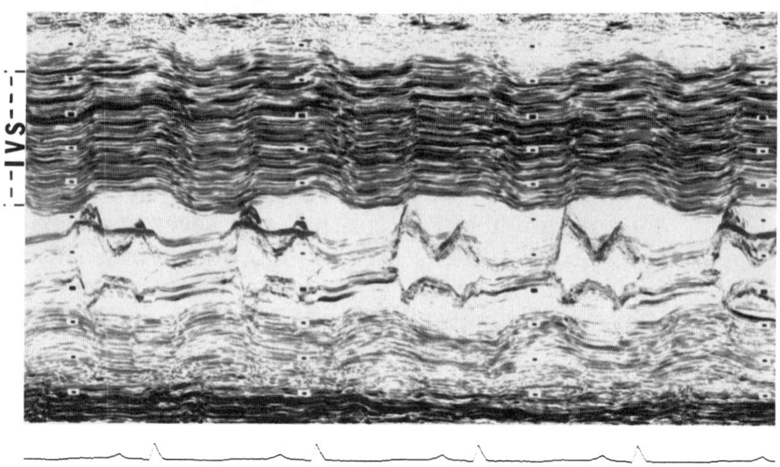

B

Figure 10.2
M-mode recording of hypertrophic cardiomyopathy, with prominent hypertrophy of the interventricular septum (IVS). A. Hypertrophic obstructive cardiomyopathy is strongly suggested in this recording, with systolic anterior motion of the anterior mitral leaflet (arrow). B. Hypertrophic nonobstructive cardiomyopathy. Note the absence of systolic anterior motion, with normal-appearing motion of the mitral valve throughout the cardiac cycle.

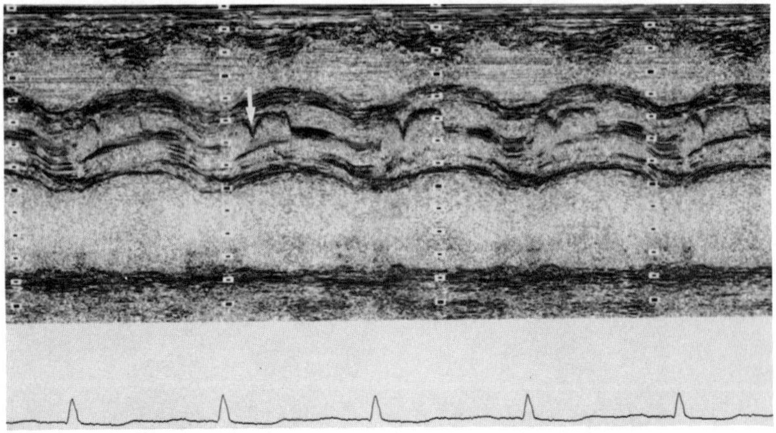

Figure 10.3
M-mode recording of aortic valve motion in hypertrophic obstructive cardiomyopathy. Note the notching of the aortic valve motion in midsystole (arrow).

In general, maneuvers that decrease venous return to the right side of the heart, and ultimately to the left side, will worsen the obstruction since left ventricular volume, as well as the width of the outflow tract, will diminish. Maneuvers that increase the resistance to ventricular emptying by increasing aortic blood pressure and systemic vascular resistance generally decrease the severity of obstruction, since left ventricular volume is slightly larger. The most important parameter that controls the severity of obstruction is myocardial contractility. A vigorously contracting ventricle causes more severe obstruction of the outflow tract than does a less dynamic ventricle. The echocardiographic examination may be used to evaluate the hemodynamic response to these maneuvers by comparing the echocardiographic findings before and after one or more maneuvers.

Doppler Ultrasound

Doppler recordings of transvalvular flow commonly reveal the hemodynamic sequelae of hypertrophic cardiomyopathy. Forward mitral flow may demonstrate abnormal diastolic inflow velocities. Peak velocity of blood flow after the atrial kick may be greater than peak velocity in early diastole, reflecting abnormal diastolic filling of the left ventricle. Various degrees of mitral regurgitation are not uncommon. Mitral regurgitant flow does not necessarily reflect intrinsic mitral valve disease. Rather, this is a reflection of the increasing tension on the supporting papillary muscle apparatus with occasional mitral valve prolapse. Occasionally,

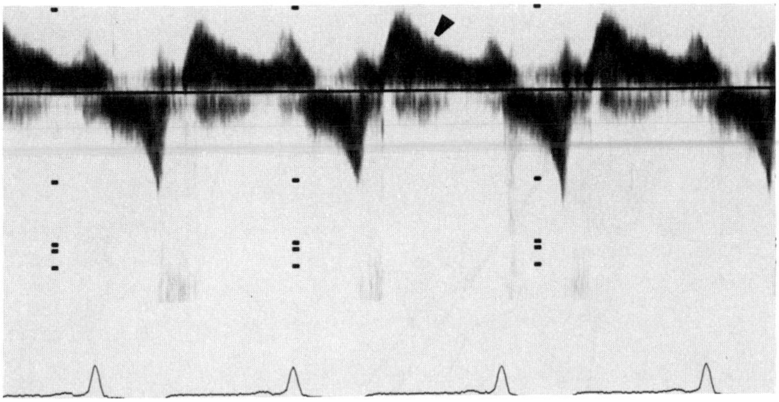

Figure 10.4
CW mode Doppler recording in hypertrophic cardiomyopathy, showing mitral regurgitation. Note the late peaking of this regurgitant flow. Abnormal ventricular diastolic relaxation predisposes to slow rate of deceleration of transmitral diastolic flow in mid-diastole (arrowhead).

mitral regurgitation may occur because of relative malalignment of the papillary muscles due to marked asymmetric hypertrophy of the left ventricle. This systolic regurgitant flow usually starts in mid to late systole, with late peaking of the velocity of regurgitant blood flow (Figure 10.4). Severe, holosystolic regurgitation is less frequently observed.

A characteristic Doppler finding typical of obstruction of left ventricular outflow is that of elevated velocities of blood flow within the left ventricular outflow tract, consistent with subaortic obstruction to blood flow (Figure 10.5). As the Doppler sample volume is moved along the left ventricular outflow tract, the velocity of blood flow suddenly increases at the level of obstruction. Similar velocity patterns would be recorded at the level of the aortic valve. This is diagnostic of subvalvular obstruction, and may be observed in patients with membranous subaortic stenosis. This abnormal velocity pattern is clearly different from that observed in aortic stenosis, where the velocity of blood flow increases only at the level of the aortic valve and downstream in the aortic root.

Peaking of the velocity of the blood flow within the left ventricular outflow tract is occasionally recorded in patients without hypertrophic cardiomyopathy. This abnormal flow pattern may be recorded in patients with prosthetic mitral valves, whereby a relatively bulky prosthesis protrudes into the outflow tract and causes mild obstruction to blood flow (Figure 10.6). Occasionally, marked hypertrophy of the papillary muscles may occur in patients with long-standing sys-

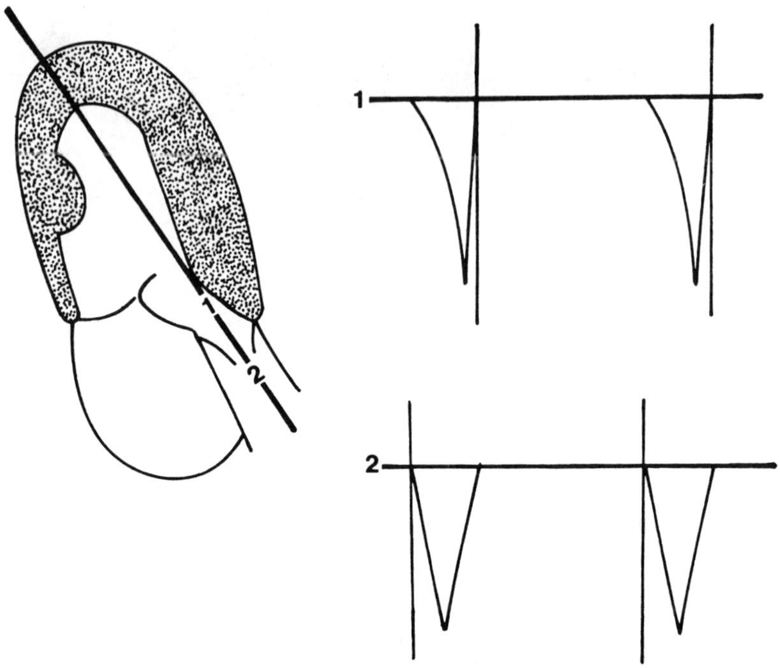

Figure 10.5
An apical long axis view in hypertrophic obstructive cardiomyopathy. The Doppler ultrasound beam is directed across the left ventricular outflow tract and aortic valve. Note the increased velocity of flow at sample location 1, with late systolic peaking and amplitude signal at the end of flow, consistent with recordings obtained upstream to the aortic valve. There is no increase of the velocity at sample location 2, with earlier peak and amplitude signal at the onset of flow, consistent with recordings obtained at the level of the aortic valve leaflets. See text for details.

temic hypertension or aortic stenosis, with severe left ventricular hypertrophy. These hypertrophied papillary muscles cause turbulence of blood flow within the left ventricular cavity that may mimick left ventricular outflow obstruction. Whatever the reason, there is usually no significant hemodynamic obstruction to blood flow in these circumstances evidenced by minimal elevation of the velocities of flow recorded by Doppler.

It is not uncommon to encounter technical difficulties during the Doppler examination of the left ventricular outflow tract. The actual location of the sample volume may not be easily identifiable within the small outflow tract in a hyperdynamic ventricle. The amplitude signal that denotes opening or closure of the aortic valve may be useful in identifying the true location of the sample volume. If the intensity of the amplitude signal is highest before the onset of flow, then

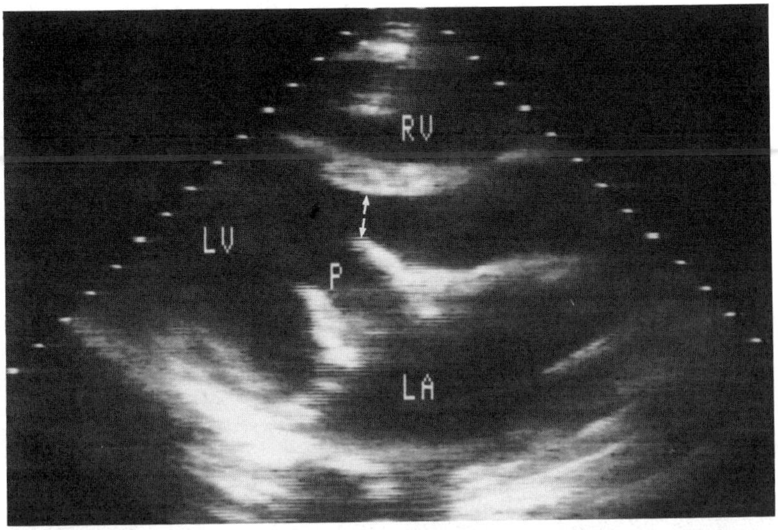

Figure 10.6
Parasternal long axis view from a patient with mitral bioprosthesis (P), normal aortic valve, and no cardiomyopathy. Note the bulky mitral prosthesis protruding into the left ventricular outflow tract (arrows) causing relative narrowing. LV = left ventricle, RV = right ventricle, LA = left atrium.

this represents opening of the aortic valve, and the respective flow is being recorded at the aortic valve level. If the intensity of the amplitude signal is highest after termination of flow, then this represents valve closure, and the sample volume is in the outflow tract. This is particularly important for accurate localization of the level of obstruction by Doppler ultrasound (Figure 10.5).

Meticulous Doppler interrogation of the left ventricular outflow tract may demonstrate mild aortic regurgitant flow. This is not a frequent finding in hypertrophic cardiomyopathy and is believed to be secondary to the chronic turbulence of flow at the level of the aortic valve, leading to leaflet dysfunction.

Similar to the effect of hemodynamic maneuvers on the echocardiogram, the Doppler velocity recording will be affected accordingly. A worsening obstruction causes earlier onset of abnormal flow with higher peak velocities, consistent with the worsening gradients.

Dilated Cardiomyopathy

In strict terms, dilated cardiomyopathy refers to a dilated heart with various degrees of impairment of contractile performance, of unknown cause. More commonly, this term is generalized to include diseased ventricles secondary to specific disorders (e.g., ischemic cardiomyopathy, denoting a markedly diseased ventricle secondary to chronic severe ischemia and multiple infarctions, alcoholic cardiomyopathy reflecting the effect of chronic alcohol abuse with cardiac dysfunction).

Echocardiographic Findings

The echocardiogram usually shows dilatation of all four cardiac chambers with generalized hypokinesia and impairment of contractility (Figure 10.7). The wall appears thinner than normal. The cardiac valves are usually normal; however, evidence of low cardiac output may be reflected as di-

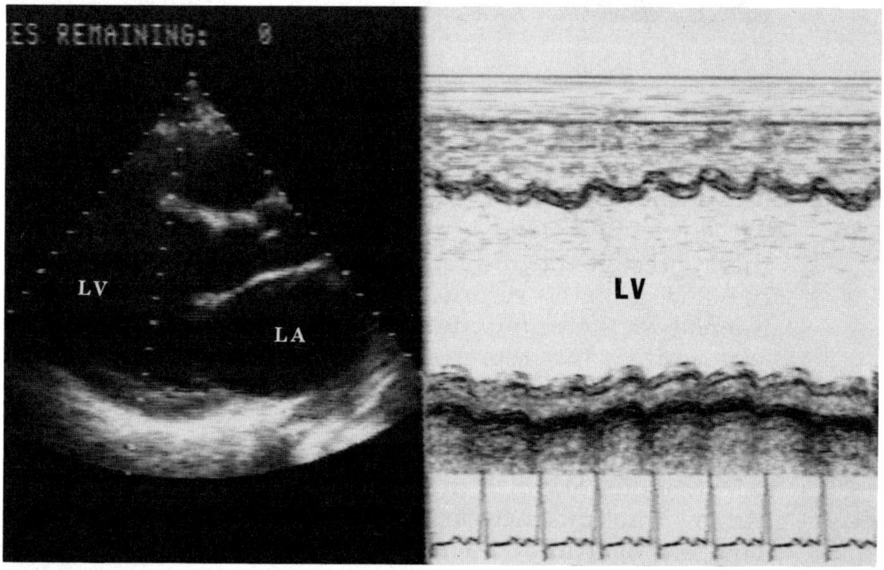

A

Figure 10.7
A. Parasternal long axis view in dilated cardiomyopathy with simultaneous M-mode recording of the left ventricular (LV) chamber. Note marked dilatation of cardiac chambers, with diminished thickness of the interventricular septum and posterior wall. Markedly impaired contractility is clearly evident on this M-mode recording. B. Apical four-chamber view in dilated cardiomyopathy demonstrating four-chamber enlargement. Dilated pulmonary veins (PV) may be occasionally seen. This dilatation may reflect the chronic elevated pressure in the left atrium (LA), commonly noted in patients with dilated cardiomyopathy. C. M-mode recording of the mitral valve in dilated cardiomyopathy, showing diminished leaflet excursion consistent with low output state. A B wave is also evident (arrowhead), suggesting elevated left ventricular diastolic pressure. LA = left atrium.

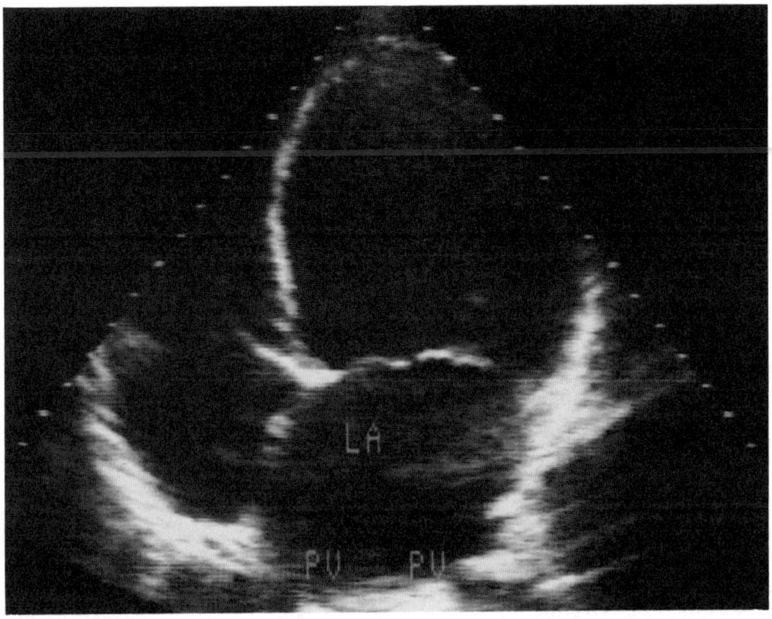

B

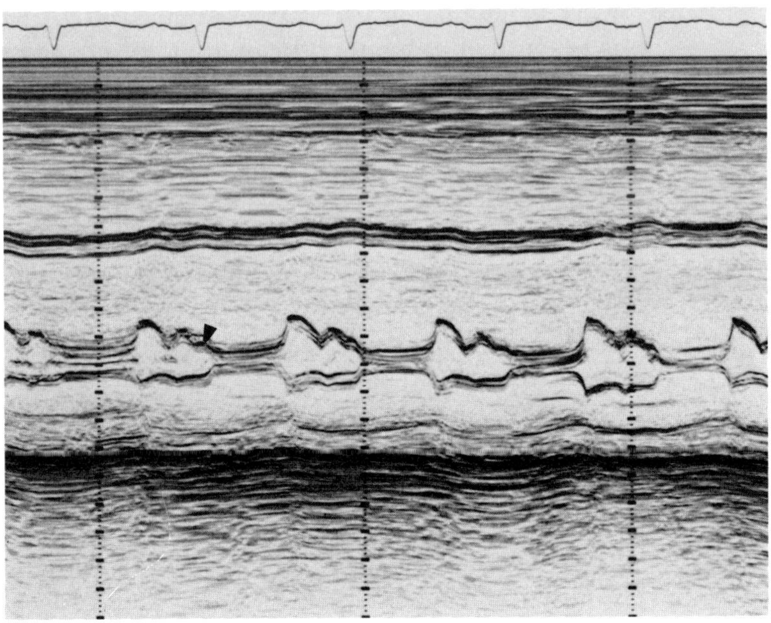

C

Figure 10.7 (continued)

minished excursion of the aortic or mitral leaflets consistent with diminished flow rate. Elevated left ventricular diastolic pressure may be reflected on the M-mode recording of the mitral valve which exhibits a B wave. Chronic severe left ventricular failure may lead to various degrees of pulmonary hypertension. This may be evident on the M-mode recordings of the pulmonary valve where there is loss of the A wave and midsystolic notching of the posterior pulmonary leaflet (Figure 11.3).

Poor left ventricular contractility, coupled with low flow state, may lead to relative blood stasis within the cardiac chambers. Mural thrombi may be detected within the left ventricular apex. Left atrial thrombi are not uncommon, but are rarely detected by conventional echocardiography because they mainly reside in the atrial appendage, which is difficult to visualize.

Doppler Ultrasound

Typically, Doppler recordings of transvalvular velocities of blood flow demonstrate diminished velocities consistent with the low flow state and decreased cardiac output.

A markedly dilated left ventricle may stretch the papillary muscles and chordae tendineae. In addition, the mitral annulus may also be dilated. Thus, various degrees of holosystolic regurgitation may be recorded by Doppler ultrasound. If the pulmonary hypertension is significant, various degrees of pulmonary and tricuspid regurgitation may also be recorded.

Restrictive Cardiomyopathy

Restrictive cardiomyopathy occurs when there is infiltration of the myocardium by abnormal material (e.g., amyloid or iron deposits). Occasionally, there is no identifiable cause for this cardiomyopathy. This results in impaired myocardial function, primarily in diastole. Systolic dysfunction results in decrease of contractile performance, whereas diastolic dysfunction results in impaired relaxation and elevated diastolic pressures. The overall effect is a diminished cardiac output with various degrees of pulmonary congestion.

Echocardiographic Findings

The echocardiogram in restrictive cardiomyopathy typically demonstrates relatively normal-sized cardiac chambers with various degrees of impairment of contractility. The most common form of restrictive cardiomyopathy is cardiac amy-

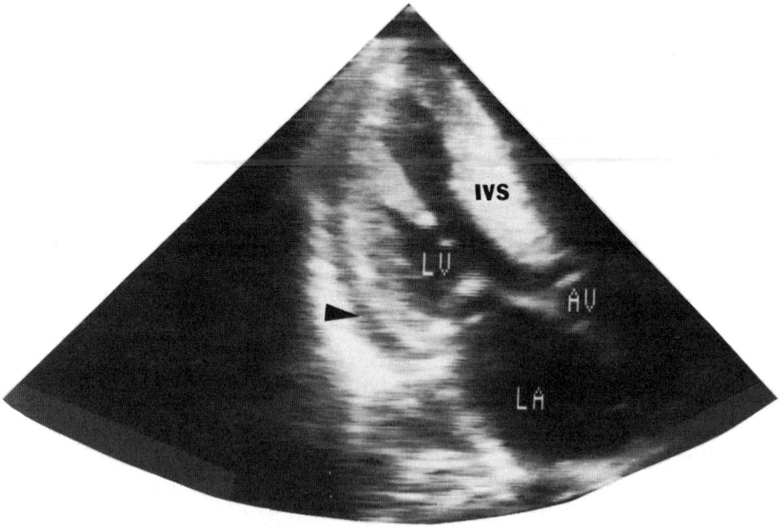

A

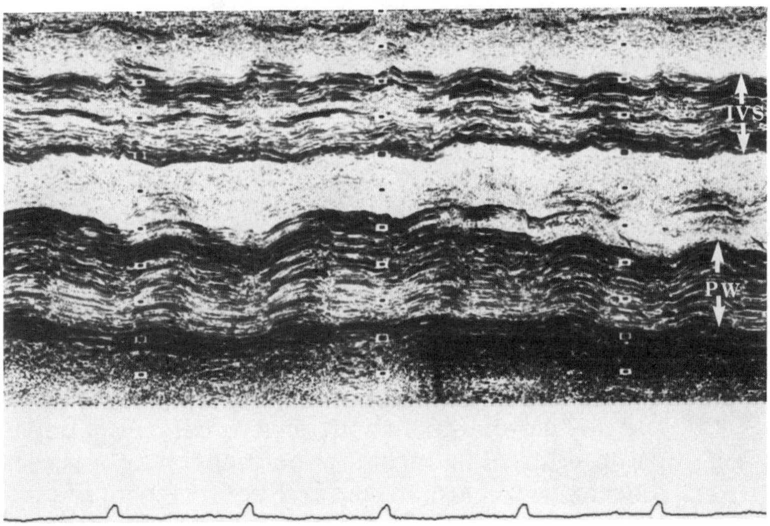

B

Figure 10.8
A. Apical two-chamber view in cardiac amyloidosis. Note the prominent echoes from the thickened myocardium, particularly the interventricular septum (IVS). A small pericardial effusion is also present (arrowhead). B. M-mode recording of the left ventricular chamber in cardiac amyloidosis. The left ventricular chamber is normal in size; however, wall thickness is increased, with prominent echoes in the interventricular septum and posterior wall (PW). Overall systolic contractility is clearly impaired. LV = left ventricle, LA = left atrium, AV = aortic valve.

loidosis. This abnormal deposition of glycoprotein causes various degrees of wall thickening and frequently produces a typical "sparkling" appearance of the myocardium on the two-dimensional echocardiogram (Figure 10.8). Abnormal deposition of amyloid may also involve the atrial myocardium and interatrial septum. When the cardiac valves are involved, the leaflets appear thickened with no restriction of mobility. Small pericardial effusion is occasionally seen.

Hemochromatosis is another form of restrictive cardiomyopathy, whereas abnormal deposition of iron occurs. Wall thickness is increased with an abnormal appearance in the myocardial echocardiographic texture, but less prominent than that observed with amyloid deposition.

Doppler Ultrasound

Doppler ultrasound velocities of blood flow may be decreased, reflecting the low cardiac output. Left ventricular diastolic abnormalities may be reflected on the transmitral velocities in the form of increased peak velocities after the atrial kick as compared to that in early diastole. Valvular regurgitation is occasionally recorded, especially with amyloid deposition in the mitral valve leaflets. However, this is nonspecific and usually of no hemodynamic significance.

Myocarditis

Myocarditis denotes inflammation of the myocardium. This is most commonly subclinical with no overt signs or symptoms. Myocarditis is commonly caused by certain viruses or toxins. Severe myocardial involvement causes dilatation of the cardiac chambers with various degrees of impairment of contractility. The cardiac abnormality may be reversible with a decrease in cardiac size and improvement of contractility. However, persistent dilatation and worsening of cardiac function may occur. The echocardiogram demonstrates dilated cardiac chambers with impaired contractility similar to that seen in dilated cardiomyopathy. Pericardial involvement at times may lead to small pericardial effusion.

Since the echocardiographic features of myocarditis cannot be distinguished from that of dilated cardiomyopathy, the diagnosis of myocarditis is a clinical one. Rapid development of left ventricular dysfunction, and at times, demonstration of regression of the abnormality on serial echocardiograms, may favor the diagnosis of myocarditis rather than idiopathic cardiomyopathy.

Doppler ultrasound findings are nonspecific and are similar to the findings in dilated cardiomyopathy.

11 Pulmonary Hypertension and Cor Pulmonale

The normal pulmonary circulation provides minimal resistance to right ventricular emptying in systole. This is in contrast to the systemic circulation, which imposes greater resistance to left ventricular ejection. Because of the difference in these resistances to blood flow, thickness of the right ventricular wall is much thinner than that of the left ventricular wall. There are many disease states that alter the pulmonary vascular resistance leading to pulmonary hypertension. The right ventricle responds to this greater work load by hypertrophy.

Pulmonary hypertension resulting from primary lung disease is commonly referred to as cor pulmonale. Secondary pulmonary hypertension is generally a result of left ventricular disease where the pulmonary circulation is affected secondarily. Congenital heart disease resulting in increased volume of blood flow into the pulmonary circulation may also cause secondary pulmonary hypertension.

Echocardiography

Hypertrophy of the right ventricular anterior free wall can be detected on the M-mode or two-dimensional echocardiogram (Figure 11.1). Usually the right ventricular cavity is normal in size. However, dilatation is not uncommon in the presence of pulmonary or tricuspid regurgitation. Dilatation of the right atrium may also be observed. Dilatation of the main pulmonary artery trunk is not uncommon in the presence of severe pulmonary hypertension (Figure 11.2).

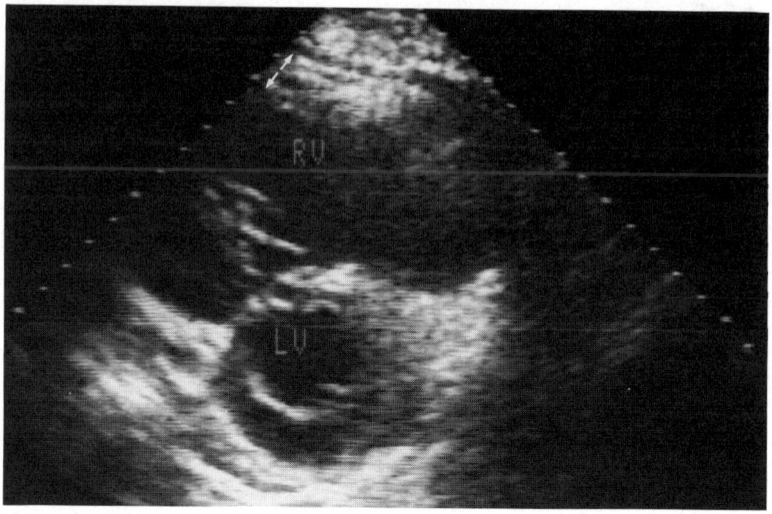

Figure 11.1
Parasternal short axis recording from a patient with pulmonary hypertension, showing hypertrophied, right ventricular, anterior free wall (arrows) and dilated right ventricle (RV). LV = left ventricle.

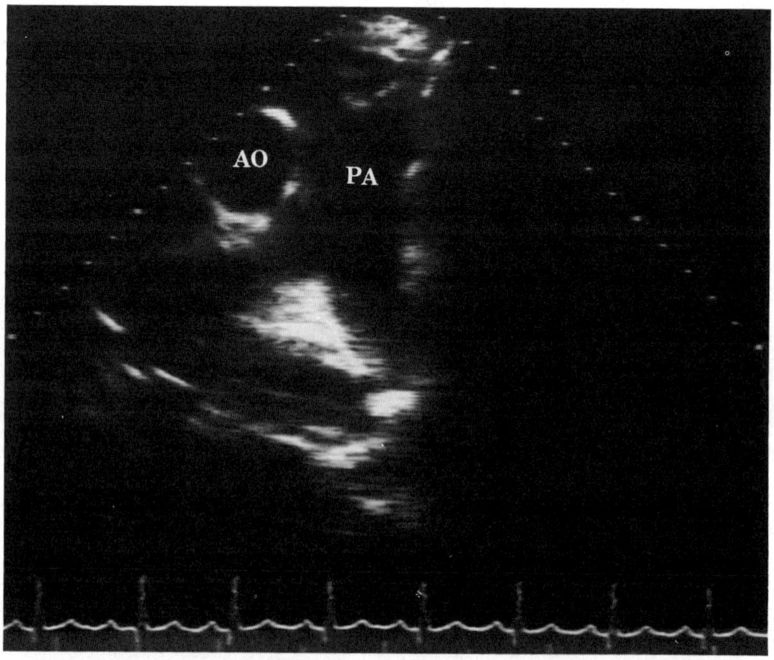

Figure 11.2
Parasternal short axis view of a dilated pulmonary artery (PA) from a patient with severe pulmonary hypertension. AO = aorta.

Frequently, abnormal motion of the pulmonary valve is noted on the M-mode echocardiogram. This represents indirect evidence of increased resistance in the pulmonary circulation. Normally, because of the relatively low diastolic pressures within the right chambers and pulmonary artery, a forceful atrial contraction induces an A bump on the M-mode recording of the posterior leaflet of the pulmonary valve. However, if the pulmonary artery diastolic pressure is elevated, the same atrial contraction does not alter the pulmonary valve motion; hence, there is loss of this A bump. Moreover, in the presence of normal pulmonary artery pressures, the posterior leaflet of the pulmonary valve exhibits gradual downsloping motion in diastole, whereas in pulmonary hypertension, the motion of this leaflet becomes flattened and horizontal. Finally, right ventricular systolic ejection is impaired due to the increased resistance in the pulmonary circulation. The reduced blood flow in mid to late systole causes partial midsystolic closure of the pulmonary valve. This can be easily observed on the M-mode recordings of the posterior pulmonary valve leaflet (Figure 11.3). It is important to note that these echocardiographic signs are not very sensitive. One or more of these ultrasound findings may be absent despite the presence of significant pulmonary hypertension. On the other hand, an absent A bump may be observed in patients with atrial fibrillation without pulmonary hypertension. This is due to the loss of an effective atrial contraction during this abnormality of cardiac rhythm.

Doppler Ultrasound

The Doppler recordings of blood flow velocities across the pulmonary and tricuspid valves may reflect the hemodynamic sequelae of pulmonary hypertension. The increased resistance to right ventricular ejection is reflected on the transpulmonic Doppler recordings. There is early peaking of the velocity of blood flow, thus resembling transaortic blood flow pattern (Figure 11.4). The higher the pulmonary resistance to flow is, the faster the acceleration of transpulmonary blood velocity is and the shorter the acceleration time. These parameters have been incorporated in mathematical equations that closely estimate pulmonary artery pressure. Midsystolic closure of the pulmonary valve as seen on the M-mode echocardiogram may be associated with Doppler recordings of sudden interruption of blood flow across the pulmonary valve.

Severe pulmonary hypertension is not uncommonly as-

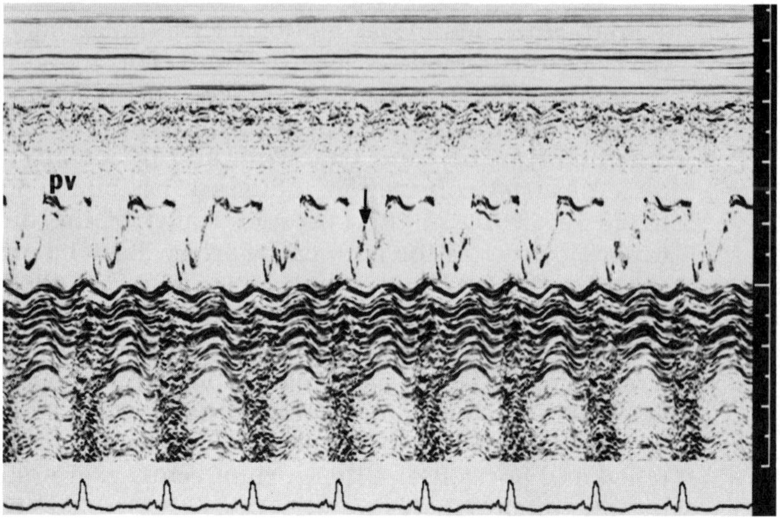

A

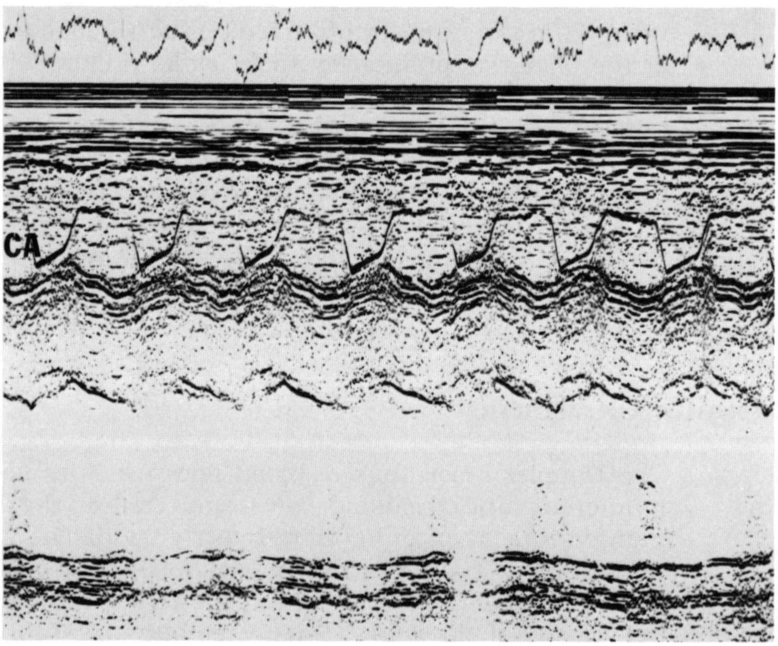

B

Figure 11.3
A. Midsystolic notching of the posterior pulmonary leaflet (arrow) is evident in this recording from a patient with severe pulmonary hypertension. B. Not uncommonly, an M-mode recording of a pulmonary arterial catheter (CA) may be confused with that of the pulmonary valve. Such catheters are commonly used in critical care units and can be easily noted on the two-dimensional echocardiogram. PV = pulmonary valve.

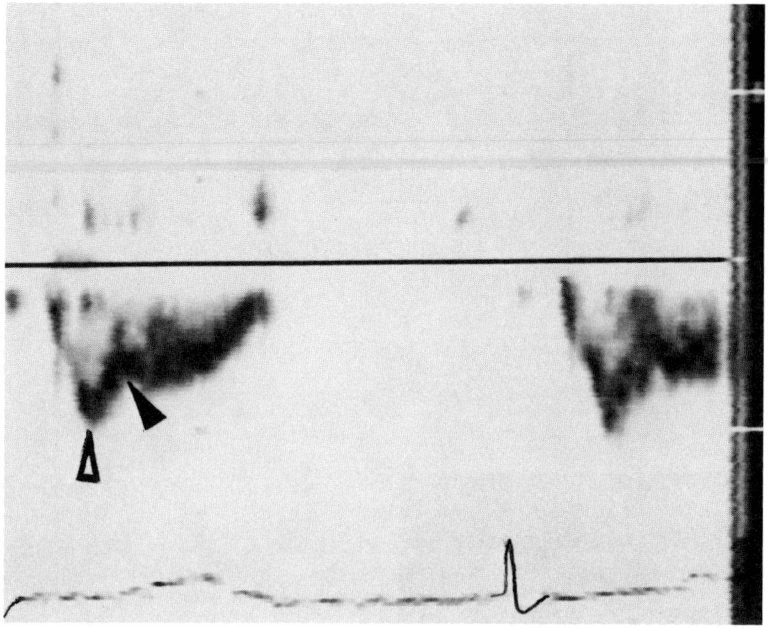

Figure 11.4
PW mode recording of transpulmonic flow from a patient with severe pulmonary hypertension. Note the early peak of transpulmonic velocity of flow (open arrowhead) and midsystolic decrease of the velocity (closed arrowhead).

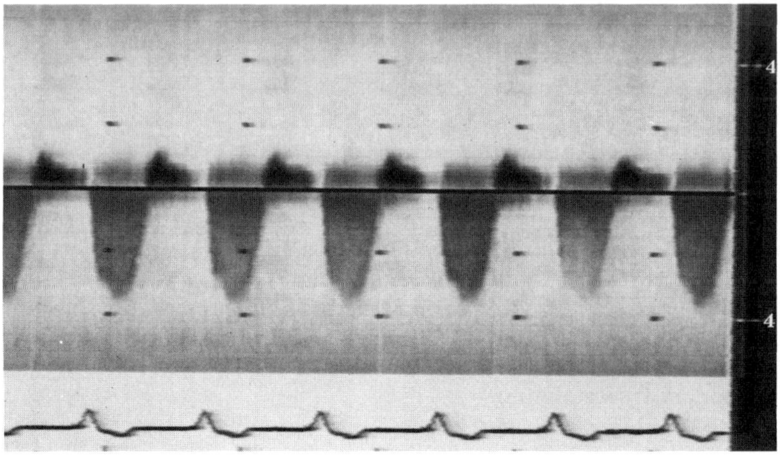

Figure 11.5
CW mode recording of severe tricuspid regurgitation from a patient with pulmonary hypertension. Note the markedly increased velocity of regurgitant blood in systole, suggesting severe pulmonary hypertension.

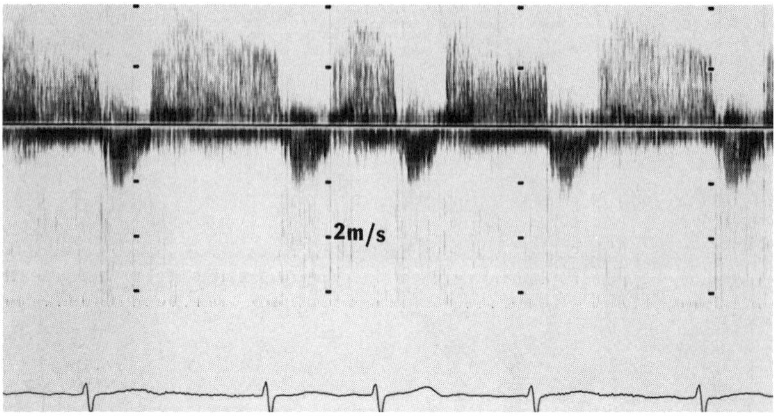

A

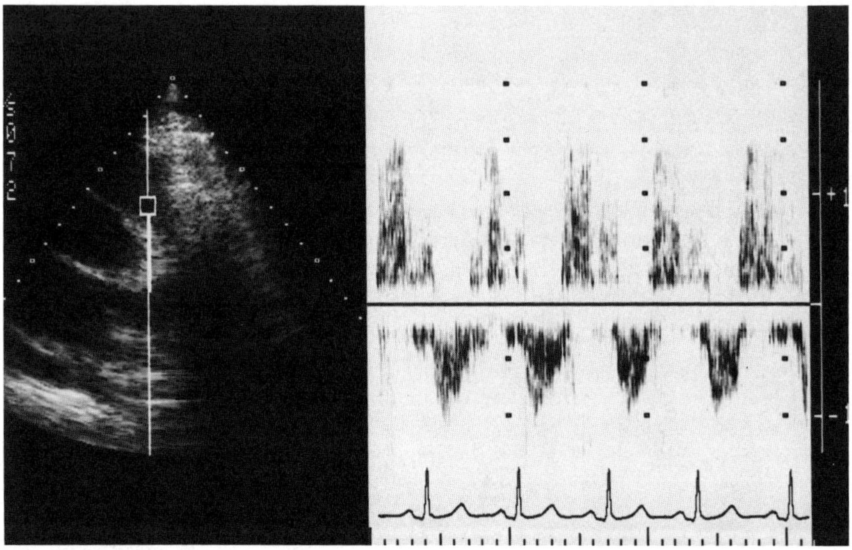

B

Figure 11.6
A. CW mode recording of pulmonic flow showing significant regurgitation, with diastolic regurgitant velocity approaching 2 m/sec, which suggests significant elevation of pulmonary arterial diastolic pressure. B. Parasternal short axis view of the aortic root and pulmonary valve with simultaneous PW Doppler recording of pulmonic regurgitation. Note the relatively low velocity of diastolic regurgitant flow in this patient with no evidence of pulmonary hypertension.

sociated with various degrees of regurgitation of the pulmonary and tricuspid valves. Hence, in the absence of any valvular pathologic states, the presence of significant pulmonary or tricuspid regurgitation represents indirect evidence of pulmonary hypertension. Peak velocity of the regurgitant blood across the tricuspid valve may be applied in the modified Bernoulli equation to estimate the peak pressure gradient between the right ventricle and atrium in systole. When added to right atrial pressure estimated by observing the degree of jugular venous distension, peak systolic right ventricular pressure may be determined (see Chapter 21) (Figure 11.5).

Similarly, the velocity of regurgitant blood across the pulmonary valve reflects the pressure gradient between the pulmonary artery and right ventricle in diastole. Greater severity of pulmonary hypertension causes increasingly higher velocities of regurgitant blood flow. This approach provides an objective assessment of the degree of elevation of pulmonary pressure. However, accurate estimation of pulmonary artery diastolic pressure is not feasible (Figure 11.6).

12 Congenital Heart Disease in Adults

Echocardiography and, more recently, cardiac Doppler ultrasound have become the best noninvasive methods to evaluate patients with suspected congenital heart disease. These procedures are frequently performed prior to cardiac catheterization and may actually provide the definitive diagnosis and obviate the need for cardiac catheterization in certain patients with congenital heart disease.

This chapter will primarily discuss the value of echocardiography and cardiac Doppler ultrasound in the evaluation of certain congenital cardiac abnormalities that are commonly encountered in adults. Several congenital anomalies, including bicuspid aortic valve, supravalvular and subvalvular aortic stenosis, mitral valve prolapse, coarctation of the aorta, and pulmonary stenosis, are discussed in other related chapters in this book.

During the intrauterine fetal development, oxygen exchange occurs in the placenta whereby maternal arterial blood, rich in oxygen, passes in close proximity to fetal venous blood. Oxygen is transferred from mother to fetus via the placenta. Hence, venous blood returning to the right atrium is well oxygenated and does not have to pass through the lungs, which are nonfunctional during the intrauterine life (Figure 12.1).

Venous blood in the right atrium can reach the systemic circulation in one of three ways:

1. The foramen ovale is a large defect in the interatrial septum that allows direct communication between the right and left atria. A major volume of venous blood returning to the right atrium travels through the foramen ovale, directly

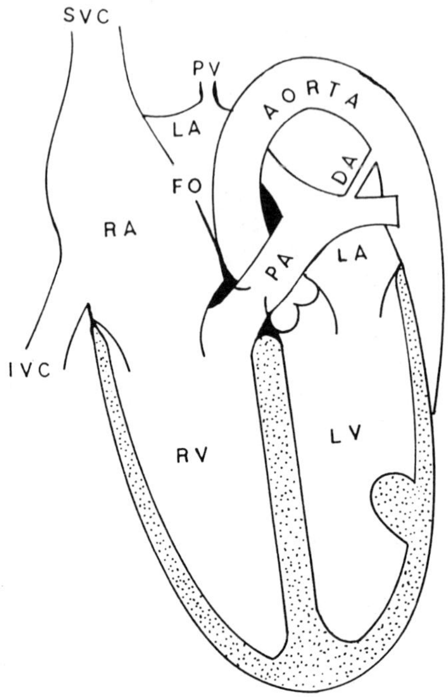

Figure 12.1
The fetal circulation. Oxygenated venous blood returning from the placenta to the right atrium (RA) may be shunted directly into the systemic circulation through the foramen ovale (FO) or the ductus arteriosus (DA), bypassing the inactive lungs. IVC = inferior vena cava, LA = left atrium, LV = left ventricle, PV = pulmonary vein, RV = right ventricle, SVC = superior vena cava. See text for details.

into the left atrium, bypassing the right ventricle, pulmonary artery, and lungs.

2. The remaining venous blood in the right atrium travels through the right ventricle and into the pulmonary artery. Another channel, the ductus arteriosus, allows direct communication for venous blood to go directly through this channel into the descending aorta, bypassing the lungs.

3. Venous blood remaining in the pulmonary artery travels through the lungs and arrives to the left atrium via the pulmonary veins.

Atrial Septal Defects

Atrial septal defects are one of the most common congenital heart diseases encountered in adults. There are several types of atrial septal defects, the most common of which is the ostium secundum, followed in frequency by ostium primum.

The remaining types of atrial septal defects are very rare and very difficult to visualize on routine echocardiography.

Ostium Secundum Atrial Septal Defect

The foramen ovale, situated at the center of the interatrial septum, functions as a direct communication between the left and right atria during intrauterine development of the fetus. Venous blood, oxygenated through the placental circulation, is shunted through the foramen ovale and ductus arteriosus, as just described, and bypasses the lungs (Figure 12.1). After birth, the foramen ovale closes in most newborns and interrupts shunting of blood into the left atrium. However, it is not unusual for a small residual opening to remain. This is referred to as patent foramen ovale and has no hemodynamic significance.

Atrial septal defect, ostium secundum type, refers to a persistent large foramen ovale with resultant left-to-right shunting of blood that persists after birth. Depending on its size, direct visualization of the defect may be seen on the echocardiogram. The interatrial septum can be seen on two-dimensional echocardiography from the parasternal short axis view at the level of the aortic valve, the apical four-chamber view, or the subcostal approach. A large defect appears as sudden interruption of the interatrial septum at its midportion, with bright echoes that delineate the edges of the defect (Figure 12.2). However, it should be noted that the direction of the ultrasound beam, in the apical and parasternal views, is almost parallel to the plane of the interatrial septum. Therefore, it is not unusual to observe echo dropout in the region of the thin membrane covering the foramen valve in the absence of any true defect. For this reason, the parasternal and apical views are not adequate to visualize small atrial septal defects, with a relatively high incidence of false-positive diagnoses (Figure 12.3). The subcostal view, showing an angulated four-chamber image of the heart, is best suited to examine the interatrial septum. In this approach, the direction of the ultrasound beam is close to being perpendicular to the interatrial septum and is better suited to visualize the defect. Routine M-mode echocardiography does not provide direct visualization of the interatrial septum.

The diagnosis of atrial septal defect can be inferred indirectly by observing the hemodynamic consequences of a large shunt on the cardiac chambers. Since left atrial pressure exceeds right atrial pressure throughout most of the cardiac cycle, a relatively large atrial septal defect allows pre-

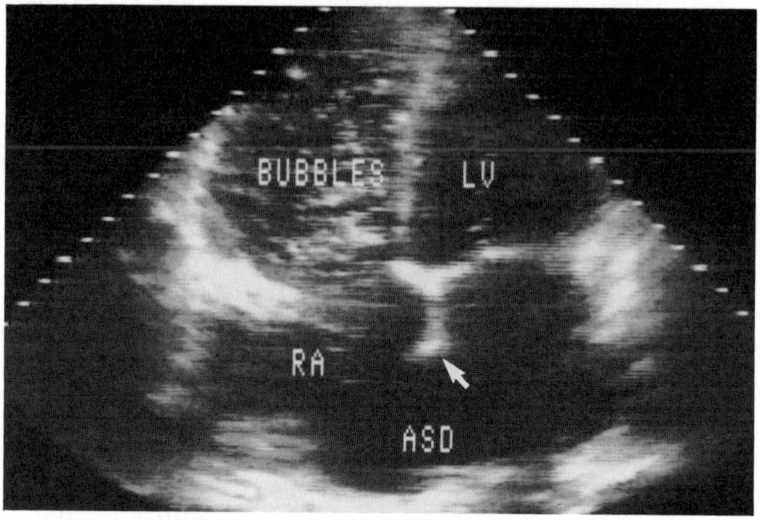

A

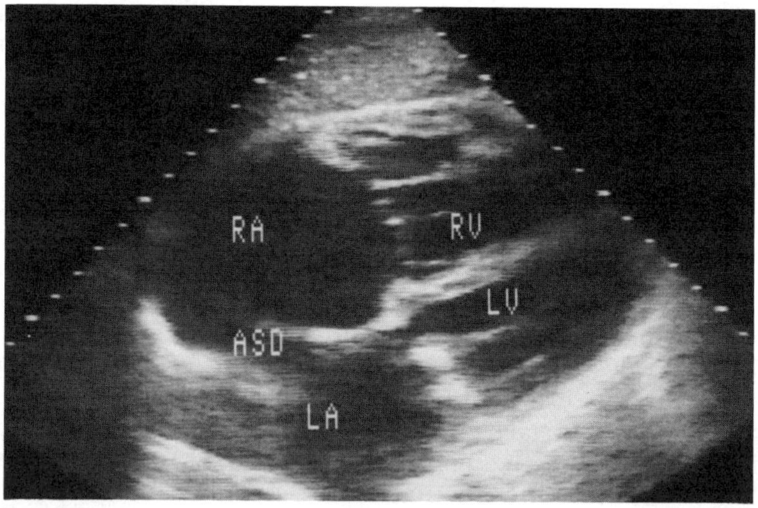

B

Figure 12.2
A. Apical four-chamber view showing a large atrial septal defect (ASD), ostium secundum type. Note the sudden interruption of the atrial septum, with broadening of the echoes at the edge of this defect (arrow). Multiple echoes (bubbles) are seen in the right ventricle secondary to contrast injection. Blood is shunted primarily from the left atrium (LA) to the right atrium (RA). However, a few bubbles are noted in the left ventricle (LV), consistent with right-to-left shunt. See text for details. B. Subcostal view of the atrial septal defect. Note the significant enlargement of the right chambers due to the large left-to-right shunt with volume overload on the right side of the heart. RV = right ventricle.

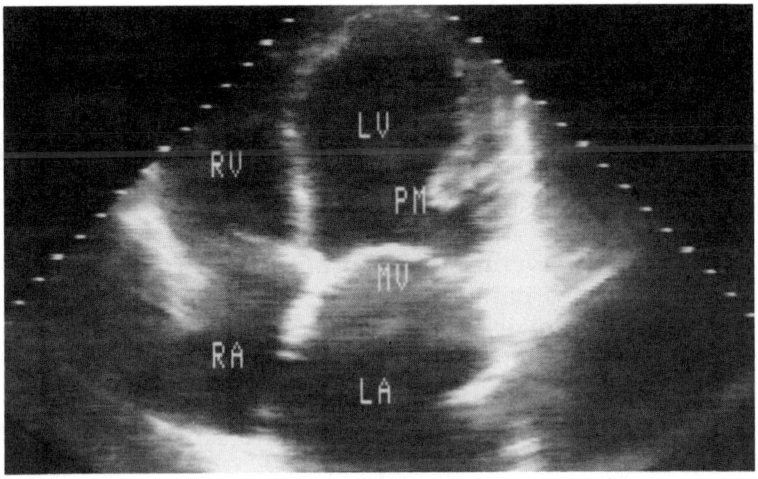

A

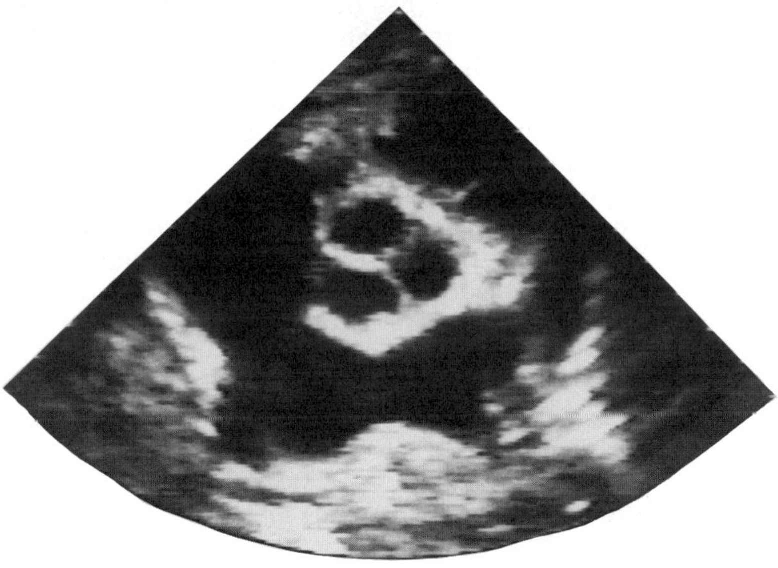

B

Figure 12.3
A. Apical four-chamber, and B. Parasternal short axis views, showing echo dropout in the region of the interatrial septum in the absence of any demonstrable true atrial septal defect. The thin membrane covering the foramen ovale may not be easily visualized in these views. Note the gradual tapering of the interatrial septum in the four-chamber view. RV = right ventricle, RA = right atrium, LV = left ventricle, LA = left atrium, MV = mitral valve, PM = papillary muscle.

dominantly left-to-right shunting of blood across the defect. This is further facilitated by the compliant right ventricle, which can accommodate the increased blood flow; minimal right-to-left shunting may be occasionally noted. This shunt causes volume overload and dilatation of both atria and the right ventricle only. Since the shunt is situated proximal to the left ventricle, this chamber is spared from the volume overload. Right ventricular dilatation causes flattening of the interventricular septum with atypical motion, which is at times paradoxical (Figure 12.4). It is important to note that similar abnormalities of chamber size and interventricular septal motion are not diagnostic of atrial septal defect and may occur secondary to any other cause of right ventricular volume overload, such as severe tricuspid or pulmonary regurgitation.

PW mode Doppler ultrasound recordings with the sample volume at the level of the atrial septum may demonstrate the abnormal flow across the defect. This is best obtained from the subcostal approach (Figure 12.5). However, the small pressure gradient across the interatrial septum may not produce adequate spectral analysis signals. In this context, color Doppler flow imaging is better suited to delineate the abnormal flow across the defect (Plate 11). The magnitude of the shunt can be estimated by comparing the velocity of blood flow across the cardiac valves. Normally, the velocity of blood across the left-sided valves is slightly higher than the velocities recorded across the corresponding right-sided valves. However, a relatively large shunt at the atrial level causes an increase in the volume of blood flow in the right chambers of the heart. This is reflected as higher velocities across the tricuspid and pulmonary valves relative to the mitral and aortic valves, respectively.

Ostium Primum Atrial Septal Defect

The interatrial septum normally extends and joins the interventricular septum at the level of the atrioventricular valves. Defects in the interatrial septum, just above the atrioven-

---

Figure 12.4
A. Parasternal short axis view showing marked right ventricular (RV) dilatation secondary to a large atrial septal defect. Note the small left ventricular (LV) size, with flattening of the interventricular septum. B. M-mode recording of the left ventricular chamber from another patient with an atrial septal defect. Note the paradoxical motion of the interventricular septum (arrowhead) as it moves anteriorly in systole.

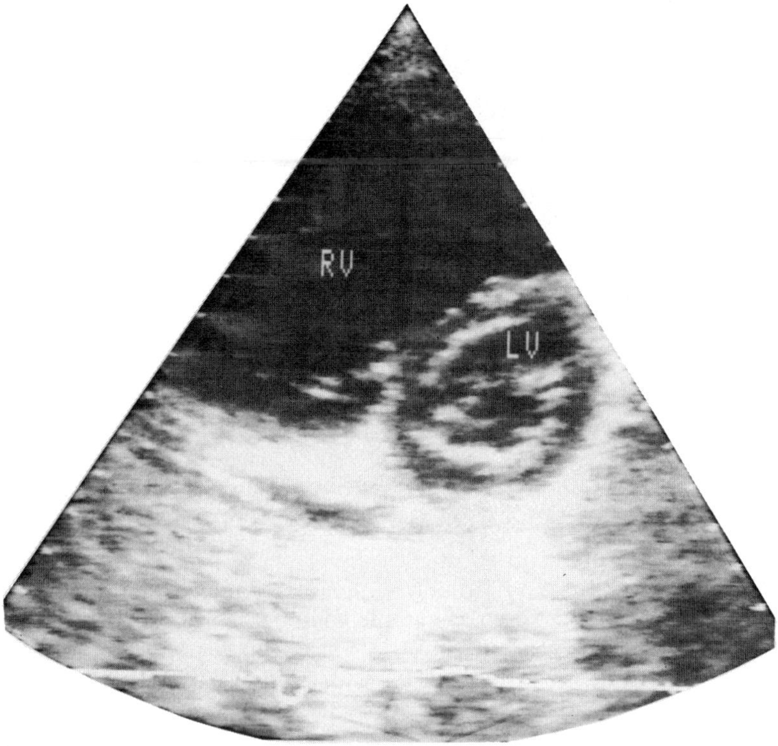

A

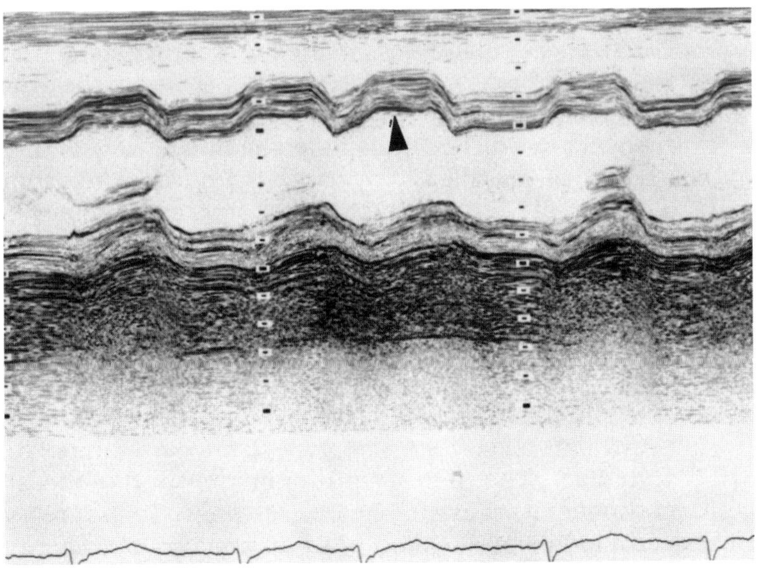

B

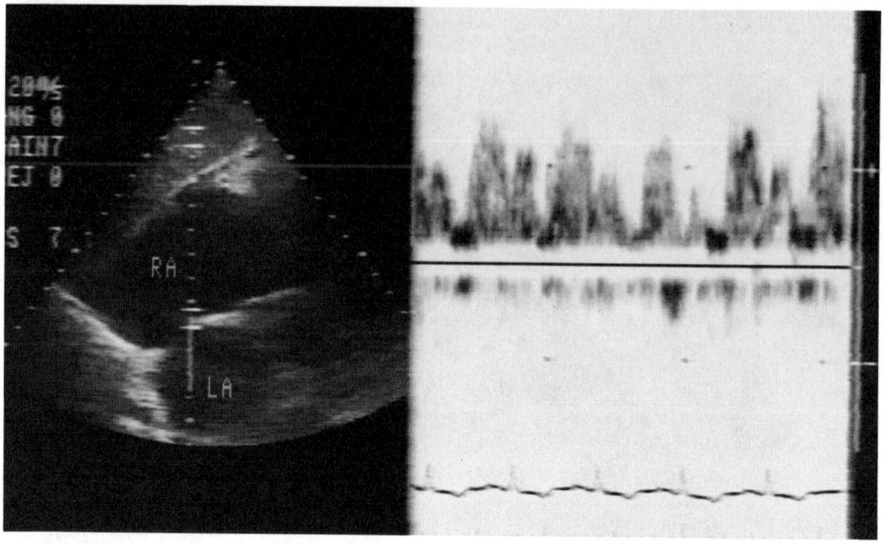

Figure 12.5
PW mode recording, obtained from a subcostal location, of flow across an atrial septal defect. Note the sample value is positioned at the site of the defect, within the right atrium (RA). The Doppler recording demonstrates continuous flow toward the transducer, consistent with left-to-right shunt. LA = left atrium.

tricular valves, are not uncommon and are referred to as ostium primum atrial septal defects (Figures 12.6, 12.7). Such defects may be associated with other congenital abnormalities, such as cleft mitral valve, whereby the anterior mitral leaflet is split, thus producing a false appearance of a trileaflet valve. The apical four-chamber view is the best approach to visualize the ostium primum atrial septal defect. The parasternal short axis view, and occasionally subcostal views, may be employed.

Sinus Venosus Atrial Septal Defect

The defect of the interatrial septum is situated close to the junction of the superior vena cava and the right atrium. Such high atrial septal defects are less common than the previously described two types, and are more difficult to visualize. The apical four-chamber and subcostal four-chamber views may be helpful at times. Such rare defects are occasionally associated with anomalous pulmonary venous drainage, whereby one or more pulmonary veins drain into the right atrium instead of the left atrium.

Other Types of Atrial Septal Defects

Rarely, defects in the coronary sinus may cause an atrial septal defect. Such defects are very difficult to visualize on

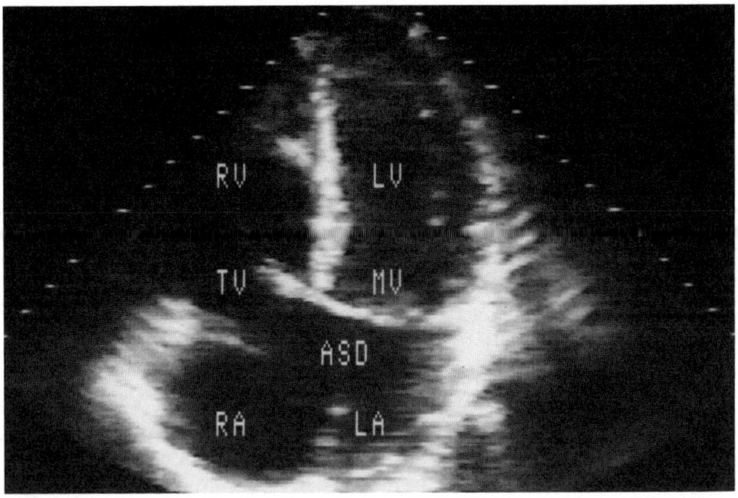

Figure 12.6
Apical four-chamber view showing a large atrial septal defect (ASD) just above the atrioventricular valves, consistent with ostium primum defect. RV = right ventricle, LV = left ventricle, TV = tricuspid valve, MV = mitral valve, RA = right atrium, LA = left atrium.

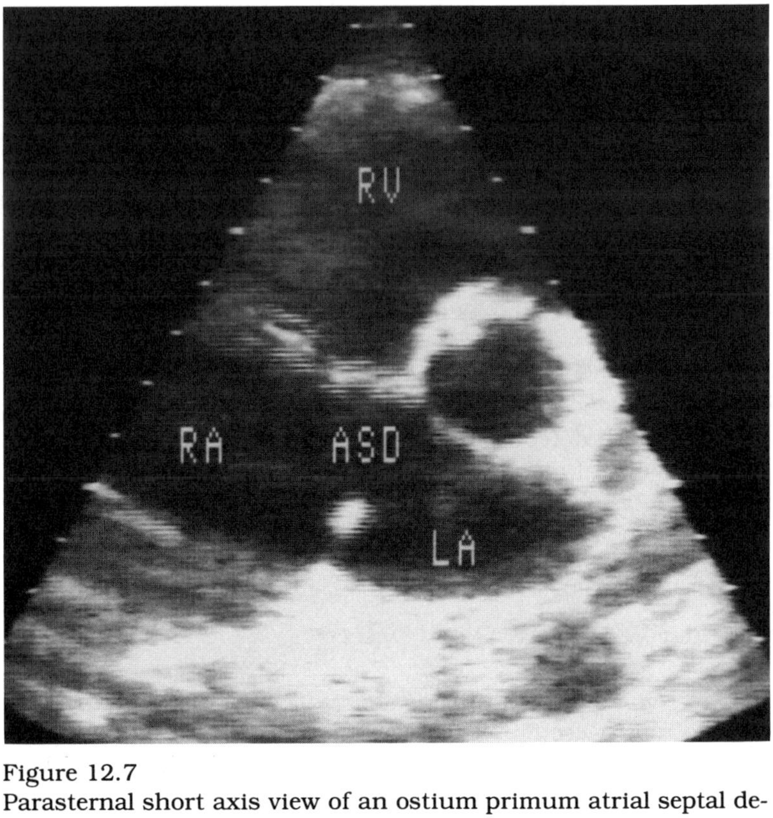

Figure 12.7
Parasternal short axis view of an ostium primum atrial septal defect (ASD). RV = right ventricle, RA = right atrium, LA = left atrium.

routine echocardiography. Common atrium with complete absence of the interatrial septum is very rarely seen in adults.

Ventricular Septal Defects

Ventricular septal defects are rather common in patients with congenital heart disease. Such defects may occur alone or may be associated with other complex congenital anomalies. There are different approaches to classify ventricular septal defects. In general, there are four types, depending on their location.

Subpulmonary Ventricular Septal Defect

As the name implies, subpulmonary ventricular septal defect occurs in the infundibular septum just below the pulmonary valve. The parasternal long axis view may demonstrate the defect along the junction of the interventricular septum and anterior wall of the aorta. The apical views may be helpful in visualizing such defects.

Perimembranous Ventricular Septal Defect

The perimembranous ventricular septal defect occurs in the vicinity of the membranous septum and is best visualized from the apical four-chamber view. The subcostal approach can also be used to identify these defects.

Atrioventricular Canal Ventricular Septal Defect

Defects in the posterior portion of the interventricular septum occur in the proximity of the atrioventricular valves. Such defects are more commonly associated with other congenital cardiac anomalies such as endocardial cushion defect. Again, the apical four-chamber view and subcostal views are more likely to identify this defect than are other routine views.

Muscular Ventricular Septal Defect

Solitary or multiple defects with finestrations may be encountered in the muscular portion of the interventricular septum close to the apex of the heart. Small defects may be hard to visualize; however, larger defects may be identified in the apical views, and at times, from a subcostal approach.

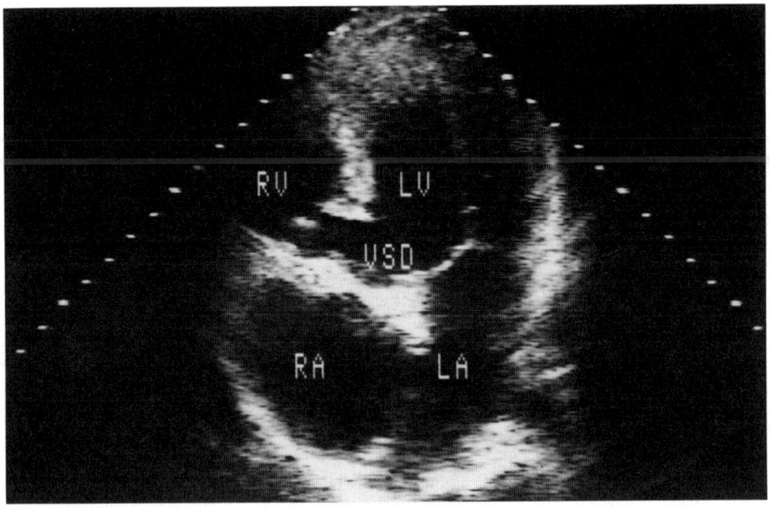

Figure 12.8
Apical four-chamber view showing a large membranous ventricular septal defect (VSD). Echo dropouts are noted in the region of the interatrial septum; however, there is no atrial septal defect. RV = right ventricle, LV = left ventricle, RA = right atrium, LA = left atrium.

Echocardiographic and Doppler Evaluation

Besides the identification of the location and size of the ventricular septal defect, echocardiography may provide evidence in regards to the magnitude of the shunt and its hemodynamic consequences. Left ventricular pressure is initially much greater than right ventricular pressure. This causes a left-to-right shunt in systole with volume overload that affects predominately the pulmonary circulation, with dilatation of the pulmonary artery and left chambers of the heart. The right ventricle is usually spared from this volume overload because the shunted blood bypasses the main portion of the right ventricular cavity, except in patients with muscular ventricular septal defect (Figure 12.8, 12.9).

A relatively large ventricular septal defect with significant left-to-right shunt will ultimately lead to pulmonary hypertension. This causes pressure overload on the right ventricle, which will undergo compensatory hypertrophy. Finally, progressive elevation of pulmonary arterial and right ventricular pressure may approach left ventricular pressure and cause reversal of the shunt with predominant right-to-left shunt. Such reversal of shunt is commonly referred to as Eisenmenger's syndrome.

Prior to the availability of cardiac Doppler ultrasonography, contrast echocardiography was helpful in the evalua-

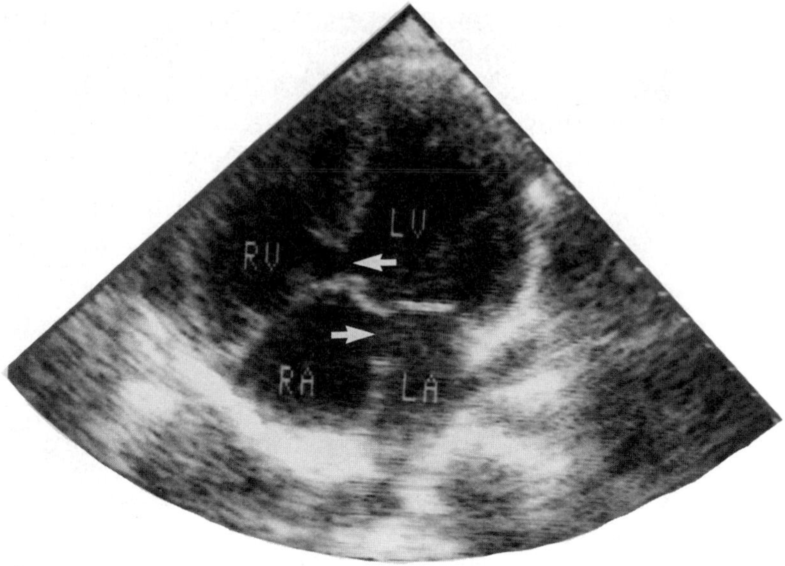

A

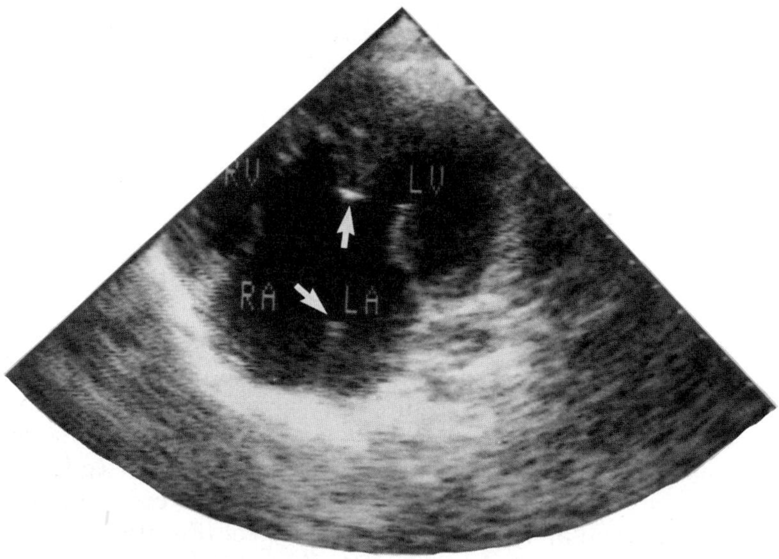

B

Figure 12.9
A. Apical four-chamber view showing endocardial cushion defect with interventricular septal defect and also ostium primum atrial septal defect (arrows). B. Apical four-chamber view from a patient with single ventricle showing a rudimentary interventricular septum (arrows), as well as ostium primum atrial septal defect. RA = right atrium, LA = left atrium, RV = right ventricle, LV = left ventricle.

tion of ventricular septal defects. The microbubbles, injected in the peripheral vein, may be seen entering the left ventricle and aorta. A "negative contrast effect" may be occasionally noted in the right ventricle or pulmonary artery. Doppler ultrasound is valuable in identifying small ventricular septal defects that are difficult to visualize on echocardiography. The location of abnormal flow pattern is dependent on the type of ventricular septal defect. Flow across the ventricular septal defect may be recorded from the four-chamber apical view; however, the parasternal approach is better suited for this purpose, as the direction of the Doppler ultrasound beam would be more parallel to the direction of the jet of flow (Figure 12.10). The sample volume, in PW mode Doppler recordings, should be positioned within the right ventricular cavity along the anterior border of the interventricular septum. Careful anterior or posterior angulation of the Doppler ultrasound beam will ultimately help localize the site of the shunt. Since associated tricuspid regurgitation is occasionally encountered in the presence of pulmonary hypertension, abnormal tricuspid regurgitant jet in systole may be recorded during the search for the ventricular septal defect by Doppler. However, the direction of the tricuspid regurgitation jet is always away from the transducer, whereas the direction of the left-to-right shunt flow is always toward the transducer. Doppler color flow imaging is a valuable new approach that may help identify small-sized ventricular septal defects with eccentric jets of flow that may be otherwise difficult to identify by other noninvasive means (Plate 12).

Depending on the magnitude of the defect, the duration of the shunt may be holosystolic or, occasionally, early systolic, with cessation of flow toward the end of systole. The severity of the shunt may be estimated by Doppler ultrasound. Similar to atrial septal defect, the velocity of blood flow across the pulmonary valve will be increased relative to the transaortic velocity, indicating a higher volume of flow across the pulmonary valve. Since the shunt occurs in the right ventricular chamber, blood velocity across the tricuspid valve is usually normal unless there is associated tricuspid regurgitation. Right ventricular and pulmonary arterial systolic pressures may be determined as the difference of systemic systolic pressure measured by sphygmomanometry and the transventricular septal defect pressure gradient estimated by the modified Bernoulli equation (see Chapter 21).

Patent Ductus Arteriosus

Similar to the foramen ovale, the ductus arteriosus establishes a communication between the left and right circu-

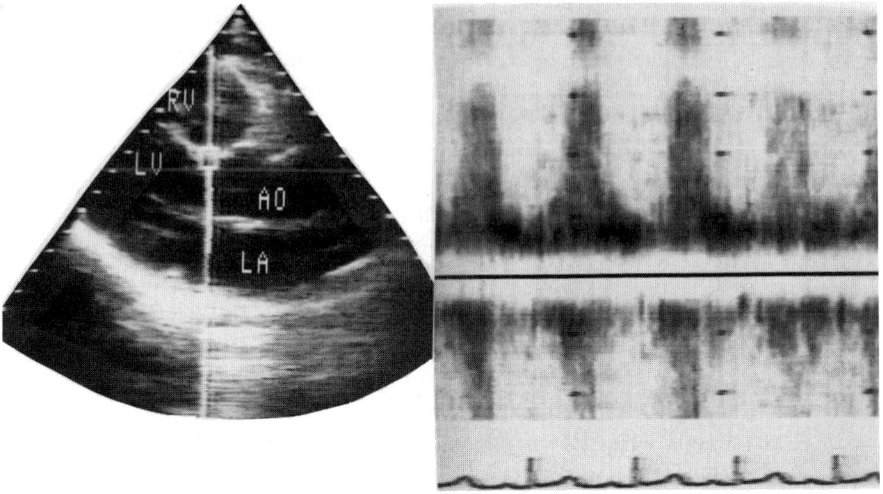

Figure 12.10
Parasternal long axis view with the Doppler sample volume situated at the level of the membranous interventricular septum. A small ventricular septal defect could not be visualized on the echocardiogram; however, a high-velocity systolic jet with turbulence and aliasing was recorded by Doppler, confirming the presence of such a defect. RV = right ventricle, LV = left ventricle, AO = aorta, LA = left atrium.

lations to bypass the lungs during intrauterine development (Figure 12.1). Soon after birth, the ductus arteriosus shrinks in size and ultimately becomes a thin, fibrous ligament. Persistence of a patent ductus arteriosus maintains a channel connecting the left pulmonary artery to the aorta.

Echocardiographic detection of this congenital anomaly is rather difficult. However, a large patent ductus arteriosus may occasionally be visualized from a suprasternal approach, or from an angulated short axis view showing the bifurcation of the main pulmonary artery. The ductus appears as a short vessel-like structure that joins the left pulmonary artery to the aorta. At times, the only notable abnormality would be a sudden interruption of echoes reflected from the aortic wall at the proper anatomic location of the ductus arteriosus.

Early in the course of the patent ductus arteriosus, there is a left-to-right shunt from the aorta to the pulmonary artery. Because aortic pressure is always higher than pulmonary arterial pressure throughout the cardiac cycle, the shunt persists in systole and diastole. Blood shunted across the patent ductus arteriosus travels through the lungs and returns to the left chambers of the heart. Consequently, the resulting volume overload causes dilatation of the left atrium and ventricle with sparing of the right chambers. However, the increased volume of flow in the pulmonary circulation may ultimately lead to pulmonary hypertension with compensatory right ventricular hypertrophy and various degrees of pulmonary and tricuspid regurgitation (Figure 12.11). On rare occasions, extreme elevation of pulmonary pressure may exceed aortic systemic pressure and cause reversal of the shunt, which becomes right-to-left, thereby establishing Eisenmenger's syndrome.

Doppler ultrasound is of great value in making the diagnosis of patent ductus arteriosus and may provide evidence of the magnitude of the shunt. Doppler recordings are best obtained from a parasternal short axis approach with the direction of the ultrasound beam maneuvered in the pulmonary artery. PW mode Doppler recordings with the sample volume positioned at the level of the pulmonary valve usually demonstrate normal flow patterns across this valve. However, a sudden increase of the velocity and duration of flow may be observed when the sample volume is gradually advanced within the pulmonary artery and approximates the site of the ductus.

The suprasternal approach is also valuable for the Doppler evaluation of persistent ductus arteriosus. Normally, blood flow in the descending thoracic aorta occurs only in systole and is away from the transducer. However, in the presence of a large persistent ductus arteriosus, it is not unusual to record in diastole reversed flow in the descending thoracic aorta distal to the persistent ductus arteriosus, reflecting reversed blood flow from the descending thoracic aorta into the ductus arteriosus (Figure 12.11).

Finally, transmitral and transaortic velocities of flow may be higher than normal, proportionate to the increased volume of flow within the left chambers of the heart.

Ebstein's Anomaly

Ebstein's anomaly is a tricuspid valve that is abnormally situated within the right ventricular cavity instead of the normal location at the atrioventricular annulus. A portion of the right ventricle becomes incorporated with the right atrium, and is referred to as the atrialized right ventricle. Thus, the right atrium would be markedly dilated, whereas the right ventricle is usually diminished in size (Figure 12.12). The abnormal location of the tricuspid valve may be readily noted on the apical four-chamber view. In this view, the normal tricuspid valve is situated within 2 to 3 mm from the level of the mitral valve. However, the tricuspid valve in Ebstein's anomaly would be further displaced into the right

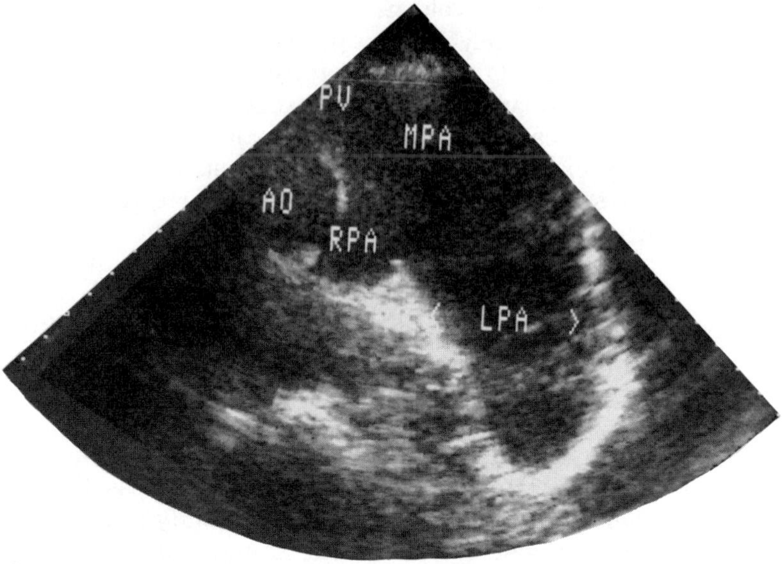

A

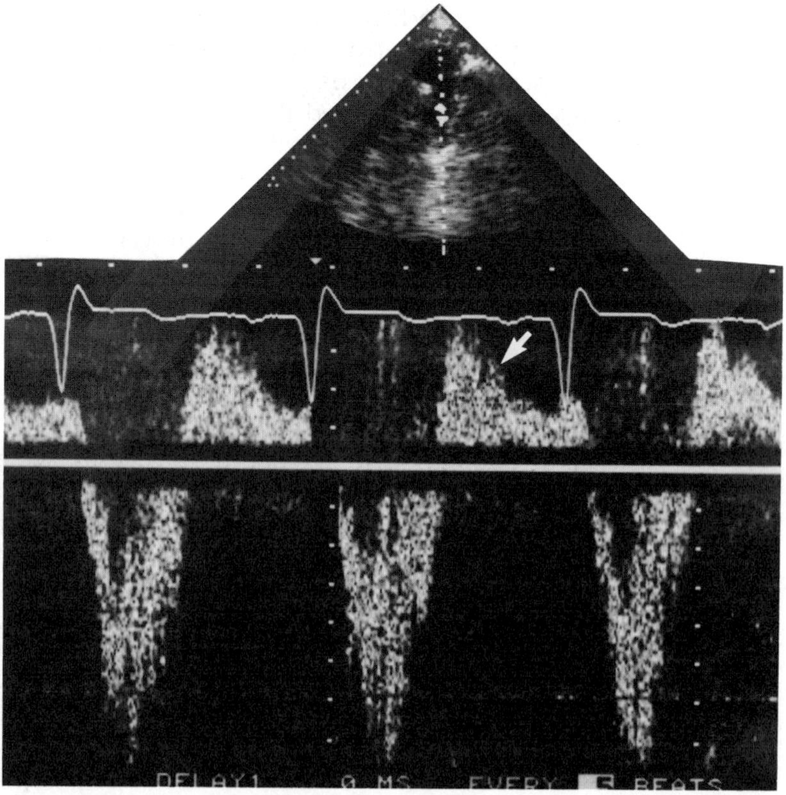

B

ventricular cavity, with greater depth relative to the position of the mitral valve. The parasternal short axis view may be helpful, at times, to disclose the abnormal location of the tricuspid valve.

M-mode recordings in Ebstein's anomaly are typical for this diagnosis. From the parasternal window, the mitral and tricuspid valves cannot be recorded simultaneously on M-mode echocardiography unless the tricuspid valve is abnormally displaced lower in the right ventricular cavity. Moreover, mitral valve closure normally precedes tricuspid valve closure by approximately 40 milliseconds, whereas in Ebstein's anomaly, tricuspid valve closure is delayed by more than 100 milliseconds relative to the mitral valve. This delayed closure of the tricuspid valve is rather characteristic of Ebstein's anomaly. Doppler ultrasound is of little value for the diagnosis of Ebstein's anomaly. However, Doppler ultrasound may provide the diagnosis of associated tricuspid regurgitation, which is frequently noted in patients with this congenital abnormality.

Tetralogy of Fallot

Tetralogy of Fallot is one of the most common complex congenital heart abnormalities encountered in adults. As the name implies, there is usually a combination of four different cardiac abnormalities: overriding aorta, ventricular septal defect, right ventricular hypertrophy, and infundibular stenosis. The ventricular septal defect constitutes a prominent abnormality in tetralogy of Fallot, with the aortic root overlying this ventricular septal defect and receiving blood ejected from both ventricles. The infundibular stenosis in the right ventricular outflow tract imposes resistance to right ventricular ejection into the pulmonary artery. This potentiates shunting of blood across the ventricular septal defect into the overriding aorta.

M-mode echocardiography commonly demonstrates discontinuity of the interventricular septum and anterior wall

---

Figure 12.11
A. Parasternal short axis view from a patient with persistent ductus arteriosus and large left-to-right shunt. The ductus arteriosus is not clearly visualized on this image. However, note the markedly dilated left pulmonary artery (LPA) (arrowheads). AO = aortic root, MPA = main pulmonary artery, PV = pulmonary valve, RPA = right pulmonary artery. B. PW mode recording in the descending aorta obtained from a patient with persistent ductus arteriosus. Note the presence of retrograde flow in diastole (arrow) up toward the transducer, which is highly suggestive of this diagnosis.

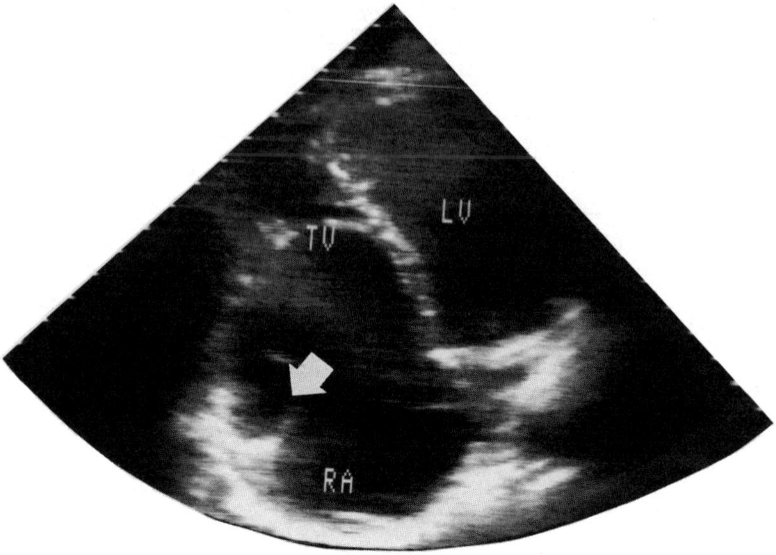

A

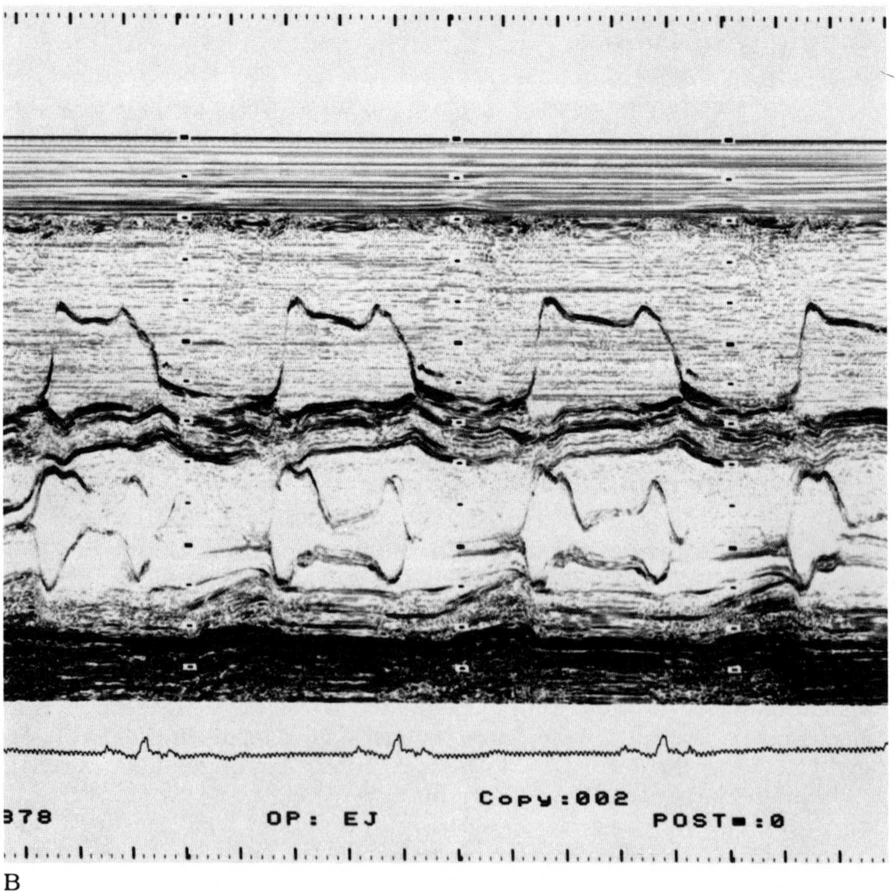

B

of the aortic root. Right ventricular hypertrophy may be evident as well. However, these findings are not diagnostic of tetralogy of Fallot and may be noted in other complex congenital cardiac anomalies. Two-dimensional echocardiography provides further description of the cardiac anatomy. The parasternal long axis view typically shows the ventricular septal defect with the overriding aorta (Figure 12.13). The apical four-chamber view with slight anterior angulation to show the aortic root is also valuable. The parasternal short axis view at the aortic level may be employed to demonstrate the narrowed right ventricular outflow tract and confirms the presence of infundibular stenosis. The pulmonary artery may be diminished in size, reflecting decreased blood flow in the pulmonary circulation. The pulmonary valve may also be stenotic at times.

Because of the multiple anomalies in tetralogy of Fallot, the Doppler examination may be confusing in view of the multiple abnormal flow patterns commonly associated with this abnormality. However, careful PW mode recordings may be valuable in confirming the diagnosis and establishing the severity of the hemodynamic abnormality. The parasternal approach, aided by simultaneous two-dimensional echocardiography, will help delineate the abnormally increased velocities of flow across the ventricular septal defect and the right ventricular outflow tract. Mild aortic and pulmonary regurgitations are not unusual in patients with this complex anomaly.

Rare Congenital Heart Disease in Adults

A single ventricle may arise from lack of development of the interventricular septum. This is commonly associated with other congenital anomalies (Figures 12.9B, 12.14). On rare occasions, aneurysmal dilatation of the interatrial septum may be noted. This exhibits exaggerated motion throughout the cardiac cycle and may simulate a masslike effect. Such aneurysmal dilatation is thought to be secondary to overstretching of a large membrane after spontaneous closure of an atrial septal defect (Figure 12.15).

Figure 12.12
A. Angulated apical view depicting the abnormal insertion of the septal leaflet of the tricuspid valve (TV) in a patient with Ebstein's anomaly. Note the location of the tricuspid valve annulus (arrow). B. The abnormal insertion of tricuspid valve in the right ventricle allows simultaneous recording of both atrioventricular valves on the M-mode recording. LV = left ventricle, RA = right atrium.

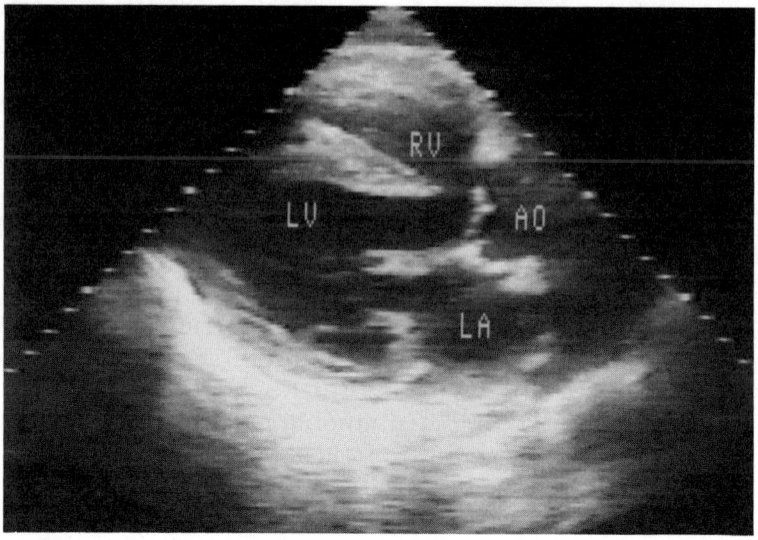

A

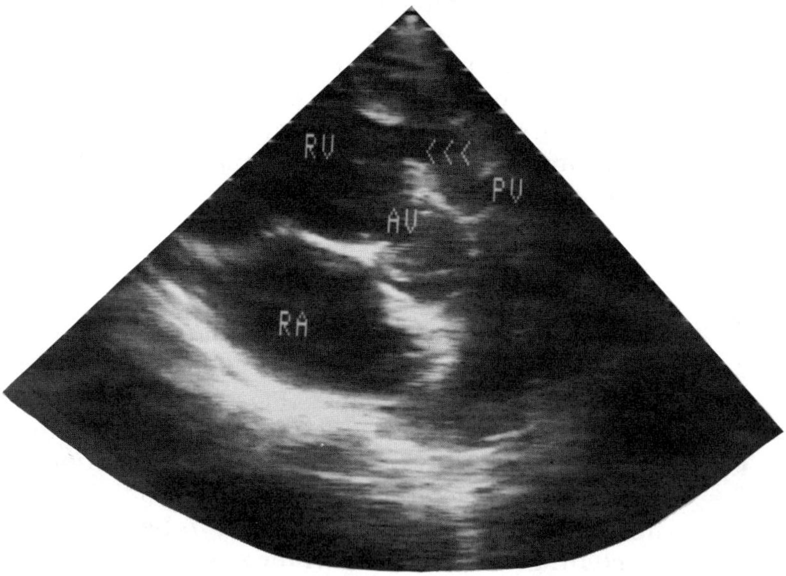

B

Figure 12.13

A. Parasternal long axis view of tetralogy of Fallot, showing the ventricular septal defect with overriding aorta (AO). B. Angulated parasternal short axis view showing the infundibular stenosis (arrowheads). AV = aortic valve, PV = pulmonary valve, RA = right atrium, RV = right ventricle, LV = left ventricle, LA = left atrium.

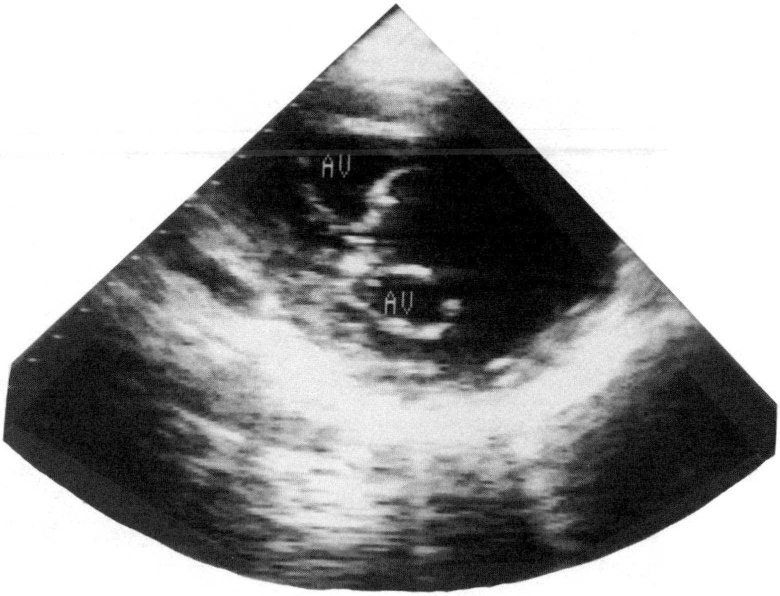

Figure 12.14
Parasternal short axis view from a patient with a single ventricle. Note the two atrioventricular valves (AV), without an interventricular septum in between.

Surgical Interventions in Congenital Heart Disease

Recent advances in cardiac surgical techniques have enhanced the survival rate of children with congenital heart disease. Increasingly, more children who have undergone palliative or corrective surgery are reaching adulthood. Conduits may be inserted in order to channel blood through alternative routes in patients with congenital anomalies that may be otherwise uncorrectable. Grafts may be inserted to close large atrial or ventricular defects. Echocardiographic examinations of such patients are best performed after the operator has thorough knowledge of the primary cardiac pathologic condition and type of surgical intervention performed prior to the ultrasound examination. In general, patches or grafts are more echo dense than normal cardiac tissue and may be easily identified. Conduits are more difficult to identify on the routine echocardiographic views. In such patients, the selection of the appropriate echocardiographic window depends on the actual congenital anomaly and type of surgery performed.

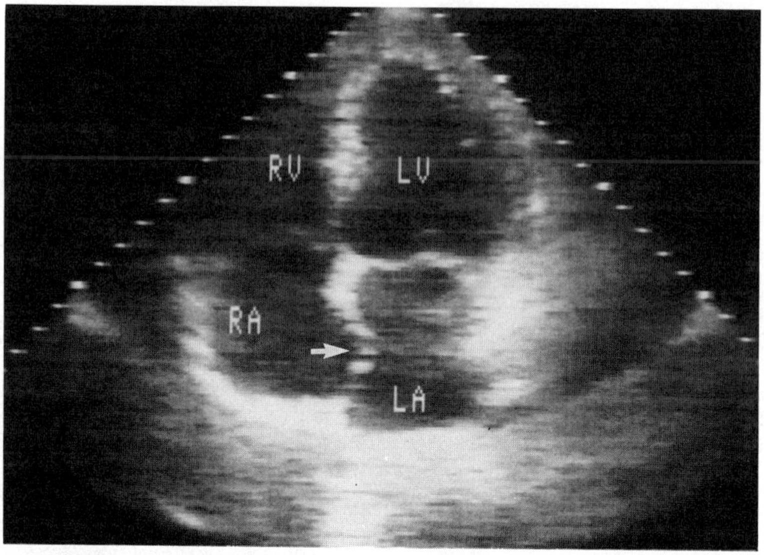

A

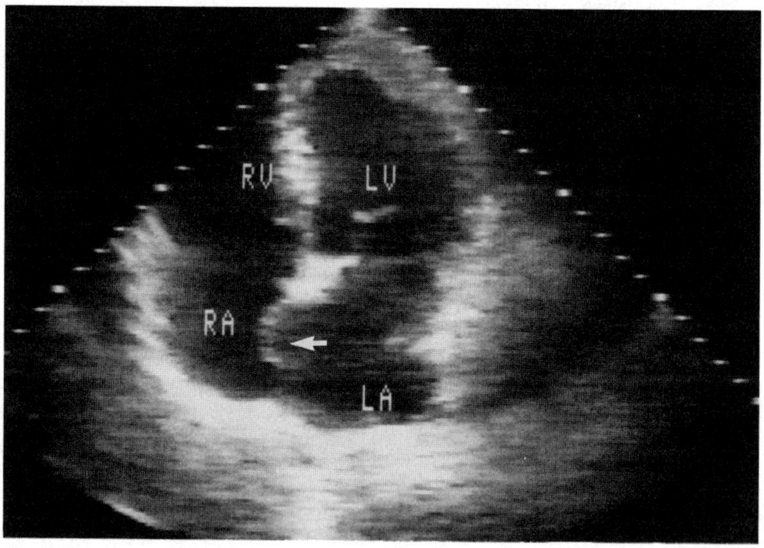

B

Figure 12.15
Aneurysmal dilatation of the interatrial septum. A. Systolic frame showing the interatrial septum (arrow) bulging into the left atrium (LA). B. Diastolic frame showing the interatrial septum (arrow) bulging into the right atrium (RA). LV = left ventricle, RV = right ventricle.

13 Pericardial Disease

The pericardium may be involved in a variety of disease processes. However, the response of the pericardium is rather limited to the production of excessive fluid that collects between the visceral and parietal layers. From there on, the progression of the disease leads to one of several avenues:

1. Resolution of the fluid with no residual abnormality,
2. Relative excessive fluid collection with increased intrapericardial pressure leading to cardiac tamponade,
3. Resolution of the fluid with residual fibrosis and thickening that lead to constrictive pericarditis,
4. Production of proteinaceous material that deposits within the pericardial fluid and produces characteristic images on the echocardiogram.

The incidence of pericardial cysts or primary pericardial tumors is rare. However, the pericardium is frequently involved when other tumors in the body metastasize to the heart.

Pericardial Effusion

Echocardiography is the best noninvasive method for the detection of pericardial effusion. Normally, there is very little fluid within the pericardial sack. This fluid may be seen as a small echo-free space, usually within the atrioventricular groove behind the mitral annulus. Occasionally, separation of the visceral and parietal layers may be noted in systole. This minimal amount of fluid is commonly referred to as physiologic pericardial effusion.

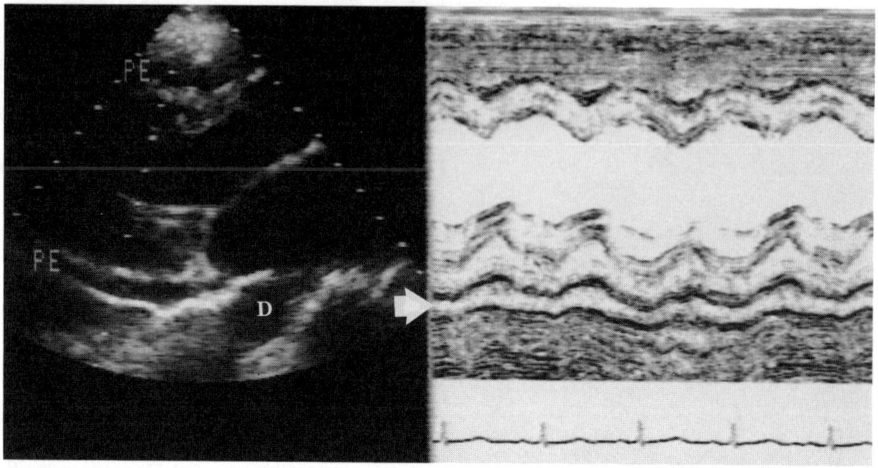

Figure 13.1
Parasternal long axis view with simultaneous M-mode recording of the left ventricle. A small pericardial effusion (PE) is evident posteriorly (arrow). D = descending aorta.

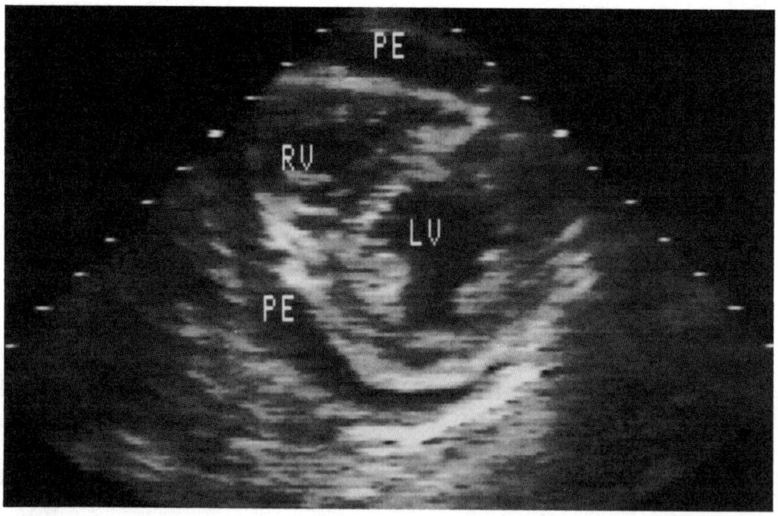

Figure 13.2
Parasternal short axis view showing a moderate anterior and posterior pericardial effusion (PE). RV = right ventricle, LV = left ventricle.

When the fluid collection within the pericardial sack increases, the separation of the pericardial layers persists throughout the cardiac cycle (Figure 13.1). This is usually detected on the anterior as well as posterior surfaces of the heart (Figure 13.2). Increasing amounts of collected fluid cause greater separation of the parietal pericardium from

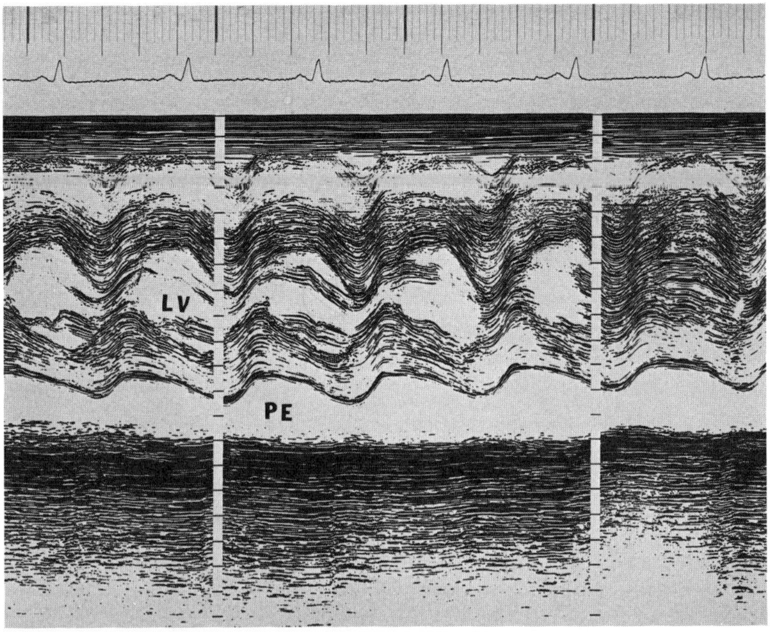

Figure 13.3
M-mode recording of the left ventricle (LV) from a patient with large pericardial effusion (PE). Note the rocking motion with exaggerated anterior and posterior motion of the heart throughout the cardiac cycle.

the visceral layer, which remains adherent to the cardiac muscle wall. Since the heart is suspended within the pericardium, it is not uncommon to observe a rocking motion of the heart throughout the cardiac cycle, as it shifts and tilts within the pericardial fluid (Figure 13.3).

M-mode echocardiography has a better spacial resolution than two-dimensional echocardiography and is better suited for the detection of very small pericardial effusion. The pericardium is made of a dense fibrous tissue that is more echogenic than cardiac muscle; therefore, decreasing the gain settings on the M-mode recordings allows selective imaging of both of the pericardial layers that appear as two parallel, wavy lines with echo-free space in between. The remaining cardiac structures are less echo-dense and would be faintly visualized (Figure 13.4).

Pericardial reflections around the four pulmonary veins prevent small amounts of effusion from collecting posterior to the left atrium (Figure 13.1). However, pericardial fluid may be occasionally observed in that region, mainly in patients with large effusions, or if the intrapericardial pressure is significantly elevated.

When the pericardial fluid contains a relatively high con-

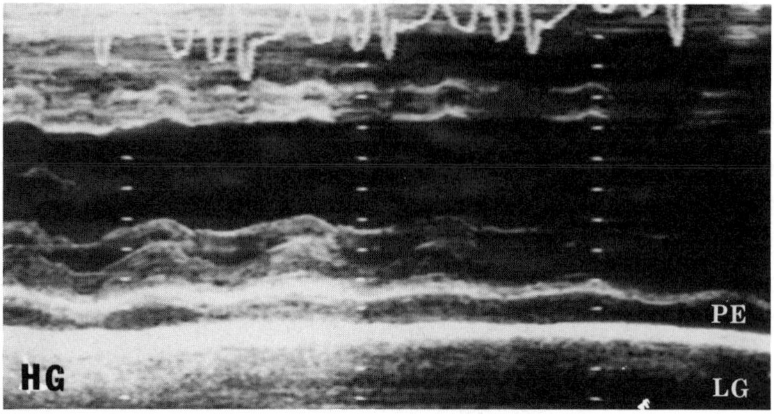

Figure 13.4
M-mode recording of the left ventricle. Gradual decrease of the gain setting allows selective imaging of the visceral and parietal pericardial layers. This maneuver is valuable in detecting small pericardial effusions (PE) that may not be readily noticed on higher gain settings. HG = high gain, LG = low gain.

centration of protein and fibrinous material, the fluid may be loculated. The fibrinous proteins may deposit and form small pockets within the pericardial sack in which fluid may be trapped. In this context, two-dimensional echocardiography is better suited than M-mode echocardiography in demonstrating such loculated pericardial effusions.

On the other hand, the fibrinous material may precipitate on the visceral pericardium. Loose strands of these fibrinous deposits may be observed by two-dimensional echocardiography floating within the pericardial effusion (Figure 13.5). Bloody pericardial effusion may cause multiple ill-defined echoes that are reflected from the red blood cell aggregates that freely float within the pericardial sack.

Finally, tumor metastasis to the pericardium may cause pericardial effusion with ill-defined dense echoes that represent the tumor masses. These masses are more commonly attached to the visceral pericardium.

Cardiac Tamponade

Chronic slow accumulation of pericardial effusion allows enough time for the parietal pericardium to distend. The pressure within the pericardial cavity may remain normal or be minimally elevated. However, when the collection of pericardial effusion is relatively rapid, such as in acute intrapericardial bleeding, significant pressure buildup may occur. Elevated intrapericardial pressures may also occur in

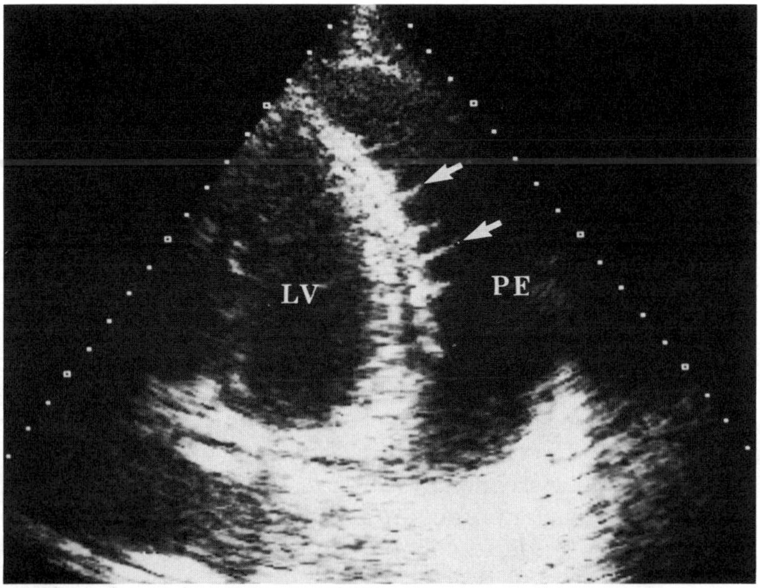

Figure 13.5
Angulated apical view showing a large pericardial effusion (PE) with fibrinous strands (arrows). LV = left ventricle.

the presence of very large pericardial effusions that exceed the capacity of stretching of the pericardial sack.

Intrapericardial pressure becomes critically important when it approaches the diastolic pressures within the cardiac chambers. Elevated intrapericardial pressure impedes venous return to the right chambers of the heart. This, in turn, leads to decreased blood return to the left ventricle and ultimately causes a drop in the cardiac output and systemic blood pressure. Thus, the clinical syndrome of cardiac tamponade ensues.

The echocardiogram typically demonstrates the presence of pericardial effusion. Massive pericardial effusions are invariably associated with cardiac tamponade; however, if the amount of fluid is not very excessive, the echocardiographic diagnosis of tamponade is more subtle. Characteristic echocardiographic signs of cardiac tamponade include early diastolic collapse of the right ventricle, presystolic collapse of the right atrium, and respiratory variations of right ventricular diastolic dimension. These changes simply reflect abnormal hemodynamics that occur in cardiac tamponade. Unfortunately, however, these echocardiographic signs may not always be present in every patient with cardiac tamponade. Minor elevations of intrapericardial pressures indicative of early tamponade may not be associated with any of these echocardiographic signs.

Presystolic Collapse of the Right Atrium

In cardiac tamponade, right atrial pressure is usually equal or slightly higher than intrapericardial pressures throughout most of the cardiac cycle. However, during early atrial diastole, which coincides with early ventricular systole, atrial relaxation may allow intrapericardial pressure to become temporarily higher than intra-atrial pressure. It is during this short interval that the right atrial free wall tends to collapse (Figure 13.6).

Early Diastolic Collapse of the Right Ventricle

Because of the relatively diminished capacities of both ventricles for diastolic filling during tamponade, the left ventricle supervenes over the right ventricle. Thus, left ventricular expansion occurs at the expense of the right ventricle, which tends to collapse during early diastole (Figure 13.7). However, if there is significant pulmonary hypertension and right ventricular hypertrophy, diastolic collapse of this chamber may not occur despite the presence of tamponade.

Respiratory Variations of Ventricular Volumes

In the normal heart, respiratory changes of intrathoracic pressures during inspiration and expiration may be associated with minor changes in venous return to the right side of the heart. Venous return to the right ventricle is slightly greater during inspiration than during expiration. This results in a slightly higher diastolic ventricular dimension as compared to the dimension during expiration. In the presence of tamponade, the respiratory variations of diastolic right ventricular dimension become exaggerated and more obvious. Because of the limited ability of both ventricles to expand, opposite changes occur in the left ventricle, whereby its dimension in diastole diminishes during inspiration as compared to that measured during expiration.

Constrictive Pericarditis

The cardiac chambers constantly change in volume throughout the cardiac cycle. The normal pericardium allows adequate expansion of ventricular chambers in diastole without any significant restraints. However, various inflammatory processes of the pericardium may cause fibrosis with thickening of the pericardial layers. When severe enough, these fibrotic changes limit the ability of diastolic expansion of the cardiac chambers, thus restricting diastolic filling.

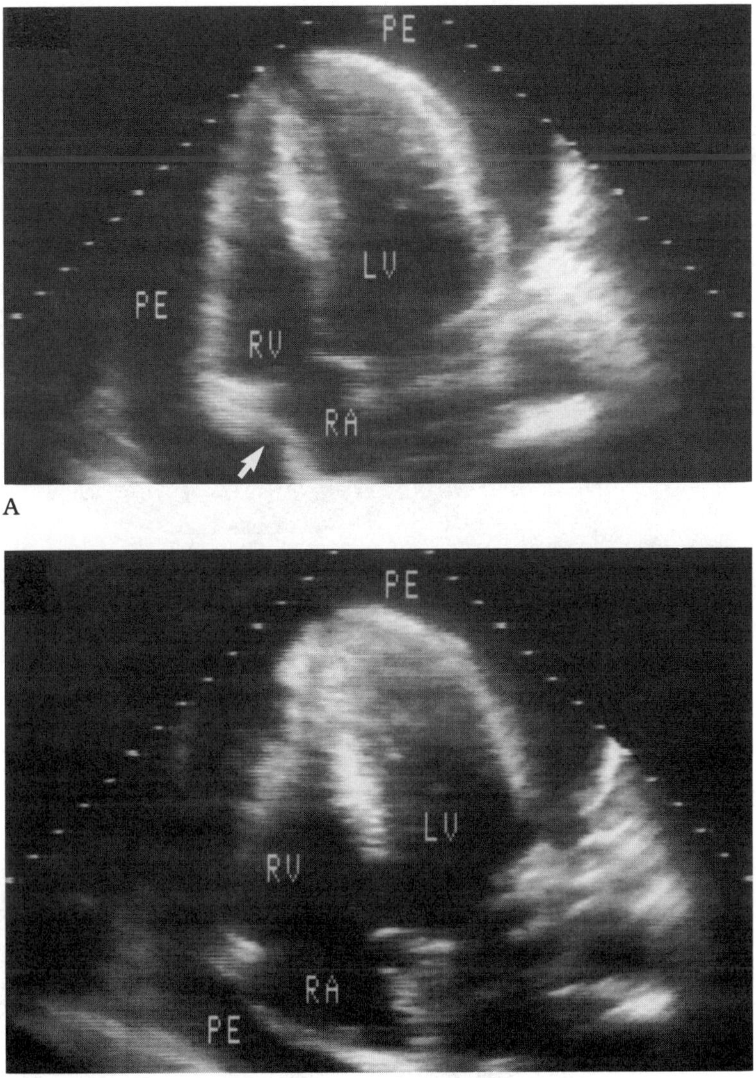

Figure 13.6
Apical four-chamber views in cardiac tamponade. A. Note the indentation of the right atrial free wall (arrow) in this presystolic frame. B. In early diastole it is normalized. PE = pericardial effusion, RV = right ventricle, LV = left ventricle, RA = right atrium.

The sensitivity of echocardiography in the diagnosis of constrictive pericarditis is very poor. Pericardial thickening, if present, may not be readily appreciated (Figure 13.8). This is dependent on the gain control setting of the ultrasound equipment. Too much gain may enhance the pericardial echoes in the absence of any true pathologic state.

Similar to the echocardiographic diagnosis of cardiac tam-

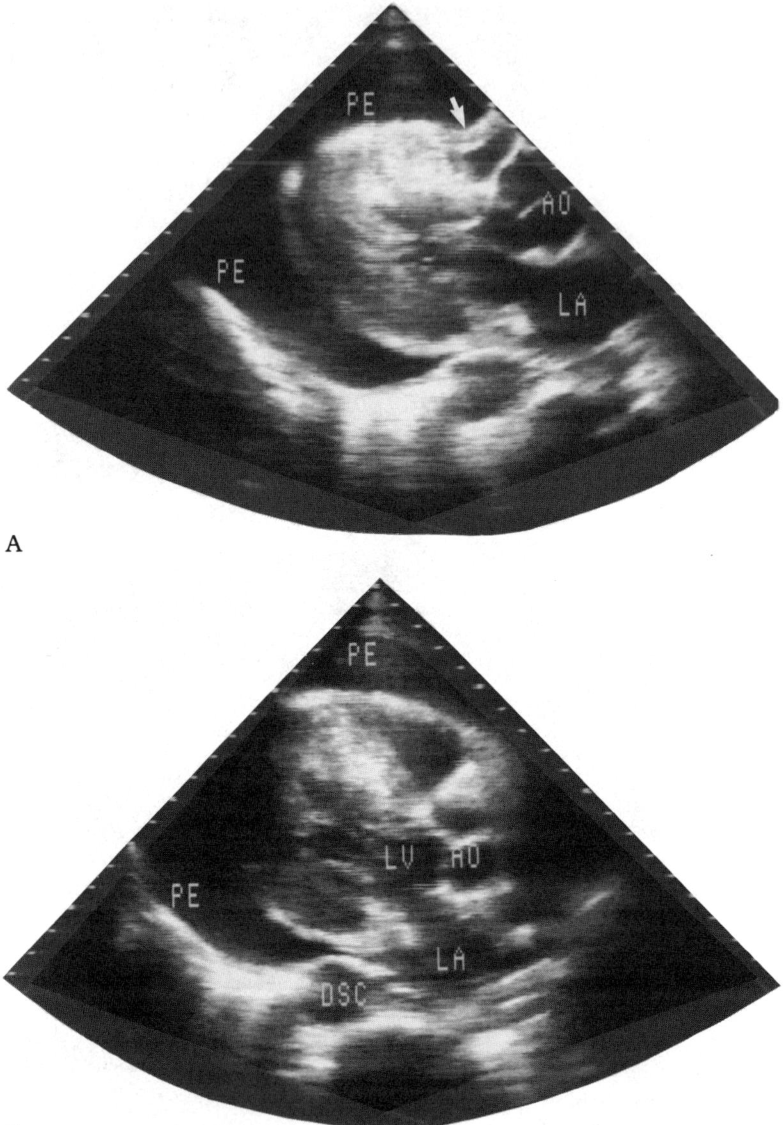

B
Figure 13.7
A. Parasternal long axis view from a patient with large pericardial effusion (PE). Note the indentation of the right ventricular free wall (arrow) in this early diastolic frame. B. In late diastole it is normalized. AO = aorta, LA = left atrium, LV = left ventricle, DSC = descending aorta.

ponade, one has to rely on indirect signs that reflect the abnormal hemodynamics caused by constrictive physiology. Markedly elevated right ventricular pressure in diastole may exceed the pulmonary artery diastolic pressure. This will cause the pulmonary valve to open prematurely, before the onset of systole. This echocardiographic sign is not very sen-

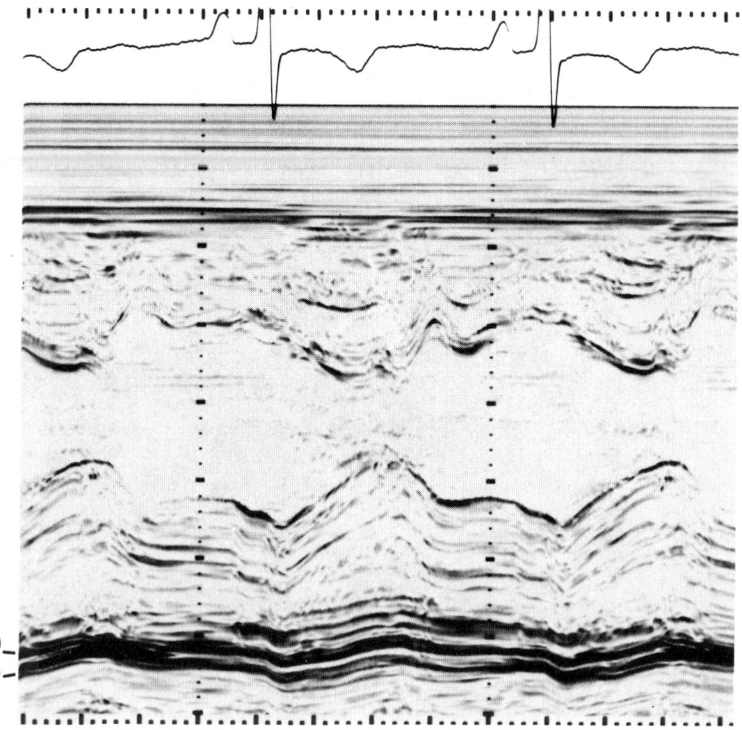

Figure 13.8
M-mode recording from a patient with constrictive pericarditis. Despite the relatively low gain setting employed to obtain this recording, note the prominent dense echoes from the visceral (vp) and parietal (pp) pericardial layers.

sitive and may be observed in patients with severe right ventricular dysfunction or volume overload in the absence of associated pulmonary hypertension.

Because of pericardial restraint to ventricular expansion, ventricular filling occurs mainly during early diastole. Close observation of M-mode recordings of the left ventricular posterior wall may demonstrate rapid posterior motion in early diastole with flattened motion afterward. Toward the end of diastole, a forceful atrial contraction may cause another brief posterior motion, which will be terminated by the onset of a new systolic cycle. Thus, ventricular filling occurs only in early diastole and after the atrial kick.

Similarly, the motion of the anterior mitral leaflet may reflect the rapid filling in early diastole. In this context, the E-F slope may be exaggerated with prominent A wave. Premature closure of the mitral valve, before ventricular systole starts, may reflect the abnormally elevated left ventricular diastolic pressure. Unfortunately, none of these echocardiographic signs are sensitive enough to establish the diagnosis of constrictive pericarditis.

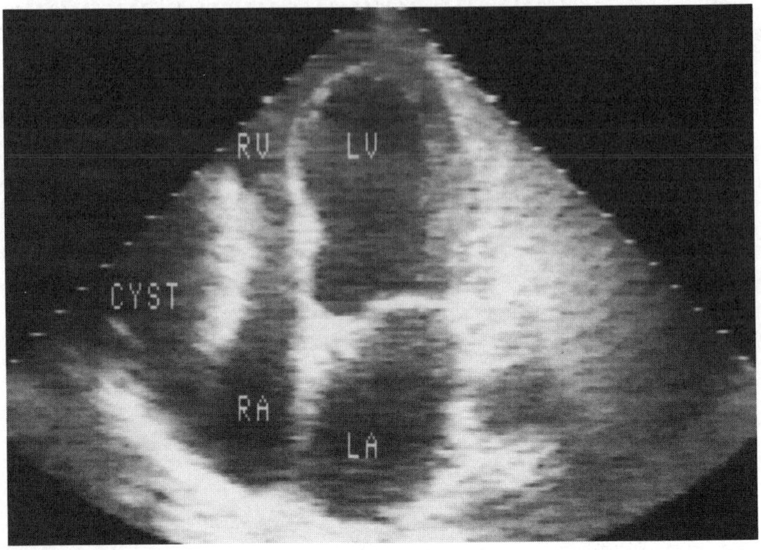

Figure 13.9
Apical four-chamber view showing a rare pericardial cyst causing partial collapse with distorted geometry of the right ventricle (RV). LV = left ventricle, LA = left atrium, RA = right atrium.

Rare Pericardial Diseases

Pericardial cysts are very rarely encountered. Such cysts with loculated fluid may cause extrinsic pressure on the adjacent cardiac chambers and restrict normal cardiac function (Figure 13.9).

Primary pericardial tumors are also very rare. Occasionally, direct invasion of the pericardium with a tumor arising from the adjacent lung or lymph nodes may cause extrinsic pressure on the adjacent cardiac chambers (Figure 13.10).

Doppler Ultrasound in Pericardial Disease

The role of Doppler ultrasonography in the diagnosis of pericardial diseases is rather limited. Abnormalities of transvalvular velocities of blood flow may reflect the hemodynamic alterations that occur in cardiac tamponade and constrictive pericarditis. Diminished flow rates may occur secondary to the decrease in stroke volume and cardiac output.

Occasionally, a patient with cardiac tamponade may demonstrate velocities of blood flow across the tricuspid and pulmonary valves that exhibit respiratory variations. These variations reflect similar changes observed on echocardiography regarding diastolic right ventricular dimensions, and

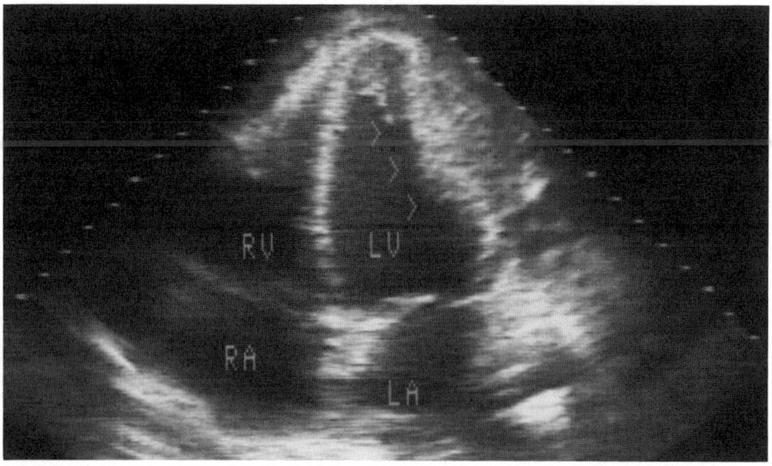

Figure 13.10
Apical four-chamber view from a patient with pericardial tumor that invaded the left ventricular (LV) lateral wall (arrowheads). RV = right ventricle, RA = right atrium, LA = left atrium.

simply occur secondary to the respiratory variations of venous return to the right side of the heart.

Pulsus paradoxus is said to occur when the systolic blood pressure measured during expiration is 10 mm Hg or more than the same pressure measured during inspiration. This may be associated with Doppler recordings of transmitral and transaortic velocities of flow that are higher during expiration than during inspiration. In this context, it is important to note that in the presence of a large pericardial effusion, the rocking motion of the heart throughout the cardiac cycle constantly changes the angle (θ) between the fixed Doppler ultrasound beam relative to the direction of blood flow across the mitral or aortic valves. Hence, any changes of the peak velocity of blood flow, as measured by Doppler ultrasound, may be related to alterations of the angle of incidence (θ) rather to variation of the true transvalvular volume of flow.

Pulsus alternans refers to the beat-to-beat variation in the stroke volume, which is occasionally noted in patients with large pericardial effusions and tamponade. Such changes may be occasionally noted on the Doppler recordings showing beat-to-beat variations in the velocity of flow across the mitral or aortic valves (Figure 13.11).

False-Positive Pericardial Effusions

The hallmark of pericardial effusion is the presence of an echo-free space that surrounds the heart. However, similar

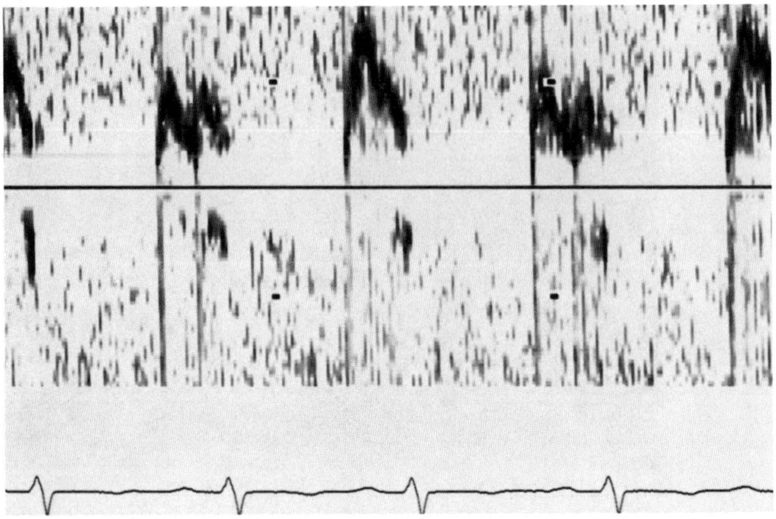

Figure 13.11
Pulsus alternans in cardiac tamponade. Note the beat-to-beat variation of transmitral Doppler recording in the presence of sinus rhythm and a regular QRS interval on the simultaneous ECG recording.

findings may be observed in the absence of any significant pericardial fluid.

Pleural Effusion

As a result of pulmonary disease, pleural fluid may collect within the left thoracic cavity. A large pleural effusion may be observed on a routine echocardiogram as an echo-free space posterior to the heart (Figure 13.12). This may be distinguished from a true pericardial effusion by the fact that nonloculated pericardial fluid is more commonly evenly distributed between the anterior and posterior cardiac borders. This is in contradistinction to the pleural effusion where the echo-free space is situated only posterior to the heart.

The descending thoracic aorta may be used as a landmark that aids in the distinction of pericardial from pleural effusions. Since the descending aorta is situated outside the cardiac border, pericardial effusion will cause an echo-free space that separates this vessel from the posterior surface of the heart. On the other hand, the echo-free space caused by a pleural effusion does not necessarily alter the anatomic relation between the descending aorta and the heart (Figures 13.12, 13.13).

Occasionally, pericardial and pleural effusion may coexist. In this context, two echo-free spaces posterior to the heart

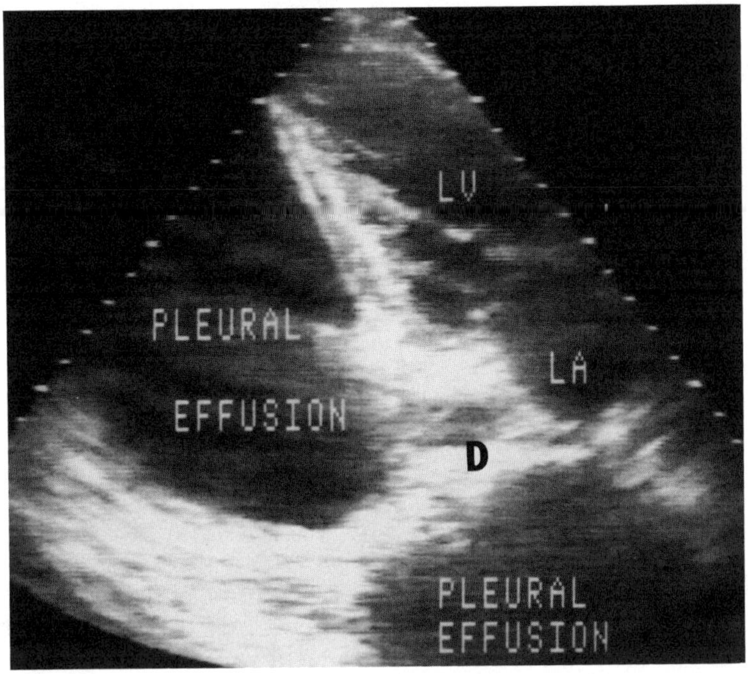

Figure 13.12
Angulated apical long axis view from a patient with large pleural effusion. Note the absence of any anterior echo-free space. This fluid lies posterior to the descending aorta (D). LV = left ventricle, LA = left atrium.

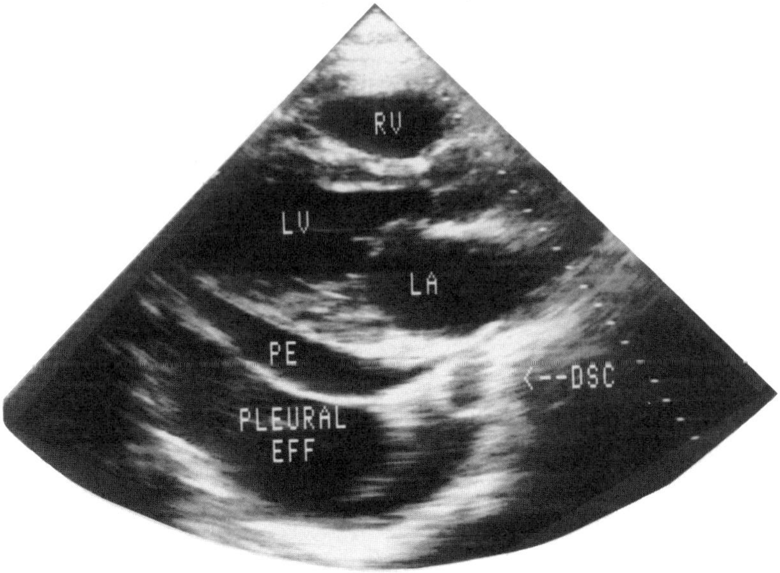

Figure 13.13
Pericardial (PE) and pleural effusions can be easily identified in this parasternal long axis view. Minimal pericardial fluid separates the posterior left atrial wall from the descending aorta (DSC), whereas the pleural effusion extends posterior to the descending aorta. RV = right ventricle, LV = left ventricle, LA = left atrium.

may be observed. The parietal pericardium serves as a boundary layer that separates the pericardial and pleural spaces (Figure 13.13).

If the pleural effusion is caused by an exudative process or is secondary to tumor metastasis, fibrinous deposits with strands may be observed within the pleural fluid. Occasionally, tumor masses or portions of collapsed lung may be noted as well.

Epicardial Fat Pad

A layer of fatty tissue normally covers the pericardium. This fatty layer is usually thickest along the anterior cardiac border and apex. Since fat is less echo-dense than normal myocardium, a relatively echo-free layer may be recorded by echocardiography, just underlying the anterior chest wall. This echo lucency could be mistaken for a loculated small anterior pericardial effusion. In general, pericardial effusion will be evenly distributed around the heart. Hence, an anterior echo-free space is more likely to represent epicardial fat in the absence of any demonstrable posterior pericardial effusion. Moreover, the serial contraction and relaxation of the cardiac chambers throughout the cardiac cycle will cause serial change in the size of the echo-free space as the pericardial fluid shifts within the pericardial cavity. However, the relatively echo-free space of the epicardial fat layer will not change in dimension throughout the cardiac cycle.

14 Cardiac Masses

Two-dimensional echocardiography is a particularly sensitive technique for the detection of intracardiac and extracardiac masses. In the evaluation of left ventricular thrombi and intracardiac tumors, it is the procedure of choice, providing a comprehensive view of the cardiac chambers and valves not available with angiography. This chapter will consider the echocardiographic assessment of the most commonly seen masses, including valvular vegetations, thrombi, and primary and metastatic tumors.

Endocarditis

Although endocarditis is not a diagnosis dependent on the echocardiographic visualization of vegetations, it is clear that echocardiography does provide very useful morphologic, anatomic, and hemodynamic information. Two-dimensional echocardiography is generally superior to M-mode echocardiography in evaluating vegetative lesions.

Patients with the highest index of suspicion for vegetative endocarditis, including those with known underlying heart disease or with a history of intravenous drug abuse, require a systematically thorough evaluation of all four cardiac chambers and valves. In general, vegetations are discrete, irregularly shaped, distinctly echogenic masses that usually attach to the valve leaflets. Without interfering with leaflet motion, vegetations generally move synchronously with the valve. Occasionally, vegetations are pedunculated and will flop around within the heart with fairly dramatic motion independent of actual leaflet motion (Figures 14.1, 7.6A).

This chapter was written by Priscilla Peters.

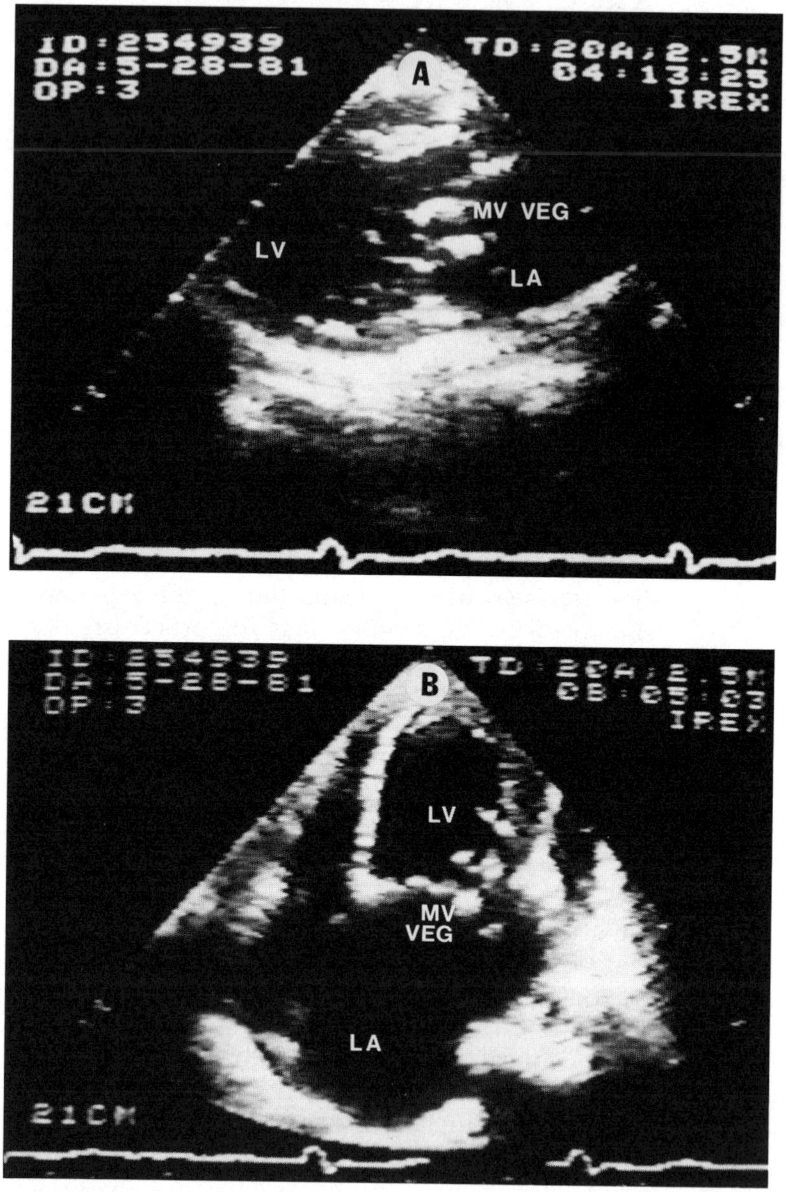

Figure 14.1
A. Parasternal long axis view, and B. Apical four-chamber view showing vegetation (VEG) on the mitral valve (MV). Note the marked dilatation of the left atrium (LA) due to significant mitral regurgitation and volume overload. C. M-mode recording of the mitral valve demonstrating a vegetation (V). The arrow denotes mitral valve prolapse. LV = left ventricle.

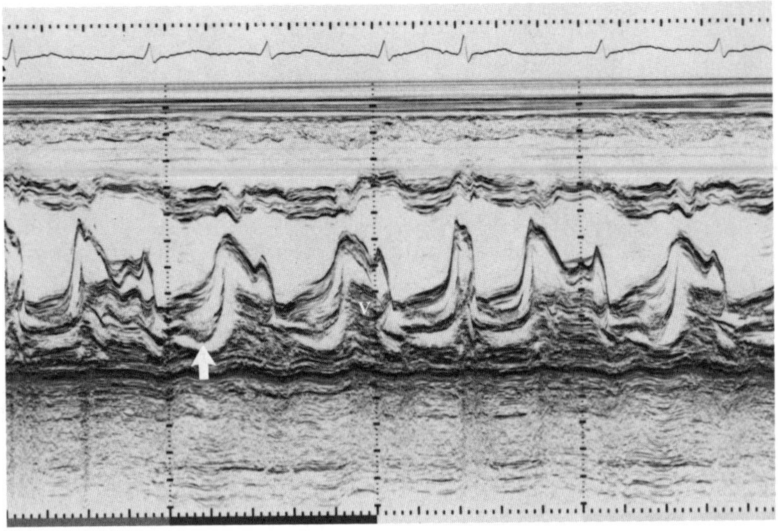

C

Figure 14.1 (continued)

Fungal vegetations tend to be larger than bacterial masses. An M-mode cursor through a vegetation usually demonstrates a smudgy, shaggy-appearing mass attached to a valve leaflet (Figure 7.6B). In addition to identifying valvular vegetations, a baseline and follow-up echocardiograms are particularly useful for the serial evaluation of ventricular function, as persistent heart failure is one indication for surgery. Important information can also be obtained concerning the extent of valvular or other surface involvement, including disruption of the leaflets (Figure 7.6C), myocardial seeding, abscess formation (Figure 7.6D), and the presence of aneurysms involving the aorta or sinuses of Valsalva.

Mitral vegetations are most likely to occur in the context of valve deformities such as leaflet prolapse (Figures 14.1C, 7.18) or rheumatic scarring, although vegetative seeding can occur in normal valves. The lesions may attach to either leaflet, and generally do not affect leaflet mobility or left ventricular inflow (although massive vegetations have been reported to cause obstruction to transmitral flow). Significant leaflet destruction can occur and it may be difficult to distinguish a mobile vegetation from a flailing leaflet.

Endocarditis of the aortic valve frequently involves congenitally malformed valves, or those that have been deformed by rheumatic fever. In the elderly, endocarditis can occur on valves with acquired sclerotic or calcific disease. Vegetations usually involve the body of the leaflet on the ventricular surface, frequently appearing as clumps of echogenic mass. As the vegetations increase in size, they can be identified prolapsing into the left ventricular outflow tract in diastole and up into the aorta in systole.

Because of the anatomic proximity of the anterior aspect of the aorta to the base of the interventricular septum, the infectious process can extend into the septum with subsequent abscess formation. Paravalvular abscesses of the aortic root can also occur. These appear as localized echolucent pouches, usually brighter than the surface from which they originate. Occasionally an aortic vegetation can extend to the base of a normal anterior mitral leaflet. Because endocarditis of the aortic valve frequently has a higher morbidity and mortality than infections of either the mitral or tricuspid valves, it is extremely important to carefully evaluate the aortic valve from as many planes as possible, and examine all structures contiguous with the aortic root, including the interventricular septum, the mitral valve, and the proximal ascending aorta. In the presence of aortic regurgitation, fluttering of the anerior mitral leaflet or the ventricular septum, or both, may be seen on the M-mode. These findings only confirm the presence of aortic regurgitation, and do not address the severity of the lesion. In acute, severe aortic regurgitation, premature closure of the mitral valve, or premature opening of the aortic valve may be noted (Figure 7.6C).

Vegetations on the tricuspid valve tend to be larger than those seen on other valves, and frequently attach to otherwise normal tricuspid leaflets. The vegetations generally attach to the atrial surface of the leaflets and can involve one or more of the three leaflets. As noted, the lesions can be quite large, and may be globular and dense, long and stringy, or bulky and frondlike in appearance. They are usually quite mobile and not particularly subtle (Figures 14.2, 7.20). The index of suspicion for tricuspid endocarditis should be high in febrile patients with a history of intravenous substance abuse. At least three views should be obtained in evaluating the tricuspid valve, as not all views provide access to all leaflets. The short axis view at the base of the heart delineates the septal and anterior leaflets, the parasternal long axis view of the right ventricular inflow tract identifies the anterior and posterior tricuspid leaflets, and the apical four-chamber view provides yet another view of the septal and anterior leaflets. Occasionally the right chambers of the heart are dilated and there is evidence of right ventricular volume overload, with or without a systolic murmur.

Pulmonary valve endocarditis, as an isolated finding, is uncommon. It is most likely to occur with underlying congenital abnormalities, especially ventricular septal defects, tetralogy of Fallot, patent ductus arteriosus, and valvular

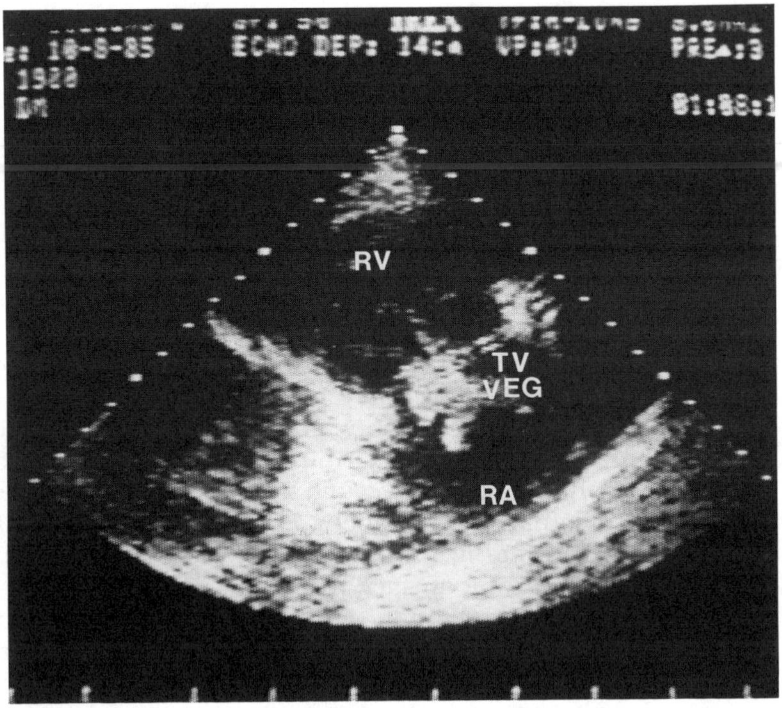

Figure 14.2
Parasternal long axis view of the right ventricular inflow tract, with a large, frondlike vegetation (VEG) of the tricuspid valve (TV). RV = right ventricle, RA = right atrium.

pulmonary stenosis. It can also be seen in intravenous drug abusers, both as an isolated finding on a normal pulmonary valve and in association with infection of the tricuspid or other heart valves. The vegetations can appear as localized clumps, or as thickening of one or more of the pulmonary valve leaflets, or as pedunculated, highly mobile masses.

Vegetation on prosthetic heart valves is frequently a difficult echocardiographic diagnosis. Mechanical valves are intrinsically highly echogenic, and distinguishing vegetative mass from valve apparatus can be difficult. Very large lesions that attach to the valve-supporting apparatus tend to exhibit motion clearly distinguishable from the ball or disc (Figure 9.15). Occasionally vegetation can actually sit within the prosthesis and impede opening or closing of the disc. Excessive motion and rocking of the prosthetic supporting apparatus can also be determined. In porcine prostheses or other bioprostheses, if attached to the leaflet, a vegetation will appear similar to one involving a native valve, usually with evident leaflet destruction.

Intracardiac Thrombi

Left ventricular thrombus formation is an important complication of myocardial infarction. The incidence of thrombus increases with the presence of aneurysm; thrombi are more likely to be seen in patients with anterior infarcts, at the apex. Thrombus formation is also common in patients with dilated cardiomyopathy; in one series, thrombi in this setting were larger than those seen in patients with coronary artery disease, probably secondary to the global nature of the left ventricular dysfunction.

Two-dimensional echocardiography is the procedure of choice for the detection of mural thrombi. Because the vast majority of clots are found at the apex of the heart, the apical planes are most important in the evaluation of thrombi. The apex should be interrogated from all three apical planes: the four-chamber, the two-chamber, and the long axis. Typically, thrombi are acoustically distinct masses that distort the endocardial surface in regions of the ventricle that are akinetic or dyskinetic (Figure 14.3). Abnormal motions of the wall are key to the diagnosis of true left ventricular thrombus; it is unlikely that a clot would form in a normally contracting ventricle. Although most apical thrombi layer the apex, occasionally some free motion can be identified. The distinction between apical clot and normal left ventricular trabeculation, so-called false tendons or heart strings, and the occasional very rare left ventricular neoplasm begins with the assessment of wall motion abnormalities. If an apical abnormality is identified and the apex tapers and contracts normally, pathologic conditions other than thrombus should be considered.

Another phenomenon that is being identified with increasing frequency is the presence of intracavitary static blood. Sluggish but still liquid blood is quite echogenic and its presence can be detected in dilated, severely hypocontractile ventricles, and occasionally in the left atrium. This static blood looks like a puff of intracardiac smoke (acoustically distinguishable from true thrombus), usually moving in a circular fashion like clothes in a dryer (Figure 6.6). Frequently, layered mural thrombus is seen in conjunction with smoke.

Thrombi in the left atrium generally occur in the setting of substantial left atrial dilatation in association with rheumatic mitral valve disease, atrial fibrillation, or both (Figure 14.4). Although clots are usually dense and globular and attached to the wall of the left atrium, they can also be freely mobile without a point of attachment. In addition, clots can layer the walls of the left atrium. These flat laminar

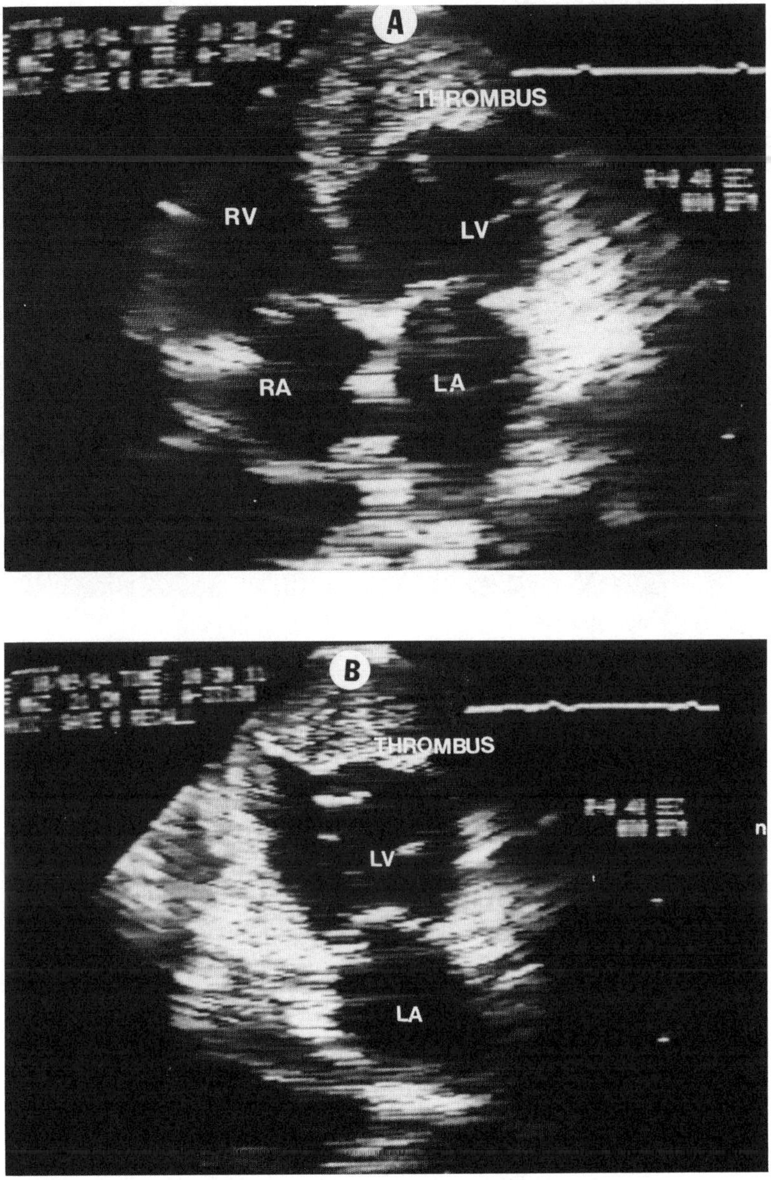

Figure 14.3
A. Apical four-chamber view, and B. Two-chamber view demonstrating a large mural thrombus layering the left ventricular apex. In real time, the apex was frankly dyskinetic. LV = left ventricle, RV = right ventricle, LA = left atrium, RA = right atrium.

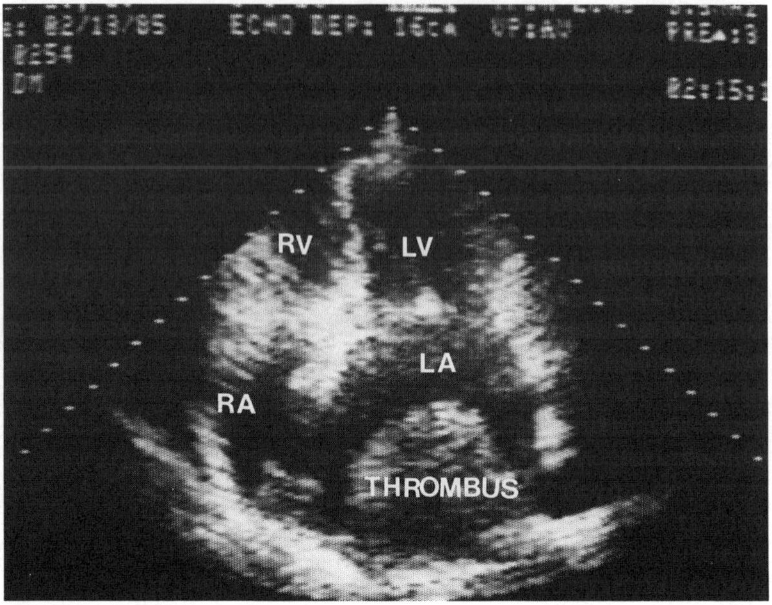

Figure 14.4
Apical four-chamber view in a patient with mitral stenosis. A large, dense thrombus layers the wall of the left atrium (LA). RA = right atrium, RV = right ventricle, LV = left ventricle.

clots may not interrupt the contour of the atrial wall and, hence, can be easily missed with two-dimensional echocardiography. Clots in the atrial appendage frequently occur with mitral stenosis; these clots are also difficult to assess because the left atrial appendage is typically difficult to interrogate with the two-dimensional beam. Occasionally, the left atrial appendage will aneurysmally dilate; it then becomes a distinctive echo target. As a left atrial thrombus is an important clinical discovery, when the index of suspicion is high, considerable care should be taken to examine the left atrium in several planes, including all the subcostal views.

Clots of the right heart, although not common, can be identified. Right ventricular thrombi can be seen in the setting of right ventricular infarction and have been reported in patients with blunt chest trauma. Clots of the right atrium are usually quite mobile and are frequently identified after a major embolic event to the pulmonary circuit has occurred. One can also identify thrombi originating in the inferior vena cava prolapsing into the right atrium. In addition to the apical four-chamber view, the right ventricular parasternal inflow view, the short axis view at the base of the heart, the subcostal four-chamber view, the inferior vena cava–right atrial junction views are especially important when looking for right atrial thrombi.

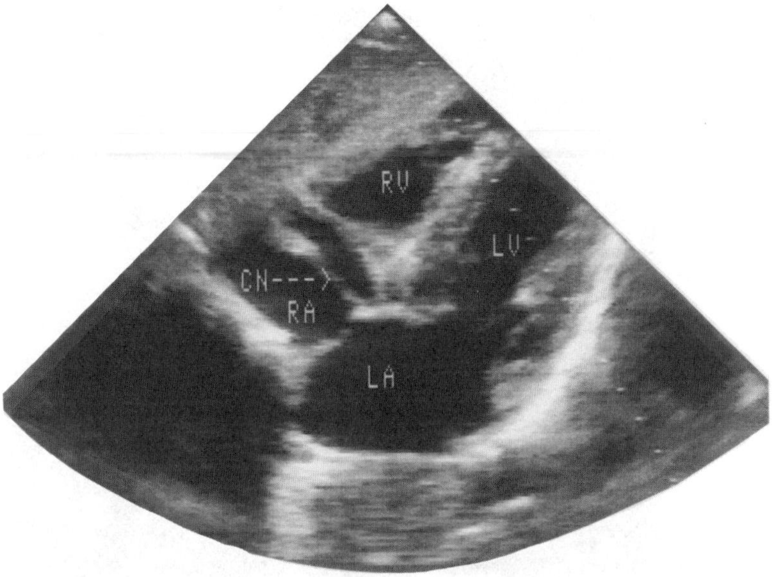

Figure 14.5
Subcostal four-chamber view of the heart, demonstrating Chiari's network (CN) in the right atrium (RA), with attachments to the interatrial septum and the right atrial wall. RV = right ventricle, LV = left ventricle, LA = left atrium.

The Chiari network, a congenital remnant of the sinus venosus, is a thin, weblike, fenestrated membrane that generally traverses the body of the right atrium from attachments at the interatrial septum and right atrial wall (Figure 14.5). It exhibits what can be quite erratic motion. This normal finding can easily be confused with floating thrombus, vegetation, or tumor, so it is important to become familiar with its appearance. The eustachian valve, which is the valve of the inferior vena cava, is generally less mobile than the Chiari network and can be recognized by its typical location, at the junction of the inferior vena cava and the right atrium. Other structures that can be identified in the right side of the heart include the moderator band of the right ventricle (Figure 1.4), hemodynamic and therapeutic monitoring lines, pacer wires, and surgically implanted conduits or shunts.

Tumors of the Heart

One of the most important applications of two-dimensional echocardiography has been the detection of intracardiac tumors. The most common cardiac tumor is the myxoma. Although myxomas usually occur singly and in the left

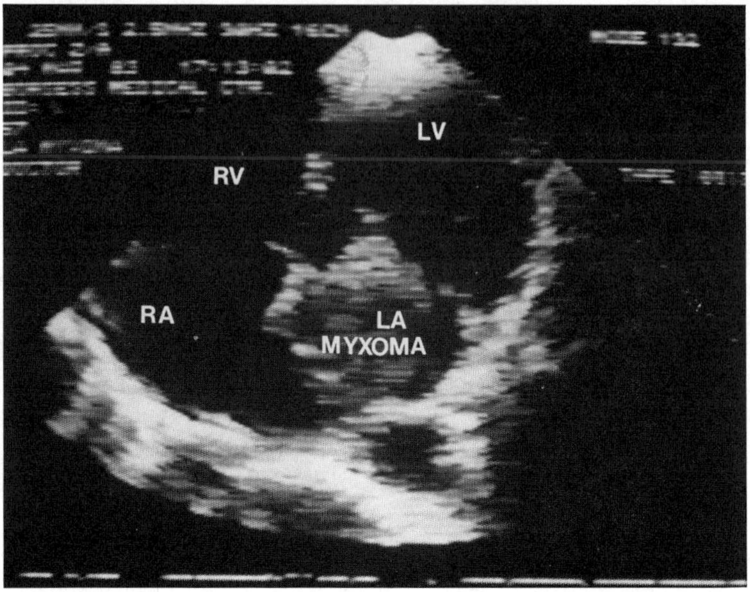

Figure 14.6
Four-chamber view of the heart, demonstrating the characteristic speckly appearance of a left atrial (LA) myxoma as it prolapses through the mitral orifice in diastole. LV = left ventricle, RV = right ventricle, RA = right atrium.

atrium, bilateral myxomas, isolated right atrial myxomas, combined left atrial and left ventricular myxomas, and right ventricular myxomas can occur. In one review, approximately 75% of myxomas occurred in the left atrium, with the remainder distributed in the right atrium (20%), left ventricle (2.5%), and right ventricle (2.5%). Typically, left atrial myxomas are pedunculated and attached to the interatrial septum at the level of the fossa ovalis. They appear speckly and well encapsulated, and most often prolapse freely through the mitral orifice in diastole and move back into the left atrium during systole (Figure 14.6). The tumors may be quite large, completely filling the left atrium and obstructing mitral inflow, or they may be small and barely moving or totally immobile.

Other primary cardiac neoplasms are rare, and most lack distinctive echocardiographic characteristics. These tumors include rhabdomyomas and rhabdomyosarcomas (usually in children); papillary fibroelastomas, which usually attach to valve surfaces; and lipomas, fibromas, teratomas, and angiosarcomas. The identification of an unexpected cardiac mass obviously warrants additional aggressive investigation. Because the heart is a common site for metastasis (usually the pericardium), attention should be paid to unusual density or thickening attached to or infiltrating the pericardium, with or without pericardial effusion (Figure 13.10), and to actual cavity invasion by the tumor. When there is valvular involvement, the tricuspid valve is most commonly affected. Tumors that most frequently metastasize to the heart are lung, breast, melanoma, lymphoma, and leukemia, so the echocardiographic exam of these patients must include assessment of all cardiac chambers and valves, in addition to the immediately adjacent extracardiac structures. Extracardiac tumors will actually erode into the myocardium and can mimic mobile thrombi and myxomas. If the tumor invades the heart by direct extension (as with lung and breast), one can frequently identify the primary extracardiac mass and the point of intracardiac erosion. Invasion of the right side of the heart by hypernephroma or hepatoma can occur. These tumors typically extend up the inferior vena cava and prolapse into the right atrium.

Two-dimensional echocardiography has become the procedure of choice for the evaluation of intracardiac masses. Its special orientation and ability to provide a view of all four chambers of the heart simultaneously make it uniquely able to identify "things that don't belong there."

15 Diseases of the Aorta

The aorta is composed of three major segments. The ascending aorta is the first segment, which starts from the aortic valve annulus and sinuses of Valsalva. This segment extends to join the aortic arch, which is the second major segment of the aorta. Three major vessels arise from the aortic arch. These are the innominate artery, the left carotid, and the left subclavian arteries. The isthmus represents the connection of the aortic arch to the descending aorta, which is the third major segment and is subdivided into the thoracic aorta, within the thoracic cavity, and the abdominal aorta, which extends below the diaphragm into the abdomen. The abdominal aorta ends in the pelvis, where it divides into two major branches (the iliac arteries) (Figure 15.1).

Because of their close association with the heart, diseases of the ascending aorta and arch commonly affect cardiac function. Aortic valvular disease may also cause secondary dilatation of the aortic root.

Aortic Dilatation

Atherosclerosis is the most common disease of the aorta. The abdominal aorta is most commonly affected; however, involvement of the ascending aorta and aortic arch may occur. Atheromatous formation with deposition of calcium is the hallmark of this disease. Weakening of the wall of the aorta predisposes for dilatation of this vessel. When there is also systemic hypertension, the aorta would be subjected to

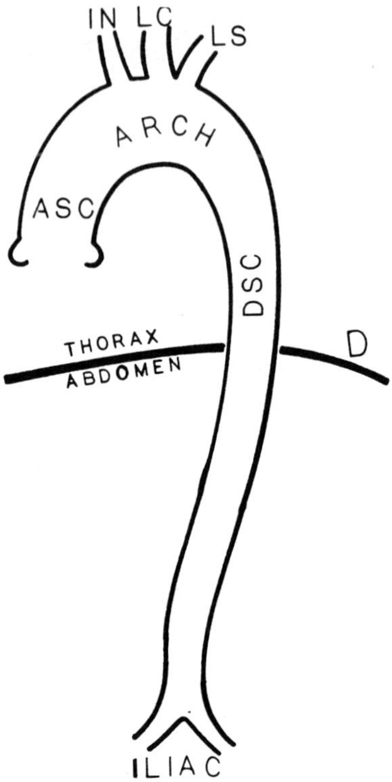

Figure 15.1
The aorta. ASC = ascending aorta, D = diaphragm, DSC = descending aorta, IN = innominate artery, LC = left carotid artery, LS = left subclavian artery.

significant shearing forces that ultimately cause more dilatation and, occasionally, formation of aneurysm.

Syphilitic aortitis, medial cystic necrosis, and connective tissue disease, such as ankylosing spondylitis, are some examples from the large list of diseases that may affect the aorta and cause dilatation. Marfan's syndrome is one form of congenital disease that weakens the aortic wall and predisposes for significant dilatation and formation of aneurysm (Figure 15.2).

Aortic dilatation may occur secondary to aortic valve disease. Poststenotic dilatation is commonly observed in patients with severe aortic stenosis. This occurs due to the high velocity of flow and turbulence of blood that occurs distal to the aortic valve obstruction. Severe chronic aortic regurgitation may also cause dilatation of the aortic root. This results from the high volume of blood ejected by the left ventricle during systole. Finally, it is not unusual to observe mild degrees of dilatation of the aorta in patients with chronic uncontrolled hypertension.

Aortic Dissection

The wall of the aorta is constantly subjected to the forceful left ventricular ejection of blood under pressure during systole. The innermost layer of the aortic wall, the intima, is most commonly affected by such shearing forces. A diseased intima, as observed in atherosclerotic disease with plaque formation, may detach from the remaining layers of the aortic wall; consequently, aortic dissection occurs (Figure 15.3).

Depending on the site of dissection, serious complications may ensue. Dissection of the aortic root may extend into the aortic valve annulus. This causes disruption of the aortic valve apparatus, leading to various severities of acute aortic regurgitation. Occasionally, one or more aortic leaflets become flail. Moreover, the dissection may involve the origin of one or both coronary arteries. If this occurs, interruption of coronary flow may lead to acute myocardial infarction.

Aortic Rupture

Traumatic injury to the chest, whether penetrating or blunt, may cause aortic dissection and, occasionally, rupture of the aortic wall. Occasionally, a large aortic aneurysm may rupture without any predisposing trauma. However, such occurrences usually prove to be fatal before the patient presents for medical attention.

A less dramatic course of events may occur when a dilated sinus of Valsalva ruptures (Figure 15.4) (Plate 13). Depending on which sinus is involved, the fistulous communication may occur between the aorta and the right atrium or ventricle, interventricular septum, and occasionally, the pericardium. Rupture of the sinus into the pericardium often leads to acute collection of blood within the pericardial sack, causing tamponade. In contrast, if the rupture occurs into one of the right chambers, a left-to-right shunt is produced. Moreover, rupture of the sinus of Valsalva commonly disrupts the aortic valve apparatus, resulting in acute aortic regurgitation as well.

Congenital Diseases of the Aorta

Marfan's syndrome is one form of congenital disease of the aorta that may cause extreme dilatation and aneurysmal formation. Coarctation of the aorta is a rare form of congenital disease, whereby there is localized narrowing of the descending aorta at the level of the isthmus. When coarctation is

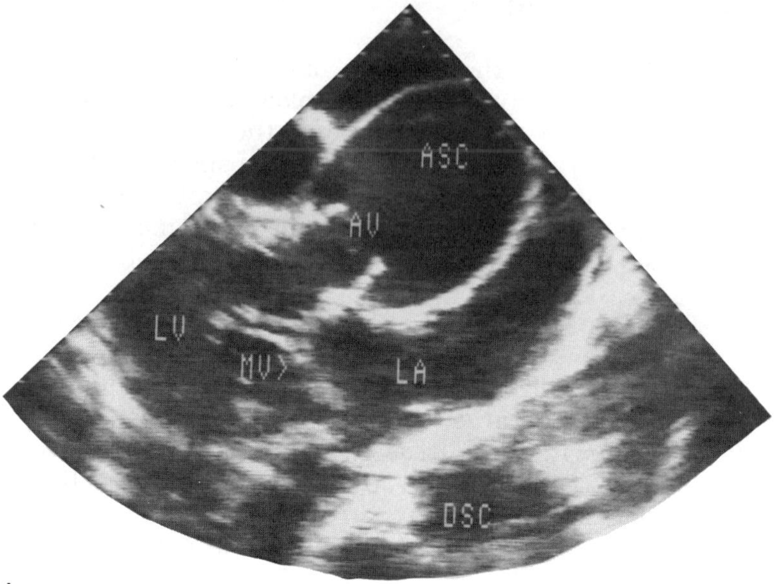

A

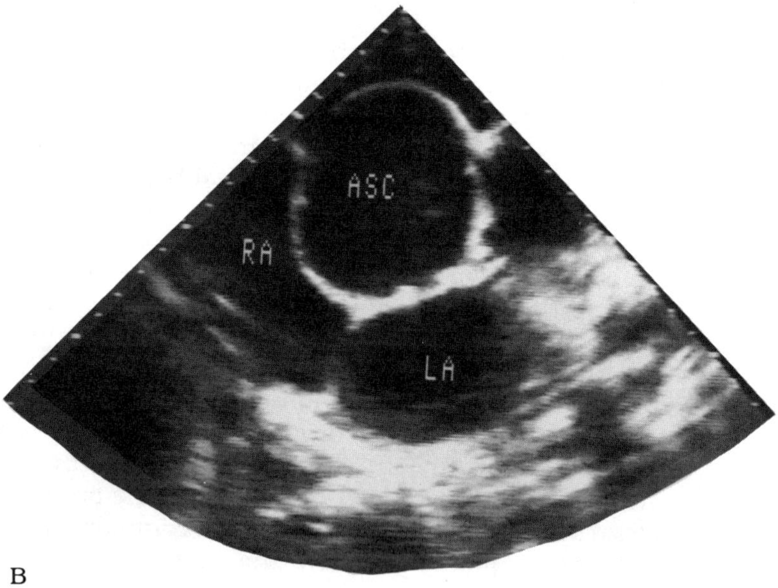

B

Figure 15.2
A. Parasternal long axis view from a patient with Marfan's syndrome. Note the extreme dilatation of the ascending aorta (ASC). The descending aorta (DSC) is also dilated. B. Parasternal short axis, and C. Suprasternal views showing the dilated ascending aorta and arch. D. M-mode recording of the aortic root, which is approximately 7 cm in diameter. MV = mitral valve, AV = aortic valve, LV = left ventricle, LA = left atrium, RA = right atrium, PA = pulmonary artery.

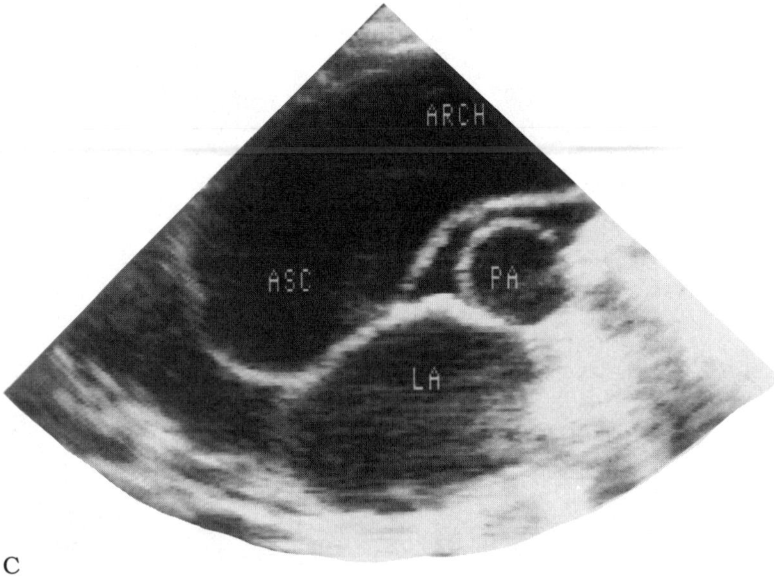

C

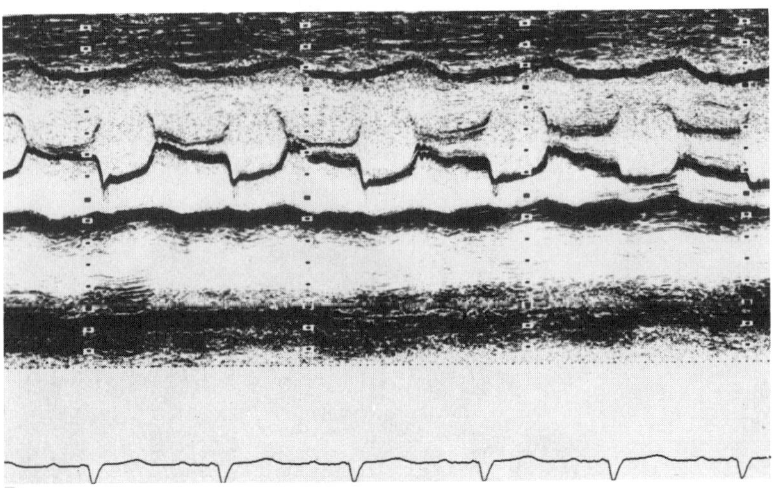

D

Figure 15.2 (Continued)

severe, arterial hypertension is not uncommon; however, because of the coarctation, the hypertension occurs only proximal to the obstruction. Thus, the blood pressure in the abdomen and lower extremities remains normal or, more commonly, diminished. The left ventricle adapts to the arterial hypertension by inducing concentric hypertrophy. There is a higher incidence of congenital bicuspid aortic valve in patients with coarctation of the aorta.

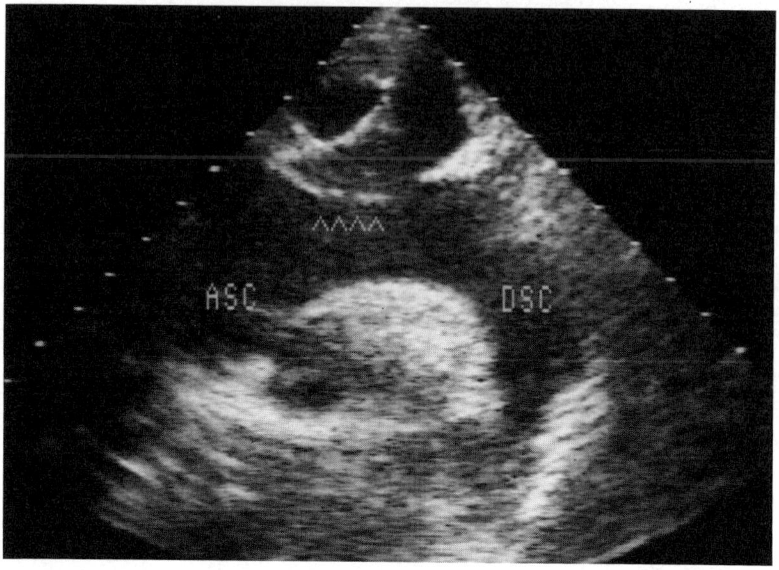

Figure 15.3
Suprasternal view from a patient with aortic dissection. Note the dilated arch with intimal flap (arrowheads). ASC = ascending aorta, DSC = descending aorta.

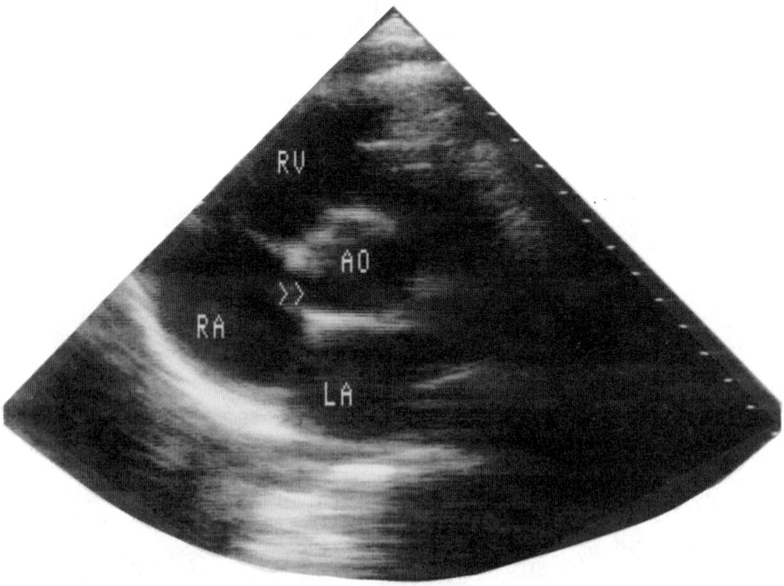

Figure 15.4
Parasternal short axis view from a patient with traumatic rupture of the right sinus of Valsalva (arrowheads), resulting in acute left-to-right shunt from the aorta (AO) to the right atrium (RA). LA = left atrium, RV = right ventricle.

Membranous supravalvular aortic stenosis is another rare congenital disease of the aorta. A membranous band of tissue may arise within the ascending aorta near the aortic valve. This anomalous tissue may cause obstruction to left ventricular ejection and will simulate aortic valvular stenosis. The aortic valve is usually normal; however, it is not uncommon to have mild aortic regurgitation due to the chronic turbulence, which ultimately leads to thickening and fibrosis of the aortic leaflets. Depending on the severity of the obstruction, compensatory left ventricular hypertrophy may occur secondary to the chronic pressure overload.

Echocardiography

Abnormal calcified deposits along the inner layers of the aortic root, as seen in patients with atherosclerosis, may produce bright echo densities.

Dilatation of the aortic root and descending aorta may be confirmed from the usual parasternal views and suprasternal approach. Occasionally, a markedly dilated ascending aorta can also be examined from a high, right parasternal view.

Establishing the diagnosis of aortic dissection is more difficult. In this context, the operator should search for the loose intimal flap, which may exhibit erratic motion relative to the wall of the aorta (Figure 15.3). Since this is a thin layer of tissue, it causes faint echoes that may be easily missed or may be confused as artifact with improper gain control settings on the ultrasound equipment. The diagnosis of aortic dissection should be confirmed by visualizing the intimal flap in at least two orthogonal views. Extension of the dissection into the aortic valve annulus may be associated with acute aortic regurgitation of various degrees of severity. Since this is rather an acute event, echocardiographic signs of aortic valve incompetence may be lacking. However, in extreme cases, one or more flail aortic valve leaflets may be observed on the echocardiogram.

Echocardiography in patients with ruptured sinus of Valsalva will demonstrate the dilatation. However, the abnormal communication caused by the ruptured sinus may not be readily apparent. In this context, a contrast echocardiographic study may demonstrate a "negative contrast effect" at the site of the left-to-right shunt.

The suprasternal view allows adequate visualization of the aortic arch and portions of the descending aorta. This is best suited to evaluate for coarctation. One may observe the dilatation of the aortic arch that suddenly decreases in diameter at the level of the coarctation. It is not unusual for patients with severe coarctation of the aorta to undergo corrective surgery during childhood. The thin narrow band at the site of coarctation is excised and the aorta is sutured again to maintain continuity of this vessel. Such patients may demonstrate bright echoes along the site of the previous surgery. However, a prosthetic conduit may be surgically inserted in some patients with severe, tunnel-like coarctation. Such conduits are occasionally identified on the echocardiogram.

A membranous supravalvular band is rarely observed on the echocardiogram; when it is severe, bright echoes may be seen along the rim of the aortic root, at the junction of the sinuses of Valsalva and the ascending aorta. The aortic dimension distal to the membranous band may be diminished.

Doppler Ultrasound

The role of Doppler ultrasound in patients with diseases of the aorta is rather limited to the identification of aortic regurgitation that commonly occurs in association with dilatation of the aortic root. In the rare patient with rupture of a sinus of Valsalva, Doppler ultrasound plays an important role in confirming the diagnosis. In this context, it is important to note that the aortic blood pressure is always higher than pressures in the right side of the heart throughout the cardiac cycle; consequently, abnormal flow patterns will be recorded in systole as well as in diastole. Depending on the site of rupture, the parasternal long axis views, as well as the short axis views, at the level of the aortic root may be utilized. Careful interrogation with the Doppler sample volume along the region of the presumed rupture will invariably detect the site of the shunt.

Doppler ultrasound may be useful in diagnosing coarctation of the aorta and establishing the severity. The suprasternal window is utilized to negotiate the Doppler ultrasound beam within the descending aorta. Increased velocities of blood flow may be recorded at the site of the coarctation. It is important to note that blood in the descending aorta flows away from the transducer. Doppler recordings will demonstrate two patterns of flow. An initial high velocity will be recorded in systole. Another high-velocity pattern will be recorded in diastole. This occurs due to the fact that blood flow distal to the coarctation is continuous throughout the cardiac cycle because of the persistent pressure gradient across the obstruction. Very high velocities across the coarctation are indicative of severe obstruction. However, in a tunnel-like obstruction, blood velocity underestimates the true gradient. Moreover, collateral blood flow may develop so that the descending aorta receives blood from collateral channels via the intercostal arteries. If this occurs, a lower pressure gradient may be recorded across the coarctation. This may further underestimate the degree of narrowing.

As with aortic valve stenosis, high velocities of blood flow will be recorded at the site of a membranous supravalvular stenosis. Since the aortic valve is not stenosed, careful PW mode Doppler recordings will demonstrate normal flow patterns at the aortic valve. It is only when the sample volume is positioned distal to the membranous band that the recorded velocity will increase. Mild aortic valve regurgitation is not uncommonly recorded by Doppler ultrasound.

16 The Heart in Systemic Disease

The heart may be affected by many systemic diseases with multiorgan involvement. Depending on the primary systemic disease, a wide spectrum of cardiac involvement may be exhibited. This varies from minimal abnormality of the heart with no clinical significance to severe abnormality whereby secondary cardiac involvement becomes life threatening. This chapter briefly discusses systemic diseases with cardiac involvement that may be detected by echocardiography.

The Heart and the Endocrine System

Diabetes Mellitus

Diabetes mellitus is a common endocrinopathy that frequently leads to heart failure. A detailed discussion of the mechanisms of cardiac involvement is beyond the scope of this book. Suffice it to mention, diabetes mellitus is a strong risk factor for coronary artery disease. When severe, it may lead to myocardial ischemia and infarction, with resulting segmental wall motion abnormalities and heart failure. The role of echocardiography in patients with coronary artery disease has already been discussed in an earlier chapter.

Occasionally, patients with diabetes mellitus present with a cardiomyopathic-like picture, diffuse hypokinesis with variable impairment of left ventricular contractile performance. This is indistinguishable from idiopathic dilated cardiomyopathy.

Hypothyroidism

Cardiac involvement in patients with hypothyroidism exhibits bradycardia with formation of pericardial effusion. Cardiac tamponade is a rare complication in hypothyroidism. Occasionally, the echocardiogram may demonstrate increased wall thickness. This represents myocardial edema and deposition of myxomatous material rather than true hypertrophy. Overall left ventricular contractility may be impaired with diffuse hypokinesis. All of these cardiac abnormalities may be reversible on treatment of this condition.

Parathyroid Disease

The parathyroid glands are important for normal metabolism of calcium. Hyperparathyroidism may alter calcium metabolism, whereby the mitral annulus is sometimes involved with excessive deposition of calcium, leading to annular calcification and various severities of associated mitral regurgitation. Moreover, calcium plays an important role in regard to myocardial contractility. In this context, the left ventricle may be hyperdynamic. On the other hand, hypoparathyroidism resulting in hypocalcemia may cause impairment of left ventricular systolic performance. Correction of the calcium blood level invariably restores normal left ventricular contractility.

Connective Tissue Diseases

Pericardial involvement is very common in a variety of connective tissue diseases, particularly rheumatoid arthritis and systemic lupus erythematosus. Pericardial effusions are rather common during active disease, and tend to disappear when the disease is controlled. Large pericardial effusions with tamponade are rare.

The coronary arteries may be involved in certain connective tissue diseases such as periarteritis nodosa and Takayasu's disease. Coronary vasculitis causing segmental involvement of the coronary arteries may result in narrowing of the vessel lumen; when the vasculitis is severe, myocardial ischemia with or without infarction may occur. Subsequently, segmental wall motion abnormalities and impaired left ventricular contractile performance may be detected on the echocardiogram. On the other hand, aneurysmal dilatation of the coronary artery may occur. Severe involvement of the proximal portions of the coronary artery may be noted on the ultrasound examination, particularly in the short axis view at the base of the heart.

Scleroderma is yet another connective tissue disease with occasional involvement of the coronary arteries that may demonstrate spasm. Myocardial infarction due to severe coronary spasm is not unusual in such patients.

Sarcoidosis may cause granuloma formation within the myocardial wall. Such myocardial involvement may cause significant abnormalities in cardiac rhythm. However, echocardiographic detection of these granulomas is very rare.

A rare cardiac complication of patients with systemic lupus erythematosus involves the mitral valve, whereby sterile, nonbacterial wartlike lesions may arise. These are commonly referred to as Libman-Sacks verrucae. The echocardiographic appearance of these vegetations is indistinguishable from the appearance of typical bacterial endocarditis, although the sterile vegetations are usually smaller.

Pulmonary involvement in connective tissue disease may lead to various degrees of pulmonary hypertension with secondary effects on the right chambers of the heart. These lead to hypertrophy or dilatation, or both, with tricuspid and pulmonic regurgitation.

Renal Disorders

Diseases of the kidneys affect the heart through many different mechanisms. Renal failure may alter adequate handling of salt and water. This results in systemic hypertension with secondary left ventricular hypertrophy. When the blood pressure is acutely elevated to dangerous levels, heart failure and acute pulmonary edema may occur. Electrolyte imbalance, primarily acidosis, causes generalized hypokinesia of the cardiac muscle with impaired contractile performance. This is usually reversible on control of the electrolyte abnormality. In addition to all of the cardiac complications just mentioned, end-stage renal failure causes accumulation of toxic metabolites that further worsen myocardial contractility. Moreover, calcium metabolism is impaired so that calcification of the mitral annulus may occur. Improvement of left ventricular function has been noted following renal dialysis of patients with end-stage renal failure. Finally, pericarditis with moderate to large pericardial effusions and, occasionally, tamponade are not uncommon in such patients.

Echocardiography may detect most of the cardiac abnormalities in patients with end-stage renal failure and can document improvement following dialysis. Typically, there is significant left ventricular hypertrophy with variable degrees of impairment of its contractile performance. The cardiac chambers may be slightly dilated. The myocardium may demonstrate a sparkling appearance almost similar to that seen in patients with cardiac amyloidosis. Pericardial effusion is frequent. Mitral annular calcification is very common. Doppler ultrasound may demonstrate mild to moderate mitral regurgitation that is commonly associated with mitral annular calcification. Regurgitation of other cardiac valves is not uncommon as well. In addition, abnormal lipid metabolism may occur in patients with chronic renal failure. This may lead to coronary artery disease with myocardial ischemia or infarction.

Hematologic Disorders

Chronic severe anemia, whether congenital or acquired, causes volume overload on the heart. This is most evident in patients with sickle-cell disease. The left ventricle may be dilated as well as hypertrophied with preserved contractile performance. Because of the abnormal aggregation of red blood cells in patients with sickle-cell disease, small myocardial infarctions have been noted in some patients. Systolic murmurs are not unusual in patients with severe, chronic anemia. This is related to the increased cardiac output and the associated increase of transvalvular flow rates. In this context, Doppler ultrasound demonstrates slightly elevated velocities of blood flow, commensurate with the increase in the cardiac output. Valvular regurgitation is infrequent. Sickle cell anemia may cause microinfarctions in the pulmonary circulation. This may lead to pulmonary hypertension and secondary effects on the right heart chambers.

Neoplastic Disorders

The heart is a common site of metastasis of various neoplastic disorders. Pericardial metastasis is most frequently observed with resultant pericardial effusions and intrapericardial tumor invasion. Intracardiac and intramyocardial tumor metastasis may also occur. This is discussed in more detail in Chapter 14.

17 Effect of Altered Rhythm or Conduction Abnormalities on the Doppler Echocardiogram

Abnormalities in rhythm as well as abnormal sequence of cardiac muscle activation result in characteristic changes of the motion patterns noted on the M-mode echocardiogram. It is important to note that these changes are often easier to detect on the M-mode echocardiogram because of its rapid sampling rate. Similar changes may be noted on the two-dimensional echocardiogram, but are less obvious because of the relatively slow sampling rate. Moreover, abnormalities in cardiac rhythm are frequently associated with changes in blood flow patterns across the cardiac valves. These changes are easily noted on the Doppler velocity recordings as well.

Abnormal Atrial Activation

Sinus Bradycardia and Tachycardia

Very slow sinus rhythm causes prolongation of diastole. This is largely reflected in a long diastasis interval. Following the E point on the M-mode echocardiogram, the mitral leaflets drift toward each other into a more neutral position. The leaflets may remain parallel to each other and occasionally exhibit undulating motion. Atrial contraction, toward the end of such a diastolic cycle, forces the leaflet to open, thus producing a distinct A wave (Figure 17.1). On the other hand, sinus tachycardia causes significant shortening of diastole. Diastasis is markedly abbreviated, or in most cases, is completely absent. Consequently, the A wave approaches

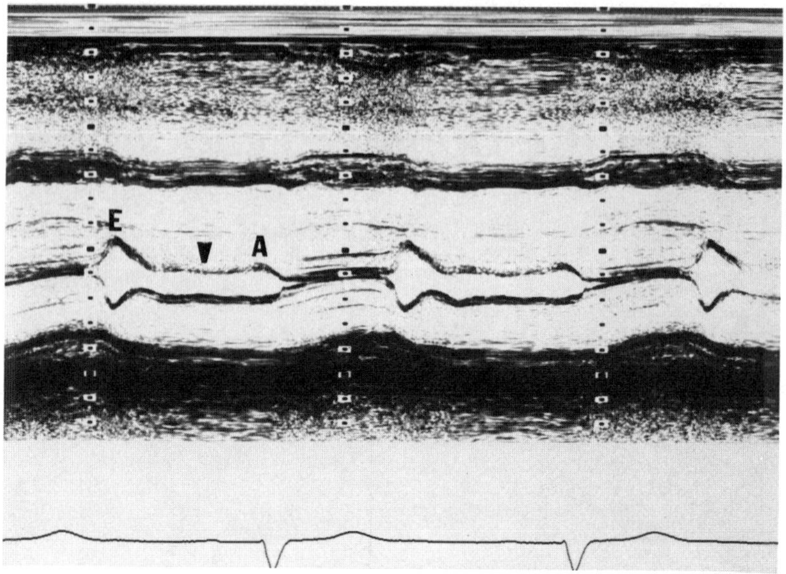

A

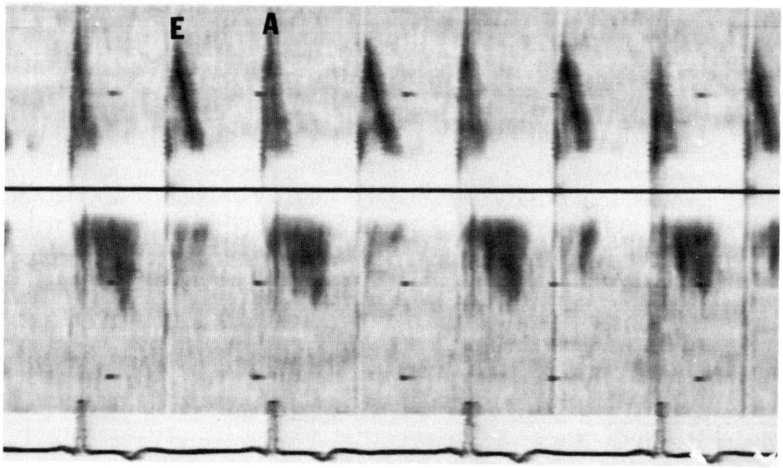

B

Figure 17.1
A. M-mode recording of the mitral valve in severe sinus bradycardia. Note the long diastasis (arrowhead). B. Doppler recording of mitral flow in sinus bradycardia. Note the absence of flow during mid-diastole, in diastasis.

the E point, and many times, both waves merge together (Figure 17.2).

Doppler recordings of transmitral flow reflect similar changes as noted on the M-mode echocardiogram. In sinus bradycardia, blood flow occurs only during early diastole and after the atrial kick. There is usually no flow during the long

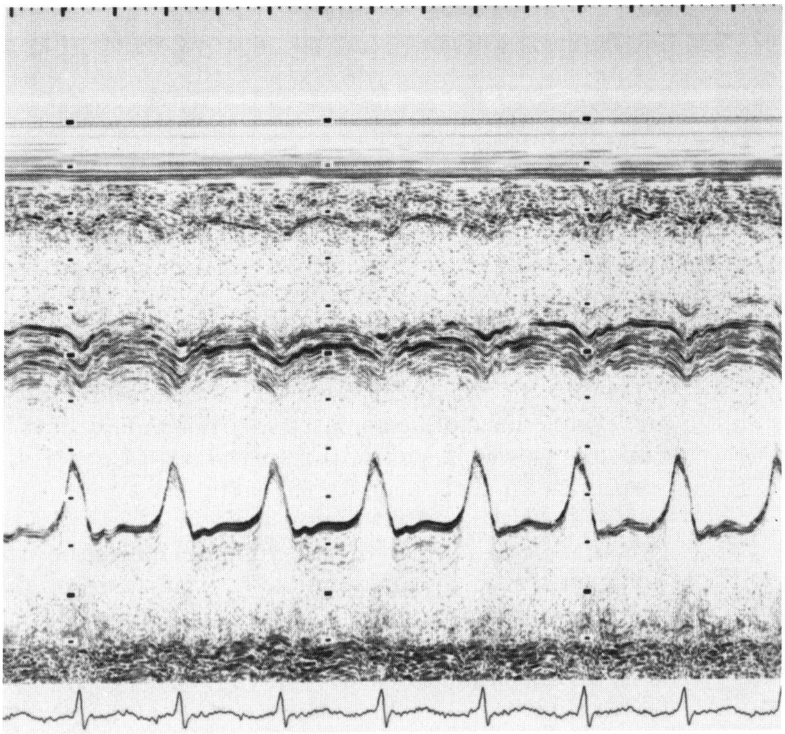

A

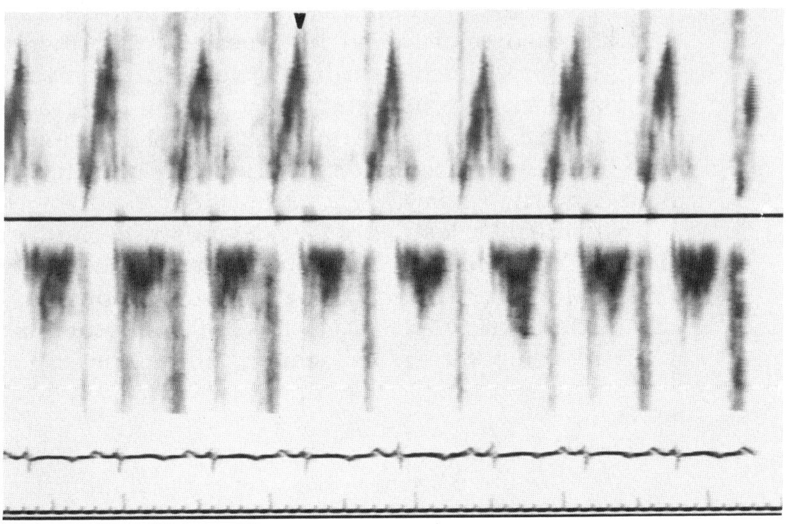

B

Figure 17.2

A. M-mode recording of the mitral valve in sinus tachycardia. Diastasis is absent, with merger of the E and A waves into a single waveform. B. Doppler recording of mitral flow in sinus tachycardia. Similar to the M-mode recording, the E and A velocities have merged into a single flow pattern (arrowhead). Flow in the left ventricular outflow tract in systole is also noted on this recording, away from the transducer.

period of diastasis. Sinus tachycardia may cause merging of the early and late diastolic flow velocities (Figures 17.1, 17.2).

Premature Atrial Contraction

Premature atrial contraction is a frequent atrial arrhythmia whereby a premature atrial activation causes atrial contraction that interrupts the normal sinus rhythm. Premature depolarization of the sinus node causes a brief pause of its electrical activity so that the onset of the next cardiac cycle is delayed.

Premature atrial contraction that occurs during ventricular systole is not associated with any echocardiographic finding. However, premature atrial contraction in diastole results in an early occurrence of the A wave on the M-mode recording of the anterior mitral valve leaflet. A very premature atrial contraction in early diastole may superimpose the A wave on the E point, similar to that observed during extreme sinus tachycardia. This occurs for one beat only. This short diastolic cycle causes reduction of ventricular filling with an associated decrease in the force of ventricular contraction in systole. The subsequent diastolic period may be associated with diminished opening of the mitral valve, probably related to abnormally elevated left ventricular diastolic pressure following the premature contraction. However, the first normal cardiac cycle is invariably associated with a more forceful ventricular systolic contraction. The mitral valve opening during the diastolic period following this forceful ventricular contraction may exhibit an exaggerated E point.

Transmitral velocities of flow demonstrate similar changes noted for mitral valve motion on the M-mode echocardiogram. Moreover, transaortic velocities of flow may demonstrate diminished velocities for the premature beat, with higher velocity for the subsequent normal beat.

Atrial Fibrillation

The rhythm abnormality called atrial fibrillation refers to the chaotic depolarization of the atrial muscle fibers with corresponding irregular activation of the ventricles. The ECG demonstrates normal QRS deflections that occur at irregular and unpredictable intervals. The P wave is lost because of the lack of synchronous electrical activation of the atria. These changes are reflected on the M-mode echocardiogram, which typically shows the erratic timing of ventricular contractions. There is no A wave on the mitral valve echocardiogram. Following the E point, the mitral leaflets drift toward

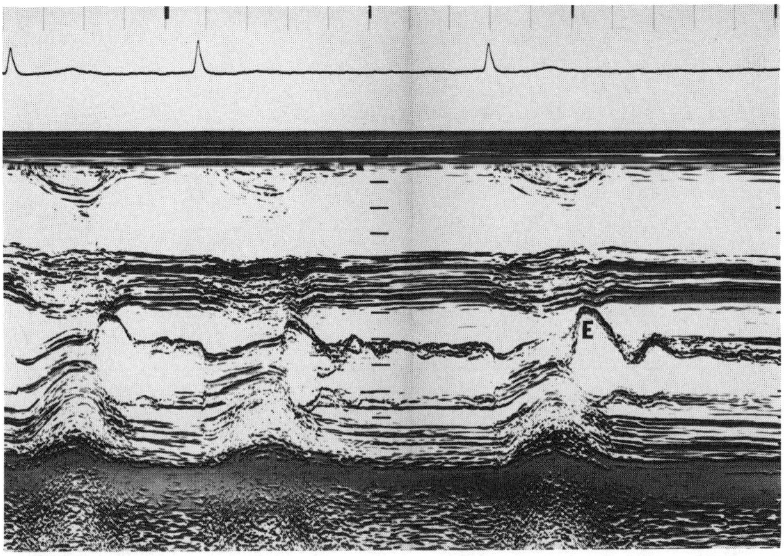

Figure 17.3
M-mode of the mitral valve in atrial fibrillation. Note the irregular cardiac rhythm. Only the E point is identifiable, followed by undulating motion of the mitral valve with no A wave.

each other and may exhibit a fine undulating motion that persists until the next systolic cycle, when ventricular contraction causes mitral valve closure (Figure 17.3).

Because of the irregular rate of ventricular contractions, there is a beat-to-beat variation in the duration of diastole. A short diastolic cycle allows little time for ventricular filling. The subsequent ventricular contraction is diminished and commonly associated with decreased stroke volume and reduced opening of the aortic valve, whereas a long diastolic cycle allows adequate ventricular filling. This is followed by a more forceful ventricular contraction, higher stroke volume, and wider aortic leaflet separation.

Doppler recordings of transmitral flow demonstrate normal velocity in early diastole with rapid deceleration afterward. The absence of any effective atrial contraction during atrial fibrillation is reflected by the loss of the normal increase of transmitral flow in late diastole (Figure 17.4). During the long diastolic cycle, there is significant reduction of transmitral flow in late diastole because of equilibration of atrial and ventricular pressures. Hence, Doppler recordings may detect flow in early diastole only.

Atrial Flutter

The rate of atrial contraction during atrial flutter is very rapid and approaches 300 contractions/min. However, be-

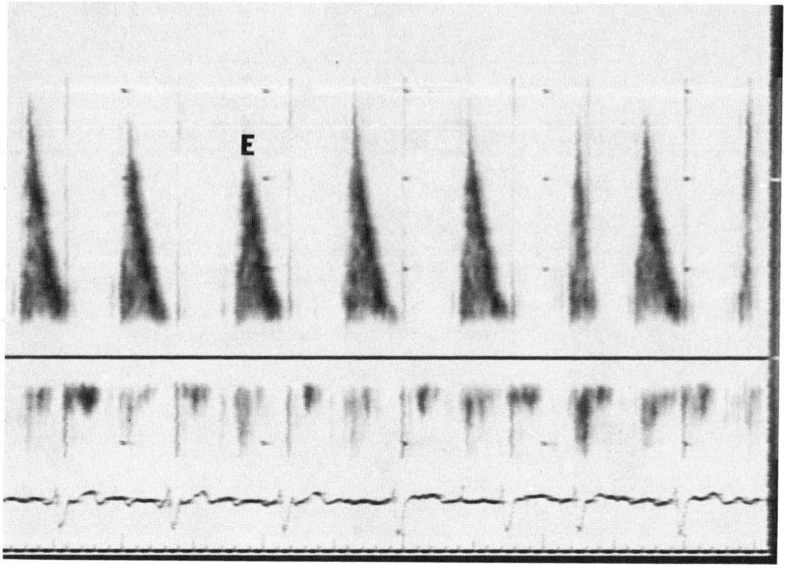

Figure 17.4
Doppler recording of mitral flow from a patient with atrial fibrillation. Note the erratic timing of ventricular contraction. Only the E velocity is noted; the A velocity is absent. Peak E velocity is variable, hence reflecting the variable degrees of left ventricular filling from one cardiac cycle to another.

cause of the limited conduction ability of the atrioventricular node, the ventricular rate rarely exceeds 150 beats/min. Medical therapy may even cause a slow ventricular rate, which is irregular at times. The ECG demonstrates frequent F waves (called flutter waves) with the intermittent QRS complexes. Each atrial activation is associated with an atrial contraction; thus, the M-mode recording of the mitral valve typically demonstrates multiple A waves that are best appreciated during long diastolic cycles (Figure 17.5).

Each atrial contraction in atrial flutter forces more blood

Figure 17.5
A. M-mode recording of the mitral valve during atrial flutter. This patient was taking medications that slowed the ventricular response, causing long diastolic intervals during which the flutter waves (F) were clearly evident on the mitral valve motion, and were intermittently interrupted during ventricular systole. B. The effect of the atrial flutter on the left ventricular M-mode recording was evident in this patient. Each flutter wave is associated with an indentation on the interventricular septum and left ventricular posterior wall (PW) (arrowheads). C. Doppler recording at a paper speed of 100 mm/sec from a patient with mitral stenosis and atrial flutter. Note the intermittent increase of the velocity of flow (arrowheads) during the flutter waves.

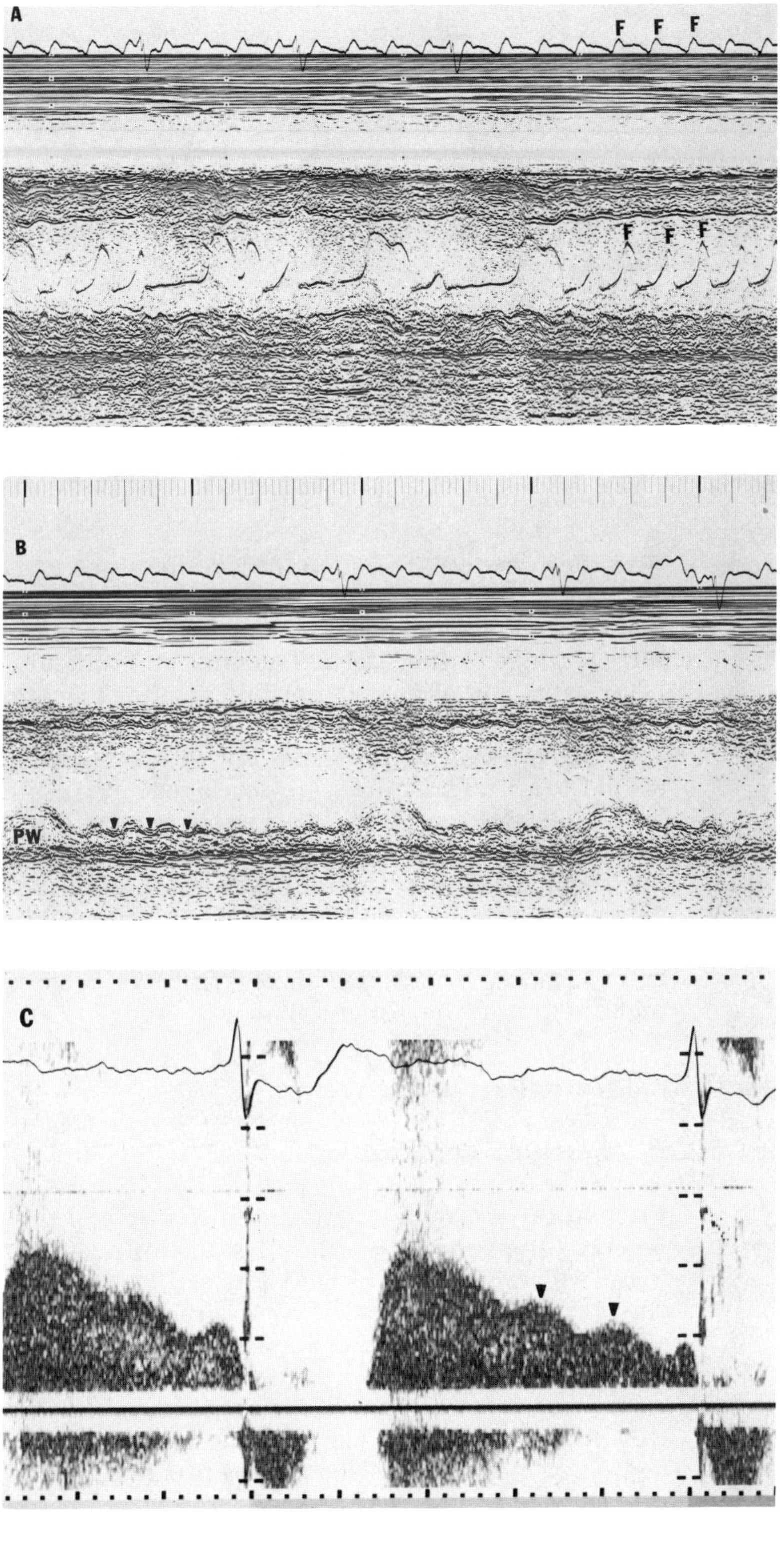
A
F F F
F F F
B
PW
C

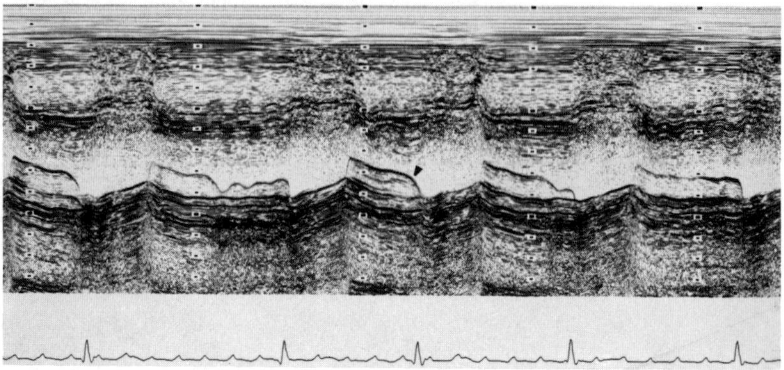

Figure 17.6
Abnormal motion of the prosthetic disc in the mitral valve position is caused by the abnormal cardiac rhythm with atrial flutter. Note the undulating motion of the disc with rounded contour in late diastole (arrowhead). See text for detail.

into the ventricle. Thus, similar to the mitral recording on M-mode echocardiography, Doppler recordings of transmitral flow will demonstrate multiple peaks in the velocity patterns with each effective atrial contraction (Figure 17.5C).

Occasionally, abnormal cardiac rhythm in patients with prosthetic valves may falsely suggest malfunction of the valve. This was evident in a patient with a disc valve prosthesis in the mitral position, who developed atrial flutter (Figure 17.6). The motion of the disc was irregular during a long diastolic cycle, with rounded contour of the disc motion in late diastole. This is thought to be secondary to the flutter waves with relative equilibration of left atrial and ventricular pressures in late diastole, hence reducing the velocity of valve closure. There was no evidence of prosthetic valve malfunction in the patient shown in Figure 17.6.

Abnormal Ventricular Activation

Premature Ventricular Contractions

Premature ventricular contraction is a frequent arrhythmia whereby the ventricular stimulus to contract starts from a focus within the right or left ventricle. This is in contrast to the normal activation of the ventricles when the stimulus for ventricular contraction originates from the sinus node in the right atrium and propagates via the atrioventricular node.

A premature ventricular contraction interrupts the preceding diastolic cycle. This causes premature closure of the mitral valve before the onset of the A wave on the M-mode recording. The force of ventricular contraction during this premature beat is usually diminished. This is commonly associated with reduced opening of the aortic valve. A very premature ventricular contraction may be so weak that the aortic valve may not open at all. The long diastolic cycle that follows this premature ventricular contraction may exhibit reduced opening of the mitral valve, probably secondary to abnormal diastolic pressure. However, in most cases, the subsequent normal ventricular contraction is more forceful as compared to other normal beats (Figure 17.7). The Doppler recordings of mitral and aortic velocities usually reflect the hemodynamic alterations described already (Figure 17.7). Transaortic velocity immediately after the premature ventricular contraction is diminished, and the subsequent normal contraction exhibits a much higher aortic velocity.

When the left ventricle is electrically stimulated through the normal pattern via the atrioventricular node, the normal propagation sequence of myocardial activation causes synchronized activation of the interventricular septum and posterior wall. However, during a premature ventricular contraction, the ectopic origin of the electrical stimulus results in an abnormal contraction sequence. This is frequently observed on the M-mode recording whereby paradoxical motion of the interventricular septum is noted. The interventricular septum typically moves anteriorly during systole, with exaggerated posterior notching in early diastole.

Left Bundle Branch Block

Diseases of the electrical conduction system of the heart may predispose an abnormal sequence of left ventricular activation. This is commonly associated with abnormal contraction patterns that can be recorded on the echocardiogram. Left bundle branch block commonly causes abnormal ventricular activation similar to that observed in ventricular premature contraction, as just described. Paradoxical or atypical interventricular septal motion is frequently observed (Figure 17.8). The interventricular septum demonstrates flattened motion during systole with occasional exaggerated notching. Usually, the motions of the mitral and aortic valves remain normal. Systolic thickening of the interventricular septum may be preserved. The sequence of mechanical contraction of the left ventricle is usually normal in patients with right bundle branch block who have no demonstrable echocardiographic abnormalities.

Atrioventricular Conduction Abnormalities

The normal sequence of atrial and ventricular contraction is separated by a physiologic delay at the atrioventricular node.

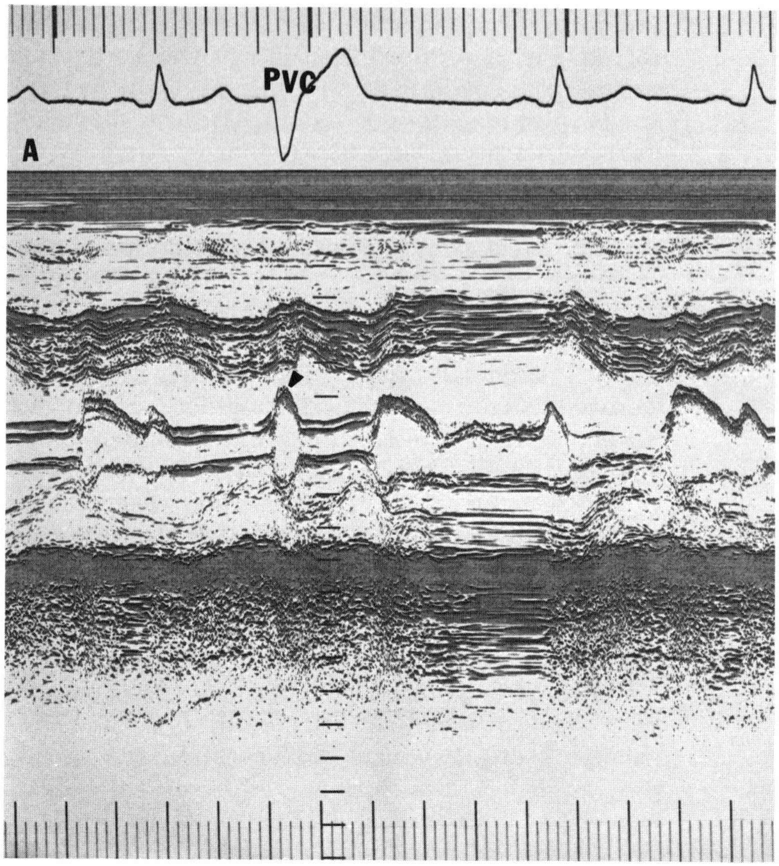
PVC
A

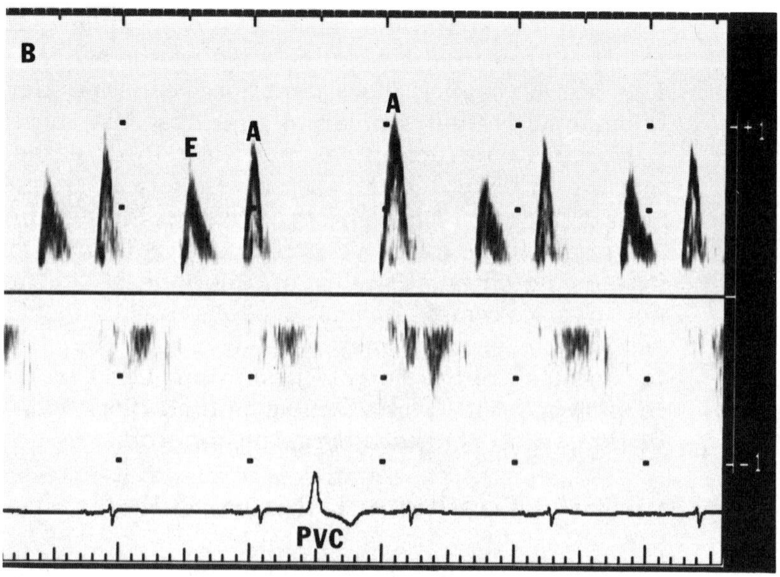
B
E
A
A
PVC

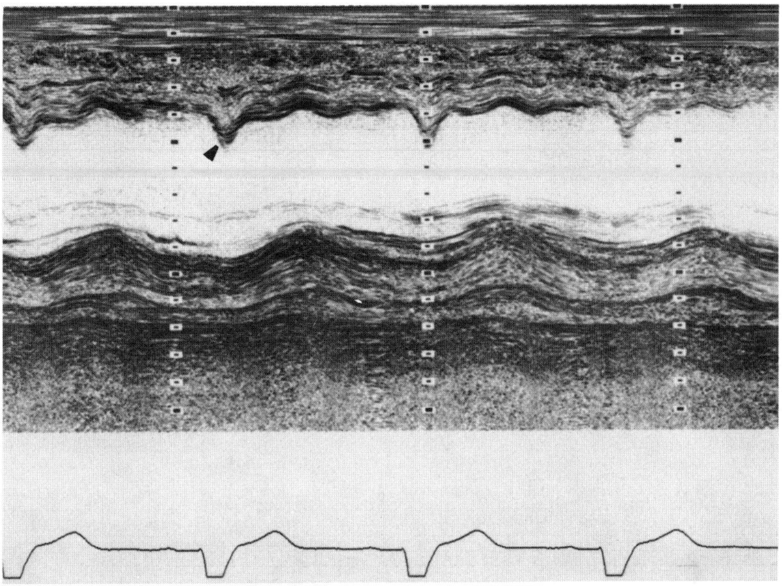

Figure 17.8
Left bundle branch block with prolonged QRS interval on the ECG. Note the abnormal motion of the interventricular septum with notching (arrowhead).

This is reflected on the ECG as the time interval between the P wave and the onset of the QRS deflection, commonly referred to as the PR interval. Diseases of the atrioventricular node may lead to delayed propagation of the electrical activity to the ventricles. This results in prolongation of the PR interval. Higher degrees of atrioventricular nodal disease may cause intermittent or, at times, complete interruption of transmission of the electrical activity to the ventricles.

First-Degree Atrioventricular Block

First-degree atrioventricular block occurs when there is prolongation of the PR interval. This is reflected on the M-mode echocardiogram; the onset of ventricular contraction is delayed relative to the A wave on the mitral valve recording. A markedly prolonged PR interval allows equilibration of atrial

---

Figure 17.7
A. A premature ventricular contraction (PVC) caused premature closure of the mitral valve (arrowhead) with a subsequent long diastolic cycle. B. Depending on when the premature ventricular contraction (PVC) occurs in diastole, transmitral flow will vary. In this example, the E velocity is absent in the diastolic cycle immediately after the premature contraction. Only the A velocity is present, and is exaggerated.

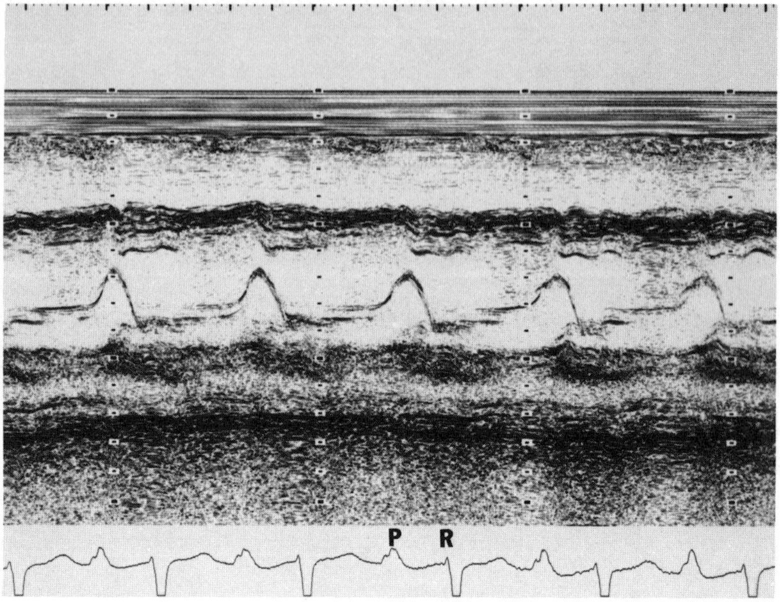

Figure 17.9
The E and A waves are merged together in this M-mode recording from a patient with first-degree atrioventricular block. Note the prolonged PR interval.

and ventricular pressures in late diastole. This may cause premature closure of the mitral valve before the onset of the next ventricular systole. Occasionally, a B wave may be noted on the M-mode recording. In this context, the B wave does not necessarily reflect an abnormally elevated left ventricular end diastolic pressure. Occasionally, marked prolongation of the PR interval may lead to merger of the E and A waves on the M-mode recording (Figure 17.9). Doppler recordings of mitral flow show similar variations as noted on the M-mode echocardiogram.

Second-Degree Atrioventricular Block

More severe atrioventricular nodal disease may lead to intermittent interruption of propagation of the electrical stimulus from the atria to the ventricles. Thus, a P wave may be recorded on the ECG and is not followed by a QRS complex. This results in a longer diastole. Such nonconducted P waves are associated with an extra A wave on the M-mode recording of the ventricle in mid-diastole. The mitral valve may close in mid-diastole only to reopen when the next P wave and atrial contraction occur.

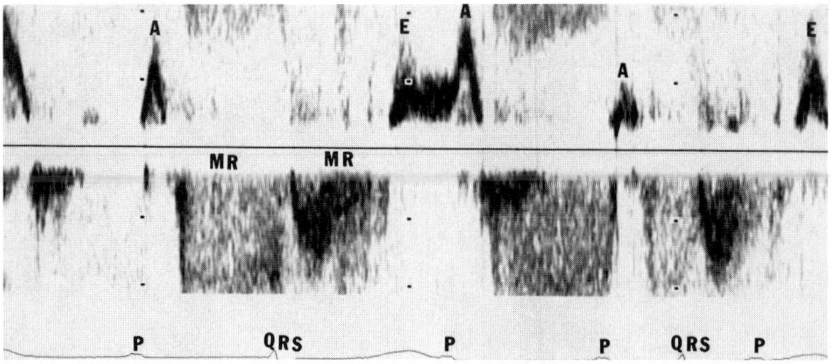

Figure 17.10
Effect of third-degree atrioventricular block on the Doppler mitral flow pattern. Forward mitral flow is chaotic with variable intervals between the E and A velocities, depending on the relative timing of ventricular and atrial contractions, which are independent of each other. Note the relation of atrial contraction (P) and ventricular contraction (QRS). This tracing also demonstrates mitral regurgitation (MR) in diastole as well as in systole.

Third-Degree Atrioventricular Block

High-grade disease of the atrioventricular node causes complete interruption of the normal propagation of electrical activity to the ventricles. Subsequently, atrial and ventricular contractions become completely independent of each other. Usually, the ventricular rate is much slower than the atrial rate. Ventricular contraction could be governed by a slow ectopic focus in the ventricles. Such contractions would simulate premature ventricular beats on the M-mode echocardiogram. Mitral valve motion would be chaotic because of the irregular timing of onset of A wave, which may occasionally occur too early in diastole and merge with the E point. The associated Doppler recordings of mitral flow will demonstrate similar chaotic velocity patterns with variable peak velocities, depending on the timing of onset of atrial contractions in diastole (Figure 17.10). Because of the relatively slow ventricular rate, diastole is markedly prolonged. Equilibration of atrial and ventricular pressures, in between atrial contractions, causes complete cessation of flow. In fact, it is not unusual for mild mitral regurgitant flow to be detected by Doppler ultrasound during such long diastolic cycles (Figure 17.10). Because of the irregular rate of ventricular filling, variable ventricular emptying in systole may cause variable velocities of flow across the aortic valve.

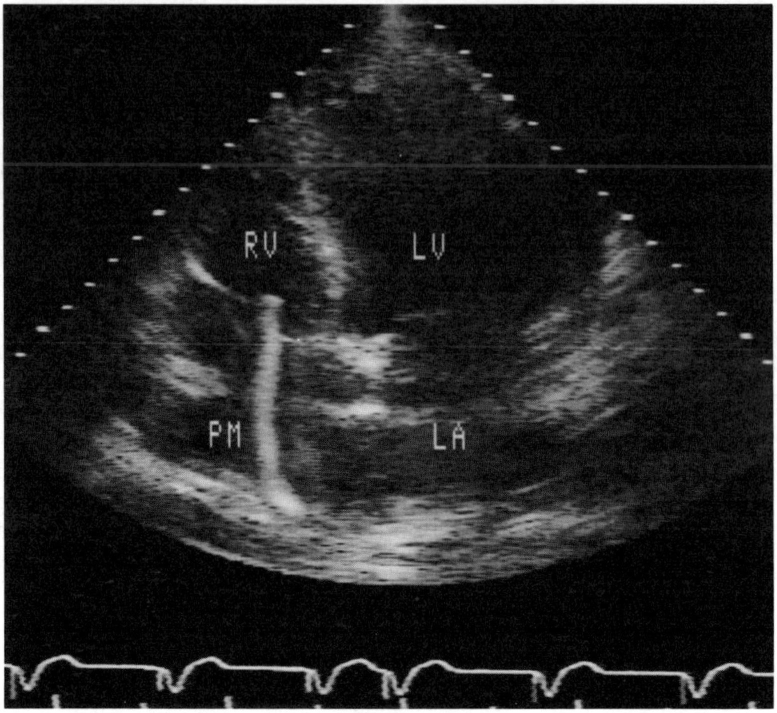

Figure 17.11
Apical four-chamber view showing a pacemaker electrode (PM) across the right atrium going into the right ventricle (RV). LA = left atrium, LV = left ventricle.

Ventricular Pacing

Echocardiograms and Doppler ultrasound recordings are frequently performed on patients with pacemakers. Ventricular pacing is most often performed through special electrodes introduced into the right ventricle (Figure 17.11). Ventricular pacing causes typical electrical deflection on the ECG. Because electrical stimulation of the left ventricle originates from within the right ventricle, it is very common to note abnormal or paradoxical motion of the interventricular septum (Figure 17.12). Intermittent normal activation of the left ventricle may occur. During such normal beats, interventricular septal motion may be normal or may reflect any intrinsic cardiac pathologic condition if present.

It is very important to know whether or not ventricular pacing is synchronized with the atrial rhythm. Atrioventricular sequential pacing with synchronized atrial and ventricular contractions will simulate left bundle branch block with sinus rhythm on the echocardiogram. However, ventricular

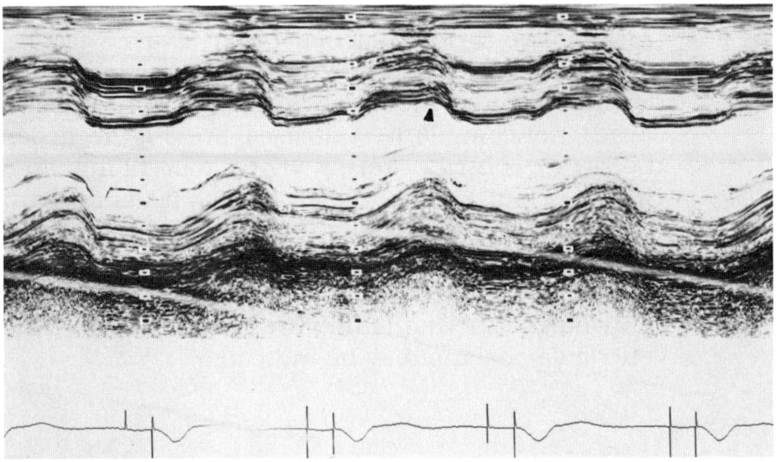

Figure 17.12
M-mode recording of the left ventricle during atrioventricular sequential pacing. Note the paradoxical motion with systolic thickening of the interventricular septum (arrowhead). Atrial and ventricular pacemaker depolarizations are noted on ECG.

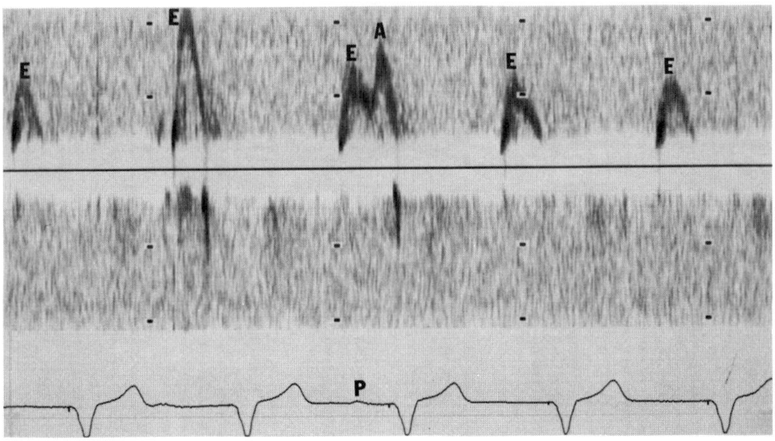

Figure 17.13
Variable transmitral flow patterns are noted in a patient with ventricular pacing and lack of synchronous atrioventricular contraction. Coincidental atrial contraction prior to the third ventricular paced beat (P) simulates a normal transmitral flow pattern.

pacing without atrial synchronization leads to variable motion of the mitral valve on the echocardiogram that is very similar to the patterns noted for third-degree atrioventricular block as described already (Figure 17.13).

Doppler ultrasound has been advocated as a valuable method to study the effect of synchronized atrial and ventricular pacing.

Asynchronous atrioventricular contractions, as noted in third-degree atrioventricular block, cause variable left ventricular filling. A normally functioning ventricle is not very dependent on adequate atrial contraction. In contrast, diseased, noncompliant ventricles are highly dependent on the atrial contribution to ventricular filling. In such patients, loss of an effective atrial kick leads to a drop in cardiac output. The demonstration of a significant difference in transaortic velocities of flow between synchronous and asynchronous atrial and ventricular pacing suggests that ventricular function is impaired, and that sequential atrioventricular pacing may be indicated.

III Doppler/Echocardiographic Applications in Cardiac Diagnosis and Management

18 Heart Failure: Finding the Cause

The heart functions as a pump to circulate blood. Oxygenated blood, returning from the lungs, is pumped by the left chambers of the heart to the peripheral tissues. And, venous blood, returning from the peripheral tissues, is pumped by the right chambers into the lungs to be oxygenated. From a clinical standpoint, heart failure denotes the inability of the heart to function as an effective pump in circulating blood between the lungs and the peripheral tissues. Common clinical symptoms of heart failure include edema (swelling of the tissues, mainly in the legs), shortness of breath, weakness, and exercise intolerance. However, such symptoms may be noted in other diseases as well. One or more of such symptoms may be present at any point in time. In general, whenever such symptoms are present, indications of cardiac dysfunction may be expected on the echocardiogram. However, it is important to note that clinical evidence of heart failure may not be readily apparent despite the presence of significant cardiac dysfunction. This is because in the early stages of disease, the heart undergoes adaptive mechanisms to adjust to the disease process and continues to pump adequate blood to the tissues. It is only with advanced disease that these adaptive mechanisms fail and clinical symptoms of heart failure ensue. Moreover, current advances in cardiac diagnosis and treatment with medications or surgery significantly alter the clinical condition, so that symptoms of heart failure may be lacking, despite the continued presence of cardiac dysfunction. Hence, it is not uncommon to realize a discrepancy between the severity of heart failure on the echocardiogram and the corresponding severity of symptoms. Occasionally, the opposite situation may be encountered, whereby symptoms of heart failure are noted despite apparently normal cardiac function on the echocardiogram.

There are four general mechanisms that may lead to clinical heart failure.

1. Impaired systolic contraction, such as dilated cardiomyopathy or coronary artery disease with myocardial infarction;
2. Impaired diastolic relaxation, such as hypertrophic cardiomyopathy or any other condition associated with significant left ventricular hypertrophy;
3. Pressure overload, such as severe aortic valvular stenosis or severe uncontrolled systemic hypertension;
4. Volume overload, such as severe mitral or aortic valvular regurgitation or congenital heart disease with large intracardiac shunt.

At any one time, one or more of these mechanisms may lead to heart failure. The echocardiographic and cardiac Doppler evaluation of the patient with heart failure should be directed to search for any such mechanisms of heart failure, and answer all of the following questions:

1. What are the mechanisms of heart failure in the particular patient being examined?
2. Are any of those mechanisms severe enough to cause heart failure?
3. If more than one mechanism is identified, which one is the main factor in causing the failure?
4. What are the associated mechanisms that alter the severity of failure symptoms?

A brief review of the mechanisms of heart failure shall be followed by hypothetical case presentations to illustrate the approach to find the cause of heart failure.

Impaired Systolic Contraction (Table 18.1)

Impaired systolic contraction is the most common mechanism encountered in heart failure. Impaired systolic contractility reduces the volume of blood ejected in systole (stroke volume) and the total cardiac output. During exercise, the diseased ventricle may not be able to meet the increased demand for oxygen and cardiac output by the

Table 18.1
Common causes of impaired systolic contraction

Left ventricle	Right ventricle
Coronary artery disease	Coronary artery disease
Dilated cardiomyopathy	Pulmonary hypertension
Myocarditis	Advanced pressure overload
Diabetes mellitus	Advanced volume overload
End-stage renal disease	
Other metabolic diseases	
Advanced pressure overload	
Advanced volume overload	

exercising muscles. Hence, shortness of breath and exercise intolerance ensue. Moreover, impaired systolic contraction is frequently complicated by elevated diastolic pressure. Elevation of left ventricular diastolic pressure is associated with elevation of left atrial pressure and congestion of the pulmonary veins and lungs. This contributes to the shortness of breath. On the other hand, elevation of right atrial pressure impedes venous return and causes peripheral edema. These diastolic pressures are further elevated during exercise, resulting in further worsening of heart failure symptoms during physical exertion.

Typical echocardiographic findings of left ventricular failure include various degrees of chamber dilatation with reduced systolic excursion of the ventricular wall and diminished fraction of shortening and ejection fraction. If left ventricular failure is secondary to coronary artery disease and myocardial infarction, segmental wall motion abnormalities may be noted, whereby reduced systolic excursion will be more prominent in the infarcted segments of the left ventricle. The remaining segments of the left ventricle may exhibit normal systolic thickening and excursion, and at times, this will be hyperdynamic, as a compensatory and adaptive response to maintain adequate cardiac output (Figure 6.1). Patients with significant coronary artery disease without myocardial infarction may present with intermittent heart failure. This is probably related to transient relative decrease of oxygen supply to the left ventricle (ischemia), resulting in transient contraction abnormality, as well as impaired relaxation. In this context, an echocardiogram, performed with the patient at rest and at a point in time remote from the ischemic episode, may not demonstrate any significant left ventricular dysfunction. Such patients are best evaluated noninvasively by performing the echocardiogram while the patient exercises. It has been clearly shown that exercise echocardiography frequently uncovers abnormal wall motion and left ventricular dysfunction in patients with significant coronary artery disease and normal left ventricular function at rest.

The echocardiographic signs of right ventricular failure include dilatation of this chamber with impaired systolic contraction of the right ventricular anterior free wall. Depending on the status of the left ventricular function, abnormal motion of the interventricular septum may be noted as well. Dilatation of the right atrium and inferior vena cava with various degrees of tricuspid regurgitation is frequently encountered.

Impaired Diastolic Relaxation (Table 18.2)

Diastolic relaxation of the left and right ventricles allows expansion of ventricular volumes with blood flowing through the atrioventricular valves. This extra blood is accumulated in the ventricles during diastole, and is ejected into the great vessels in systole. Hence, any condition that prevents adequate ventricular relaxation results in relative decrease in diastolic filling with a net result of decrease of stroke volume ejected in systole, decreasing cardiac output and leading to heart failure. Furthermore, impairment of ventricular filling leads to secondary elevation of pressure in the atria. Similar to elevated atrial pressure due to systolic dysfunc-

Table 18.2
Common causes of impaired diastolic relaxation

A. Coronary artery disease
   1. Ischemia
   2. Infarction
B. Cardiac tamponade
C. Constrictive pericarditis
D. Restrictive cardiomyopathy
E. Significant left ventricular hypertrophy
   1. Hypertrophic cardiomyopathy
   2. Hypertensive heart disease
   3. Aortic valve stenosis
F. Extrinsic cardiac compression

tion, pulmonary congestion, peripheral edema, or both, are frequently encountered. During exercise, such symptoms of heart failure are worsened due to progressive increase in diastolic filling pressures and inability to increase the cardiac output. Finally, increased heart rate during exercise leads to significant decrease in the duration of diastole. This further reduces ventricular filling and limits the increase in stroke volume and cardiac output.

Echocardiographic features of impaired diastolic relaxation are variable, depending on the primary disease process. The most obvious findings may be seen in patients with cardiac tamponade (Chapter 13) with large pericardial effusion. Other echocardiographic features of impaired diastolic relaxation include a prominent A wave and occasional B wave on the M-mode recordings of the mitral valve (Figure 6.7). The prominent A wave signifies a forceful atrial contraction to force blood into a noncompliant ventricle. The B wave reflects elevated diastolic filling pressure. The Doppler recording of transmitral flow frequently demonstrates a prominent velocity after atrial contraction (A) higher than the early diastolic velocity (E). It has been suggested that the ratio of E/A less than unity may be consistent with impaired diastolic relaxation of the left ventricle (Figure 18.1). However, this finding is frequently noted in elderly normal subjects. Variations in preload, afterload, and associated valvular pathologic states significantly alter the E/A ratio so that this abnormality is not consistently observed in patients with suspected impaired diastolic relaxation.

Other echocardiographic features of impaired diastolic relaxation may be easily overlooked. Some subtle findings include:

1. Decreased rate of left ventricular filling, as evident by flattened motion of left ventricular posterior wall in diastole due to lack of adequate filling;
2. Diminished rate of wall thinning in early diastole with relatively slow return of left ventricular posterior wall to its presystolic dimension due to slow relaxation;
3. Prolonged isovolumic relaxation time (Figure 1.7) due to a relatively slow decline of left ventricular pressure at end systole;
4. Reduced rate of change of left ventricular volume in early diastole.

Unfortunately, most of these parameters are not consistently observed in patients with suspected impaired diastolic relaxation, and several parameters necessitate the use of

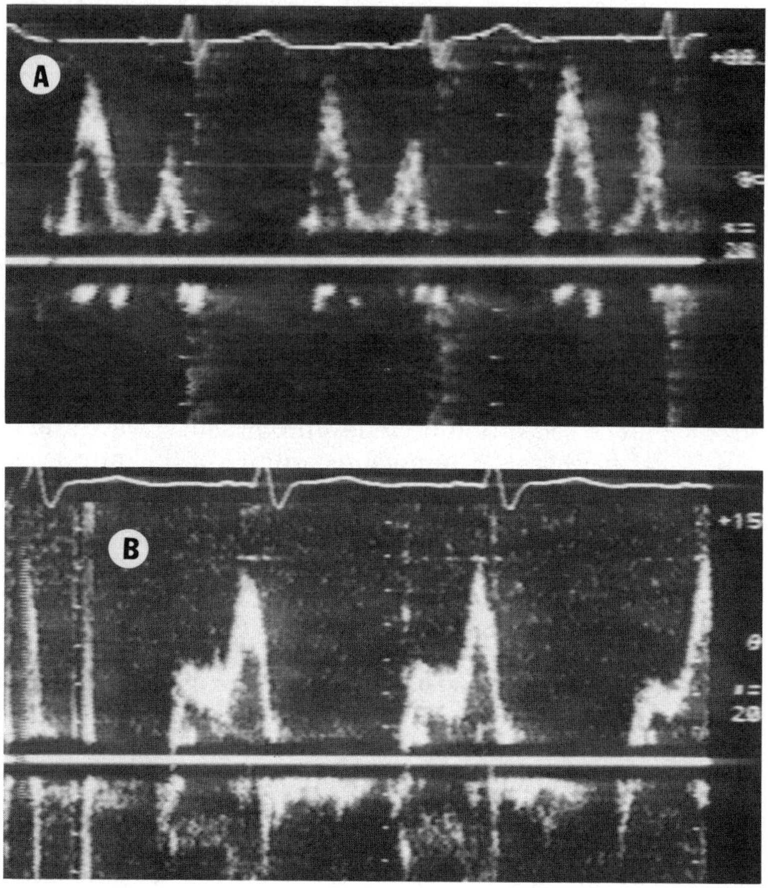

Figure 18.1
A. Normal transmitral flow with E/A ratio greater than one.
B. Reversed E/A ratio, which is less than one, in the same patient shown in A during an attack of angina with myocardial ischemia.

sophisticated computerized measurements that may not be readily available.

Chronic Pressure Overload (Table 18.3)

Valvular stenosis represents a common cause of pressure overload. Aortic valve stenosis imposes resistance to left ventricular ejection in systole. In order to overcome this extra resistance, the left ventricle undergoes adaptive changes with progressive hypertrophy to generate higher systolic pressure and eject blood across the narrowed aortic valve orifice. In uncontrolled systemic hypertension, the resistance to left ventricular ejection lies within the aorta and peripheral circulation whereby the increased peripheral re-

Table 18.3
Common causes of chronic pressure overload

Left ventricle	Right ventricle
Aortic valve stenosis	Pulmonary hypertension
Systemic hypertension	Pulmonary valve stenosis
Coarctation of the aorta	Pulmonary artery stenosis
Obstruction of the left ventricular outflow tract	Infundibular stenosis

sistance necessitates progressive left ventricular hypertrophy. In this context, symptoms of left ventricular failure may occur due to one or more of several factors:

1. Stroke volume and cardiac output may be significantly reduced due to an inability of the left ventricle to eject blood against severe outflow obstruction by aortic stenosis or marked elevation of peripheral resistance in systemic hypertension. This leads to shortness of breath, fatigue, and exercise intolerance. At this stage of heart failure, systolic contractility may be normal or minimally impaired.
2. Persistent severe pressure overload will ultimately exceed the adaptive capacity of the left ventricle with gradual progression of impairment of contractility. This leads to further decline of stroke volume and cardiac output.
3. With progressive hypertrophy, impaired diastolic relaxation due to the hypertrophy leads to progressive increase in diastolic pressures.

The echocardiogram frequently demonstrates various degrees of left ventricular hypertrophy commensurate with the severity of pressure overload. Moreover, echocardiographic features of impaired diastolic relaxation or impaired contractility, or both, are frequently encountered. Occasionally mild ventricular dilatation is encountered in late stages of the disease. The Doppler ultrasound frequently demonstrates reversed E/A ratio suspicious for impaired diastolic relaxation.

Acute Pressure Overload

Acute pressure overload is occasionally encountered in patients with systemic hypertension due to excessive salt intake or noncompliance with medications who may develop rapid acceleration of blood pressure. This represents a sudden change of the resistance to left ventricular ejection. In this context, left ventricular adaptive changes are inadequate to cope with this sudden elevation of blood pressure. Stroke volume and cardiac output drop, and diastolic pressures rise, leading to pulmonary congestion and acute pulmonary edema.

Echocardiographic evaluation of the patient with such "malignant hypertension" frequently demonstrates significant left ventricular hypertrophy with various degrees of impairment of contractility, depending on the severity and duration of the hypertension.

A less frequently encountered cause of acute pressure overload occurs in patients with a malfunctioning mechanical prosthetic valve whereby the disc or ball valve remains stuck in the closed or semiclosed position due to thrombus formation. Fortunately, such a complication is rare. Occasionally, intermittent failure to open may occur. In this context, a malfunctioning aortic mechanical prosthesis will impose sudden restriction to left ventricular ejection and cause acute heart failure and pulmonary edema. A malfunctioning mitral mechanical prosthesis will impose sudden restriction to left atrial emptying with similar hemodynamic consequences.

Acute right ventricular pressure overload may be encountered in patients with acute pulmonary embolization whereby a large thrombus may occlude one or more major branches of the pulmonary artery. This causes sudden increase of resistance to right ventricular ejection with associated decrease of stroke volume and cardiac output. The echocardiographic findings are nonspecific, since the left ventricle may exhibit normal systolic function. Such an acute process does not allow enough time for compensation by the right ventricle, which may exhibit normal chamber size with variable degree of impairment of contractility.

Chronic Volume Overload (Table 18.4)

Valvular dysfunction with significant regurgitation is the commonest form of chronic volume overload encountered in adults. The affected ventricle will dilate in order to accommodate the increase of blood flow imposed by the incompetent valve. During the early stages of disease, ventricular adaptation allows for progressive ventricular dilatation with hyperdynamic motion of the wall. This allows the ventricle to continue to provide adequate cardiac output to the peripheral tissues. However, progressive increase of the volume overload will ultimately cause significant chamber dilatation

Table 18.4
Common causes of chronic volume overload

Left ventricle	Right ventricle
Aortic regurgitation	Pulmonary regurgitation
Mitral regurgitation	Tricuspid regurgitation
Patent ductus arteriosus	Atrial septal defect
Ventricular septal defect	Muscular ventricular septal defect
High output state	High output state

with gradual decrease of contractility and cardiac output. A gradual increase of diastolic pressures will also occur. At this stage of disease, clinical symptoms of heart failure ensue.

The echocardiogram typically exhibits dilatation of the cardiac chambers or great vessels that are in immediate proximity to the disease process leading to the volume overload. Hence, in severe chronic mitral regurgitation, the left atrium and ventricle will dilate due to the increased volume of regurgitant blood going back and forth into these chambers. In aortic regurgitation, the aortic root and left ventricle will dilate. In atrial septal defect with left-to-right shunt, the left and right atria will be dilated. However, the increase of blood flow into the right atrium will ultimately increase the blood flow in the right ventricle and pulmonary artery, which will also dilate. In membranous ventricular septal defect with left-to-right shunt, the increase of blood flow across this defect, in systole, will be directly transmitted to the pulmonary artery, which will dilate. This shunted blood will ultimately increase the volume of blood flow into the left atrium and ventricle, which will also dilate. The right ventricle may not dilate during the early stages of disease, since the shunted blood almost bypasses this chamber and flows directly into the pulmonary artery. During the latter stages of a chronic large ventricular septal defect, pulmonary hypertension will ensue. When the hypertension is severe, right ventricular dilatation and hypertrophy will be noted.

Metabolic conditions, such as thyrotoxicosis and severe anemia, or mechanical abnormalities such as a systemic arteriovenous fistula create a situation whereby there is increased volume of blood flow across all four cardiac chambers, which will gradually dilate. High-output cardiac failure occurs when the adaptive ventricular changes are inadequate with progressive increase of left ventricular diastolic pressure and pulmonary congestion. However, it is important to note, as the name implies, the cardiac output remains normal or high during high-output failure.

Acute Volume Overload

Sudden rupture of a cardiac valve or its supportive apparatus, or sudden failure of a prosthetic valve creates an acute regurgitant state which, when severe, will exceed the capacity of the affected cardiac chambers to cope with the increased volume of flow. Because this is an acute process, the affected cardiac chambers do not have enough time to dilate. This leads to rapid severe elevation of diastolic pressures.

In acute mitral regurgitation, left ventricular contraction in systole will cause a major volume of blood to regurgitate back into the left atrium. Hence, the volume of blood ejected into the aorta will be reduced with decrease in the total cardiac output. In acute aortic regurgitation, a major volume of blood ejected by the left ventricle into the aorta will regurgitate back into the left ventricle, reducing the total blood flow to the peripheral circulation.

Echocardiographic features of acute volume overload will demonstrate various degrees of dilatation of the cardiac chambers affected. The left ventricle may be hyperdynamic. The valvular pathologic condition leading to the acute volume overload may be noted on the echocardiogram. Cardiac Doppler study will frequently demonstrate significant valvular regurgitation.

Case Presentations

The following case presentations will serve to illustrate the value of echocardiography and cardiac Doppler ultrasound in the evaluation of heart failure. This is achieved by answering all of the questions detailed earlier in this chapter.

Patient 1

A 60-year-old diabetic woman was admitted with acute large inferoposterior myocardial infarction. On admission, she had pulmonary congestion and mild hypotension, presumed to be secondary to left ventricular failure due to the myocardial infarction. An echocardiogram performed on the first day of hospitalization demonstrated a slightly dilated left ventricle, with an akinetic inferoposterior wall and apex. Overall contractility was moderately impaired with an estimated left ventricular ejection fraction of 45%. The A wave on the M-mode recording was prominent. There was no evidence of mitral regurgitation on the Doppler recording; however, the E/A ratio of transmitral flow was reversed. Appropriate therapy was instituted, with gradual improvement of the symptoms. On the third hospital day, the patient developed abrupt hypotension and acute pulmonary edema. She was noted to have a loud holosystolic murmur at the left sternal border. A repeat echocardiogram demonstrated an akinetic inferoposterior wall, same as in the previous study; however, the anterior left ventricular wall was hyperdynamic. Overall contractility appeared to be slightly improved. Again, there was no evidence of mitral regurgitation on the Doppler ultrasound. However, the transpulmonic velocity of blood flow was slightly increased. Careful investigation of the interventricular septum by PW mode Doppler ultrasound demonstrated abnormal high velocity of flow, with marked turbulence in the right ventricle close to the cardiac apex, consistent with a ventricular septal defect. The diagnosis of ruptured interventricular septum secondary to acute myocardial infarction was made.

The first echocardiogram and Doppler study demonstrated two common mechanisms of heart failure, both of which may be implicated as cause of failure on the first day of hospitalization. Impaired systolic contraction contributed to reduced cardiac output and hypotension. Impaired diastolic relaxation led to pulmonary congestion. Despite the absence of any evidence for further myocardial infarction, sudden worsening of the symptoms of heart failure and the Doppler finding of a ventricular septal defect strongly pointed to an additional mechanism of failure on the third hospital day. The new ventricular septal defect created a state of acute volume overload. Whereas the actual volume of this left-to-right shunt may not have been very large, it was sufficient to induce heart failure on a previously compromised ventricle.

Patient 2

A 35-year-old man presented with a history of exercise intolerance, intermittent shortness of breath, and atypical chest pain of many years' duration. His physical examination demonstrated hyperdynamic cardiac apical impulse, loud fourth heart sound, and loud midsystolic murmur in the left lower sternal border that worsened and occurred earlier in systole during Valsalva's maneuver. Hypertrophic cardiomyopathy was suspected and later confirmed on the echocardiogram, which demonstrated marked hypertrophy of the interventricular septum and a hyperdynamic ventricle. The left atrium was moderately dilated. The cardiac Doppler study demonstrated a midsystolic flow velocity of 4 m/sec with late peaking and turbulence in the left ventricular outflow tract. Appropriate therapy was instituted, with moderate improvement of exercise tolerance. Six months later the patient presented with acute onset of chest pain and pulmonary edema. He was noted to have irregular fast pulse, which was not present on a previous examination. A new echocardiogram demonstrated similar findings as in the previous study. However, a velocity of 5 m/sec was noted at the left ventricular outflow tract by Doppler ultrasound. The cardiac rhythm was atrial fibrillation with a ventricular rate of 140 beats/min.

Hypertrophic cardiomyopathy is a known cause of impaired diastolic relaxation with pulmonary congestion secondary to elevated diastolic pressures. Worsening of the symptoms was associated with the onset of atrial fibrillation. In this context, the loss of an effective atrial contraction led to a reduction of left ventricular filling, with worsening of the obstruction in the left ventricular outflow tract. Moreover, the diastolic filling period was markedly shortened due to the rapid ventricular rate. This caused further reduction of left ventricular filling and increase in diastolic pressures with worsening symptoms of heart failure. In this patient, the mechanism of heart failure was still the same. However, it was exaggerated with the onset of rapid irregular cardiac rhythm and loss of effective atrial contraction.

Patient 3

A 72-year-old man presented with shortness of breath and was noted to have a harsh systolic murmur at the aortic area. The echocardiogram demonstrated severe stenosis of the aortic valve with marked left ventricular hypertrophy. Overall contractility was borderline impaired with fractional shortening at 27% and estimated ejection fraction at 50%. Cardiac Doppler ultrasound demonstrated high velocity of flow across the aortic valve with a peak velocity of 5 m/sec and estimated mean pressure gradient of 80 mm Hg. There was no evidence of aortic regurgitation. The transmitral E/A ratio was reversed. Severe stenosis of the aortic valve was confirmed by cardiac catheterization; the coronary arteries were normal. He later underwent aortic valve replacement with a mechanical disc prosthesis, and had no immediate postoperative complications. On the third postoperative day, he developed acute hypotension and pulmonary edema. The ECG did not demonstrate any ischemia or infarction. The echocardiogram demonstrated a hyperdynamic ventricle with fractional shortening at 45% and estimated ejection fraction at 65%. There was no abnormal wall motion. The aortic prosthesis exhibited exaggerated motion with rocking of the valve ring, suspicious for dehiscence of the sutures. There was premature closure of the mitral valve. Doppler ultrasound demonstrated severe prosthetic regurgitation.

This patient presented with symptoms of heart failure primarily due to severe pressure overload resulting from severe stenosis of the aortic valve. In the presence of marked left ventricular hypertrophy, impaired diastolic relaxation was suspected; however, this was probably of secondary importance in regards to the symptoms of heart failure. Worsening of heart failure in the postoperative period is largely due to severe regurgitation at the aortic prosthesis with acute volume overload. In this context, the previously hypertrophied left ventricle could not accommodate the increased volume load. The symptoms were worsened by the impaired left ventricular diastolic relaxation, which was further exaggerated by the increased volume load on a noncompliant ventricle. This was evident by the premature closure of the mitral valve in late diastole due to marked elevation of left ventricular diastolic pressure. An interesting observation was the normal motion of the interventricular septum postoperatively. It is common to observe paradoxical motion of the interventricular septum in the first 6 months after cardiac surgery. Absence of paradoxical motion of the interventricular septum in the early postoperative stage represents a subtle sign of prosthetic valve malfunction and volume overload.

19 Left Ventricular Dysfunction: Determining the Severity

The purpose of any echocardiographic examination is, first, to establish the diagnosis of cardiac pathology, and second, to determine its severity. An integral task in this process is to determine the effect of the cardiac pathologic states in question on left ventricular performance. Clinical decisions for medical therapy or surgical intervention frequently depend on the status of left ventricular function as determined by initial examination or subsequent follow-up studies. The efficacy of the medical therapy or surgical intervention relies on serial estimates of left ventricular performance (Tables 19.1, 19.2).

Left Ventricular Size

M-mode and two-dimensional echocardiography have largely replaced the routine chest x-ray for the evaluation of cardiac size. Echocardiography is superior to the radiologic approach in distinguishing enlargement of the cardiac chamber from hypertrophy. Moreover, echocardiography is more suited to identifying which chamber is enlarged, and to what extent.

Internal Dimensions

Internal dimensions are usually obtained at end diastole and end systole. These measurements can be obtained from the M-mode tracings at the level of the left ventricle. The begin-

Table 19.1
Normal range of m-mode derived measurements of cardiac chamber dimensions and valve excursion in adults[a]

	Range[b]
Aortic root diameter	20–37 mm
Left atrial diameter	19–40 mm
Right ventricular diameter	10–26 mm
Left ventricular diameter at end diastole	37–56 mm
Left ventricular % fractional shortening	30–45%
Mean ventricular circumferential fiber shortening	1.02–1.94 circumference/sec
Interventricular septal thickness at diastole	6–11 mm
Interventricular septal excursion at systole	6–9 mm
Posterior wall thickness at diastole	6–11 mm
Posterior wall excursion at systole	9–14 mm
Aortic cusp separation	16–20 mm
Anterior mitral leaflet excursion	20–35 mm
Mitral diastolic E-F slope	80–150 mm/sec

[a]Values for children vary depending on age, weight, and body surface area.
[b]These values vary depending on source of reference.

Table 19.2
Normal range of ventricular volumes and performance obtained by cardiac catheterization normalized to body surface area[a]

	Range
Left ventricular volume at end diastole	50–90 ml/m^2
Left ventricular mass	76–108 g/m^2
Stroke volume	32–48 ml/beat/m^2
Cardiac output	2.8–4.2 liter/min/m^2
Ejection fraction	58–75%

[a]These values vary depending on source of reference.

ning of the QRS complex on the simultaneous ECG is used to identify the point in time during which the left ventricle has achieved its maximal dilatation at end diastole. The point in time during which the interventricular septum achieves its maximal systolic posterior excursion denotes the end of ventricular ejection. At this time, the left ventricle is at its smallest dimension during the cardiac cycle.

Depending on the ultrasound equipment and the gain setting used to obtain the M-mode tracing, broadening of the echoes reflected from the endocardial surface of the left ventricle may occur. To avoid confusion and to maintain consistency, measurements of left ventricular internal dimensions are commonly performed by the leading edge–to–leading edge method (Figure 19.1). Care should be made to distinguish the echoes originating from the chordae tendineae of the mitral valve apparatus from those of the endocardial surface of the left ventricular posterior wall; otherwise, dimensions of the left ventricle may be falsely underestimated.

Accurate and reproducible measurements of left ventricular internal dimensions rely heavily on the location of the transducer on the chest wall relative to the position of the left ventricle within the chest cavity (Figure 19.2). The path of the ultrasound beam must be almost perpendicular to the plane of the interventricular septum and left ventricular posterior wall. Otherwise, the ultrasound beam oriented in an oblique direction relative to the left ventricular cavity may seriously affect the validity of these measurements. Patient positioning is also important. With the transducer fixed at the same location of the chest wall, chamber dimensions measured from M-mode tracings obtained with the patient in the supine position are slightly different from those obtained from M-mode tracings obtained with the patient in the left lateral decubitus position.

M-mode measurements of left ventricular internal dimensions adequately reflect overall size of the left ventricular cavity. This is particularly true in subjects with normal ventricular size or those with generalized left ventricular dilatation. However, these measurements are less reliable in reflecting overall left ventricular size in patients with abnormal segmental wall motion. Paradoxical septal motion, apical dyskinesia, or both, seriously underscore the validity of the M-mode echocardiogram as a measure of global left ventricular size, particularly during ventricular systole. This problem can be resolved by two-dimensional echocardiography whereby measurements of left ventricular internal dimensions can be performed at multiple levels within the cavity and from different two-dimensional views.

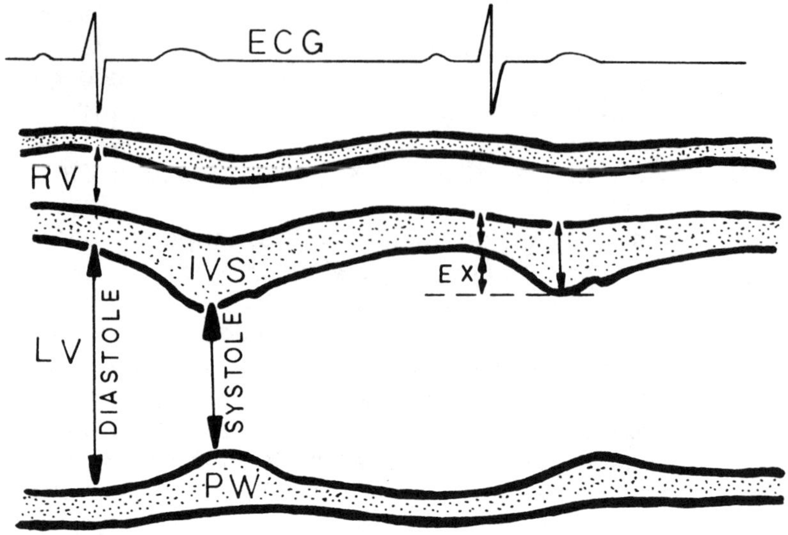

A

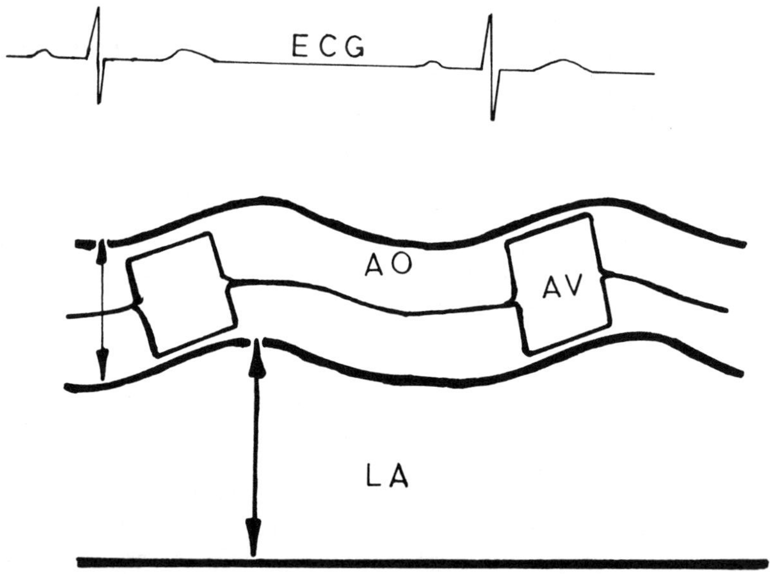

B

Figure 19.1
Schematic M-mode recording depicting the methods applied to measure dimensions of the chambers. A. Left ventricular (LV) diastolic diameter is measured during the time of inscription of the R wave on the simultaneous ECG recording. Following the leading edge–to–leading edge method. Left ventricular end diastolic dimension is measured from the internal edge of the echoes generated from the endocardial surface of the interventricular septum (IVS) to the external edge of the echoes generated from the endocardial surface of the posterior wall (PW). Left ventricular end systolic diameter is measured at the time of maximal systolic excursion of the interventricular septum, in the same manner de-

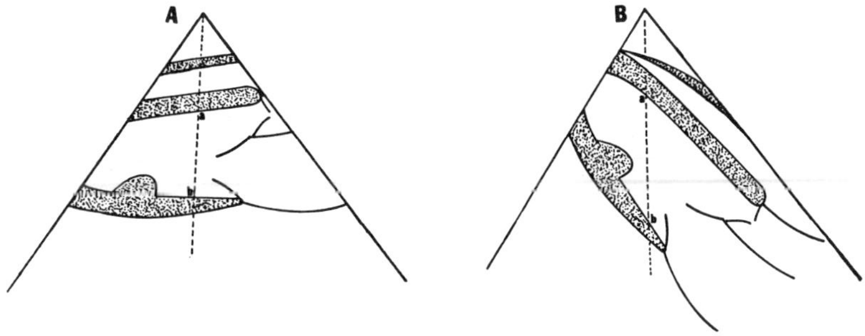

Figure 19.2
A parasternal long axis view showing the path of the M-mode ultrasound beam traversing the left ventricle. A. The M-mode beam bisects the left ventricle perpendicular to the interventricular septum and posterior wall. This is the ideal method to determine left ventricular internal dimensions. B. From a transducer position in the fourth or fifth intercostal space, the parasternal long axis view is angulated. The M-mode ultrasound beam bisects the left ventricular cavity at an oblique angle. Estimate of the resulting left ventricular interval dimension is less accurate.

Ventricular Volume

Volume estimates of the left ventricle represent a better index of its overall size than simple measurements of the diameter at its base. The left ventricular cavity can be simulated to a geometric model whose volume can be determined mathematically from its dimensions. A prolate ellipsoid is a three-dimensional figure whose major axis is equal to twice the

---

scribed above. Diastolic and systolic thickness of the interventricular septum and posterior wall are measured during the same time intervals used to measure end diastolic and end systolic dimensions, respectively. The method to determine systolic excursion (EX) of the interventricular septum is also shown in this illustration. This is measured as the vertical distance between the relative positions of the interventricular septum endocardial echoes from end diastole to end systole. See text for details. B. Aortic root (AO) diameter is measured from the leading edge of echoes generated from the anterior wall of the aorta, to the leading edge of echoes generated from the posterior wall of the aorta. This measurement is obtained during the inscription of the R wave on the simultaneous ECG. Left atrial (LA) diameter is measured from the leading edge of echoes generated from the posterior wall of the aorta, to the leading edge of echoes generated from the posterior wall of the left atrium. In this method of measurement, the thickness of the posterior wall of the aorta is included in the left atrial dimension. This measurement is obtained in early diastole. RV = right ventricle, AV = aortic valve.

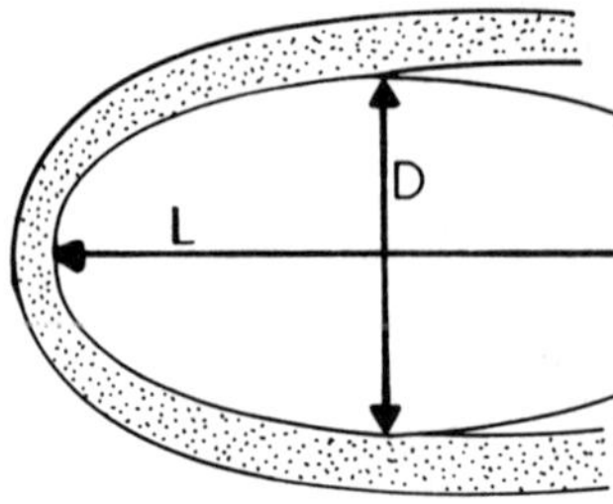

Figure 19.3
Simulation of the left ventricular cavity as a prolate ellipsoid. The major axis L is equal to twice the minor axis D.

minor axis (Figure 19.3). The volume (V) of this geometric model is determined as follows:

$$V = \frac{4\pi}{3} \times \frac{L}{2} \times \frac{D}{2} \times \frac{D}{2}$$

Since the major axis (L) is twice the minor axis diameter (D), then the volume is:

$$V = \frac{4\pi}{3} \times \frac{2D}{2} \times \frac{D}{2} \times \frac{D}{2}$$

$$V = \frac{\pi}{3} D^3$$

$$V = 1.047\ D^3$$

$$\text{or } V = D^3 \qquad \text{(Equation 19.1)}$$

where $\pi = 3.14$.

This mathematical approach can be applied to estimate left ventricular volume from its internal dimension at its base, measured by M-mode echocardiography. However, since left ventricular major axis is not always equal to twice its minor axis, a modified formula has been developed by Teicholz:

$$V = \frac{7}{2.4 + D} \times D^3 \qquad \text{(Equation 19.2)}$$

A similar approach can be employed using measurements of left ventricular dimension from two-dimensional echocardiographic recordings.

The left ventricular cavity has been simulated to many different geometric models or combinations of multiple geometric figures. Unfortunately, volume measurements obtained through any of these approaches are acceptable only

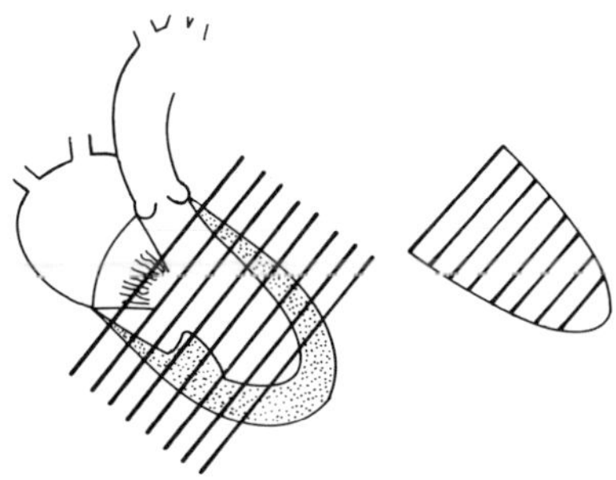

Figure 19.4
Simpson's method to estimate left ventricular volume. The left ventricle is divided into multiple sections of equal width. The volume of each section is measured. Total left ventricular volume is equal to the sum of volumes of each smaller section.

for ventricles that are normal in size or are slightly dilated. Alterations of left ventricular geometry encountered in patients with severe coronary artery disease and significant abnormalities in wall motion greatly reduce the validity of most of these geometric models. This has prompted investigators to search for a newer method that does not rely heavily on left ventricular geometry to estimate its volume.

Simpson's method to estimate left ventricular volume is based on a different approach that divides the left ventricle into small sections. Hence, left ventricular volume is determined by adding the volumes of each individual section measured by two-dimensional echocardiography (Figure 19.4). For this purpose, multiple short axis views of the left ventricle are needed at multiple levels along the long axis. Theoretically, this approach is advantageous because the left ventricular cavity is not simulated by any geometric model. However, technical difficulties are frequently encountered when one is attempting to record multiple short axis views because of the boney rib cage and poor acoustic windows. The modified Simpson's method employs the same principle but necessitates the use of a computer to simulate the multiple cross sections of the ventricle. For this purpose, the apical two-chamber view and the parasternal short axis view at the level of the papillary muscles are obtained. The endocardial surface is outlined and digitized into the computer, which will then electronically perform the analysis and estimate the volume.

Simpson's method and the modified Simpson's method have been shown to be highly accurate in the estimation of left ventricular volumes. However, during clinical applications of these methods, excellent quality echocardiograms with well-defined endocardial borders are crucial in the successful estimation of left ventricular volumes. Unfortunately, echocardiograms of such excellent quality may not be obtained in many patients with various technical limitations. Hence, volume measurements may not be as accurate as previously thought to be, if the endocardial surfaces were not well visualized.

Left Ventricular Mass

Concentric left ventricular hypertrophy is frequently encountered as a response to pressure overload such as systemic hypertension or aortic valve stenosis. This form of hypertrophy can be easily noted as an increased thickness of the echoes reflected from the ventricular septum and left ventricular posterior wall on the M-mode echocardiogram. This is determined using the leading edge–to–leading edge method (Figure 19.1), whereby the measurement is obtained from the most anterior echoes along the right border of the interventricular septum to the beginning of endocardial echoes along the left border of the septum. Thickness of the posterior wall is measured from the most anterior endocardial echoes to the beginning of the dense pericardial echoes. All of these measurements are best obtained at the point of onset of the QRS complex on the simultaneous ECG recording, coinciding with late diastole. Measurements of wall thickness obtained in systole are expected to increase due to contraction and thickening of the myocardium during this period of the cardiac cycle.

Ventricular hypertrophy may be present without any significant increase in wall thickness. This situation may be encountered in patients with significant ventricular dilatation, and is commonly referred to as eccentric hypertrophy. In this context, the degree of left ventricular hypertrophy may be underestimated as determined by wall thickness only. Estimation of left ventricular muscle mass is the best noninvasive indicator of hypertrophy, whether concentric, eccentric, or a combination thereof.

Left ventricular mass can be estimated using the same principles employed to estimate left ventricular volume. For this purpose, one estimates the volume with and without incorporating wall thickness in the analysis (Figure 19.5). The difference of these two volume measurements represents the volume of left ventricular muscle only. Mass is equal to the product of volume and density. Hence, left ventricular muscle mass would be equal to the product of the estimated muscle volume and the density of muscle, approximately 1.05 g/cm^3.

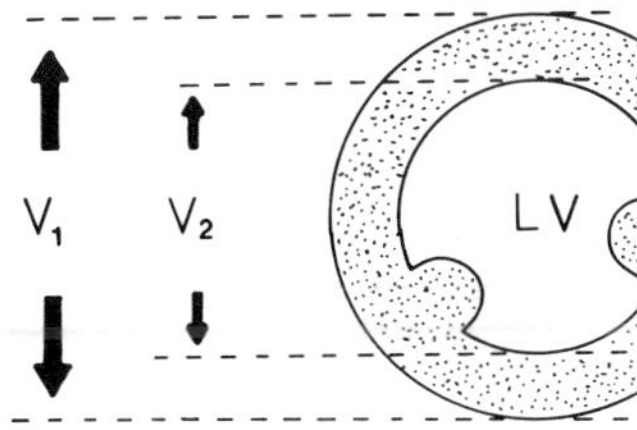

Figure 19.5
The method applied to estimate left ventricular mass. V_1 represents estimates of left ventricular volume, including the thickness of the interventricular septal and posterior wall. V_2 represents estimates of true left ventricular volume using internal dimensions only. True left ventricular muscle volume is the difference between V_1 and V_2. When true ventricular muscle volume is multiplied by the density of cardiac muscle tissue, left ventricular mass is obtained.

Left Ventricular Contractile Performance

There are many ways to evaluate left ventricular contractile performance. Each of these methods has certain practical advantages and limitations. The following discussion will briefly describe the more common approaches to evaluating left ventricular function noninvasively.

Systolic Excursion of the Wall

Ventricular contraction causes the interventricular septum and posterior wall to thicken and encroach on the left ventricular cavity, which becomes smaller in dimension as it ejects blood into the aorta. Using the M-mode tracings of the left ventricle, systolic excursion of the interventricular septum is determined as the distance of systolic posterior motion relative to its position at end diastole. This is determined by plotting two horizontal lines on the M-mode tracing. The first line is drawn at the level of the endocardial surface of the interventricular septum at end diastole (beginning of the QRS complex on the ECG), and the second line is drawn at the level of the endocardial surface of the interventricular septum at end systole (peak posterior excursion in late systole). The vertical distance between these two lines represents the degree of systolic excursion of the interventricular septum (Figure 19.1). A similar approach is performed to determine the systolic excursion of the left ventricular posterior wall. A hyperdynamic ventricle exhibits exaggerated systolic excursion, whereas a poorly contractile ventricle causes minimal excursions in systole.

Fractional Shortening

This parameter reflects the relative change of left ventricular internal dimension throughout the cardiac cycle. The fractional shortening is measured as the ratio of the difference between end diastolic (EDd) and end systolic (ESd) internal diameters to the end diastolic internal diameter. This ratio is multiplied by 100 to obtain the percent fractional shortening (FS).

$$\%FS = \frac{EDd - ESd}{EDd} \times 100 \qquad \text{(Equation 19.3)}$$

The fractional shortening is the most commonly applied M-mode-derived measure of left ventricular systolic function. Increased fractional shortening is observed in patients with hypercontractile ventricles, whereas a poorly contracting ventricle exhibits diminished values of this parameter. However, in the presence of regional wall disease, the fractional shortening may not reliably reflect overall systolic performance.

Ejection Fraction

Ejection fraction is similar to the fractional shortening. However, it employs the percent change of left ventricular volume instead of the percent change of left ventricular internal dimension. Using any of the methods described to estimate left ventricular volumes, by M-mode or two-dimensional echocardiography, the ejection fraction (EF) is calculated as the percent ratio of the difference between end diastolic (EDv) and end systolic volumes (ESv) to the end diastolic volume.

$$\%EF = \frac{EDv - ESv}{EDv} \times 100 \qquad \text{(Equation 19.4)}$$

The ejection fraction is the most common parameter employed during cardiac catheterization or nuclear cardiac imaging to evaluate left ventricular systolic function. It is less widely used on routine echocardiography because of the limitations described earlier in estimating left ventricular volumes by echocardiography.

Mean Velocity of Circumferential Fiber Shortening

Mean velocity of circumferential fiber shortening (V_{cfm}) determines the mean rate of change of left ventricular circumference in systole relative to its circumference at end diastole. In order to determine this value, one has to measure the left ventricular internal dimensions at end diastole and end systole, as well as the duration of left ventricular ejection time (LVET) measured as the duration of aortic valve opening from the M-mode echocardiogram. Given that end diastolic circumference equals $\pi \times$ EDd and end systolic circumference equals $\pi \times$ ESd,

$$V_{cfm} = \frac{(\pi \times EDd) - (\pi \times ESd)}{LVET \times (\pi \times EDd)}$$

$$V_{cfm} = \frac{EDd - ESd}{LVET \times EDd} \qquad \text{(Equation 19.5)}$$

Cardiac Output

The main function of the heart is to pump oxygenated blood to the peripheral tissues. The volume of blood ejected by the left ventricle during each systolic contraction is referred to as the stroke volume (SV). The cardiac output (CO) is the volume of blood ejected by the ventricle during a 1-minute interval; thus, the cardiac output is equal to the product of stroke volume and heart rate (HR).

$$CO = SV \times HR \qquad \text{(Equation 19.6)}$$

The stroke volume can be estimated as the difference between end diastolic and end systolic volumes measured by M-mode or two-dimensional echocardiography. Hence, this measurement suffers the same limitations as described earlier for estimating left ventricular volumes by echocardiography.

The stroke volume and cardiac output can be estimated by Doppler recordings of transvalvular velocities of flow. This approach will be discussed in more detail in Chapter 21.

Diminished cardiac output causes reduction of flow rate across the mitral and aortic valves. This may be reflected as diminished amplitude of excursion of the anterior mitral leaflet in early diastole (Figure 10.7C). Diminished separation of the aortic leaflets in systole may also occur.

Doppler Evaluation of Systolic Ejection Dynamics

Doppler recordings of transaortic velocities of flow allow adequate evaluation of left ventricular ejection dynamics. Several parameters have been examined: peak ejection rate, which is simply the peak velocity of blood flow during systole; acceleration time, which is the time interval from onset of flow to peak ejection velocity; and acceleration rate, which is the ratio of the peak velocity to acceleration time. All of these parameters have been shown to correlate with the ejection fraction and, thus, reflect left ventricular systolic function. However, such measurements are affected by preload and afterload and may not closely reflect left ventricular contractile status.

Left Ventricular Diastolic Performance

Left ventricular relaxation in diastole is a dynamic process that requires energy utilization. In most instances, diseases of the left ventricle cause impairment of both systolic as well as diastolic function, as seen in patients with dilated cardiomyopathy. However, certain conditions affect diastolic relaxation properties primarily in the presence of normal systolic function. Such diseases include early myocardial ischemia, systemic hypertension, and hypertrophic cardiomyopathy. Therefore, the need arises to develop noninvasive parameters to evaluate left ventricular diastolic function.

Isovolumic Relaxation Period

Isovolumic relaxation period is the time interval, very early in diastole, when the aortic valve is closed but the mitral valve has not yet opened. During this interval of the cardiac cycle, the left ventricular myocardium is relaxing without any change in ventricular volume because its inlet and outlet valves are closed. Impaired ventricular relaxation frequently causes delay of mitral valve opening, with prolongation of the isovolumic relaxation time (Figure 1.7).

Isovolumic relaxation time can be measured by M-mode echocardiography in several ways. The earliest methods employed simultaneous phonocardiographic recording of the aortic closure sound and M-mode recordings of the mitral valve. The isovolumic relaxation time is measured from the first high-frequency deflection of the sound of aortic valve closure on the phonocardiogram to the onset of mitral valve opening on the M-mode tracing. Newer ultrasound equipment allows simultaneous recordings of two M-mode tracings derived from the two-dimensional echocardiogram. In this approach, simultaneous recordings of the mitral and aortic valves can be obtained and the isovolumic relaxation time is measured as the time interval from aortic valve closure to onset of mitral valve opening. The isovolumic relaxation time can also be estimated by determining the time interval between the maximal systolic excursion of the left ventricular posterior wall to the onset of mitral valve opening. Finally, isovolumic relaxation time can be estimated, from a simultaneous recording of the phonocardiogram and Doppler transmitral velocity of flow, as the time interval from the first high-frequency deflection of the aortic closure sound to the onset of transmitral flow by Doppler.

Because of the differences in methodology, measurements of isovolumic relaxation time may differ slightly depending on the approach employed.

Analysis of Mitral Valve Motion

In the absence of mitral valve disease, abnormal left ventricular diastolic relaxation may cause abnormal motion patterns of the anterior mitral leaflet on the M-mode echocardiogram. Because of impaired relaxation in early diastole, left atrial emptying during the rapid filling period is delayed with resultant decrease in the E-F slope. Atrial contribution of left ventricular filling is increased so that a forceful atrial contraction may cause an exaggerated A point on the M-mode recordings of the mitral valve. The amplitude of excursion of the anterior mitral leaflet during atrial contraction may exceed the amplitude achieved in early diastole during the E point.

Finally, abnormal diastolic relaxation frequently causes significant elevation of left ventricular pressure at end diastole. This tends to interrupt transmitral flow in late diastole with partial closure of the mitral valve prior to ventricular contraction. This may cause a characteristic pattern on the M-mode tracing whereby a small notch is observed on the anterior mitral leaflet recording (B notch) immediately before its closure (Figure 6.7).

Analysis of Transmitral Velocity

Abnormal diastolic relaxation of the left ventricle may alter transmitral velocities of flow in the same manner noted for mitral valve motion on the M-mode echocardiogram. The most prominent abnormality noted is the reversal of the ratio of E and A velocities. Normally, the E velocity is higher than the A velocity, with an E/A ratio greater than one. In patients with abnormalities in left ventricular diastolic relaxation, reduced filling rates in early diastole tend to decrease the E velocity with a secondary exaggeration of the A velocity; thus, the E/A ratio becomes smaller than one (Figures 6.9, 18.1). Whereas many studies have confirmed these findings in a multitude of clinical conditions, it is important to note that the reliability of a reversed E/A ratio in identifying abnormal left ventricular diastolic relaxation has not been clearly established as yet. The presence of mitral regurgitation may normalize the E/A ratio despite the presence of impaired ventricular diastolic properties. Moreover, more recent studies have suggested that changes in preload and afterload will also alter the E/A ratio despite the presence of impaired diastolic relaxation.

20 Heart Murmur: Establishing the Diagnosis

Heart murmurs are caused by turbulence of blood as it crosses a narrow path relative to the volume and rate of flow. Heart murmurs caused by rapid flow rates across normal cardiac valves are called functional murmurs. This is because there is no true valvular abnormality. Such murmurs are common in children and young adults. Pathologic murmurs are those caused by turbulence of blood flow across diseased cardiac valves or abnormal communications such as a ventricular septal defect in congenital heart disease. In general, a careful physical examination provides clues as to whether a murmur is functional or pathologic. Moreover, the physical examination may define the cardiac abnormality causing a pathologic murmur.

Echocardiography and Doppler ultrasound are important in confirming the presence and cause of a cardiac murmur, especially when multiple pathologic states with different murmurs coexist. At the start of the ultrasound study, the operator should examine the patient to identify the characteristics of the murmur in question. Based on these initial observations, the operator can direct the ultrasound study to obtain the best echocardiographic and Doppler recordings for proper diagnosis. In general, cardiac murmurs are either systolic, diastolic, or continuous throughout the cardiac cycle.

Systolic Murmurs

These murmurs occur during the time interval between S_1 and S_2, during ventricular systole (Figure 1.7). Functional flow murmurs across the pulmonary and aortic valves are low in intensity. The ultrasound examination usually demonstrates normal semilunar valves with adequate mobility. Doppler recordings are also normal, or may demonstrate slightly increased velocities of blood flow commensurate with the increased flow rate. Systolic functional murmurs almost always occur in the context of normal cardiac valves, except in patients with aortic valve sclerosis whereby the thickened aortic leaflets may be slightly restricted, frequently causing a mild turbulence of blood flow. However, the degree of leaflet restriction is minimal and causes no significant obstruction to flow.

Pathologic systolic ejection murmurs start shortly after S_1 and are usually encountered in patients with pulmonary or aortic valve stenosis. Obstruction to left ventricular outflow tract, such as in hypertrophic obstructive cardiomyopathy and congenital subvalvular or supravalvular stenosis, also causes systolic ejection murmurs.

Besides obstruction to forward flow, pathologic systolic murmurs commonly occur secondary to turbulence of blood as it regurgitates across an incompetent atrioventricular valve. These regurgitant systolic murmurs usually start immediately after S_1. However, regurgitant murmurs secondary to mitral valve prolapse or papillary muscle dysfunction may start in mid to late systole.

Finally, ventricular septal defect with left-to-right shunt typically causes a pathologic, systolic murmur. The intensity and duration of these murmurs depend on the severity of the shunt and also on the relative pressure gradient between the left and right ventricles.

The echocardiogram will invariably identify the valvular or congenital abnormality that may be the cause of the systolic murmur in question. This can be further confirmed by Doppler ultrasound recordings across an anatomic abnormality noted on the echocardiogram. Doppler recordings are best suited to localize the site of turbulence of blood, and thereby represent the best noninvasive method to establish the diagnosis.

Multiple systolic murmurs can be confusing on the physical examination. The echocardiogram may detect multiple valvular pathologies, such as combined aortic stenosis and mitral regurgitation. Hypertrophic cardiomyopathy commonly causes two murmurs that represent the obstruction to left ventricular outflow tract and the commonly associated mitral regurgitation. Doppler ultrasound can easily identify the origin of such multiple murmurs. In this context, the operator should orient the Doppler ultrasound beam along one direction to obtain the best recordings of one pattern of flow; tilting the transducer with a different angulation of the ultrasound beam may detect another flow pattern of a completely different timing-of-onset and velocity profile. Simultaneous two-dimensional recordings with PW mode Doppler ultrasound will greatly aid the operator in defining the site of origin of each abnormal pattern of flow.

Diastolic Murmurs

Diastolic murmurs occur during the time interval between S_2 of one cardiac cycle and S_1 of the subsequent cardiac cycle (Figure 1.7). Few clinical settings are associated with functional diastolic murmurs. Patients with large left-to-right shunts, whereby there is a large volume of blood flow across an atrioventricular valve, may have a functional diastolic murmur across that valve. Subsequently, a persistent ductus arteriosus may cause increased transmitral flow with a functional diastolic murmur across this valve, whereas an atrial septal defect with left-to-right shunt may cause a functional diastolic murmur across the tricuspid valve. In some rare instances, a large left atrial myxoma may prolapse into the mitral valve in diastole and cause relative obstruction to transmitral flow. Austin Flint murmur is a functional diastolic murmur occasionally heard at the apex and left sternal border in patients with significant aortic regurgitation. This murmur is different from the true murmur of aortic regurgitation. Moreover, due to its location, it may be confused with the diastolic murmur of mitral valve stenosis. However, Austin Flint murmur is actually a functional murmur generated by vibratory motion of the anterior mitral leaflet as it is trapped in between two jets of blood flow in diastole: the aortic regurgitant jet and the normal transmitral flow (Figure 7.10A). The echocardiogram and Doppler recordings can easily demonstrate the absence of mitral stenosis with normal transmitral velocity of flow. Thus, from the preceding discussion, it is noted that functional diastolic murmurs may occur, but only in the setting of another cardiac abnormality.

Pathologic diastolic murmurs are caused by turbulence of forward flow across a stenotic atrioventricular valve such as in mitral valve stenosis. In this setting, the murmur starts shortly after S_2, but not before opening of the mitral valve.

Regurgitant flow across an incompetent semilunar valve may frequently cause pathologic diastolic murmurs. Such murmurs typically start immediately after the onset of S_2.

Multiple diastolic murmurs are not uncommon. A typical

example is that observed in patients with rheumatic heart disease who have mitral stenosis and aortic regurgitation.

The echocardiogram frequently identifies the anatomic cardiac abnormality causing a diastolic murmur. In addition, Doppler ultrasound aids in confirming the diagnosis, particularly when multiple murmurs are heard. Combined two-dimensional echocardiography and careful PW mode Doppler recording greatly enhance the validity of ultrasound in evaluating these murmurs.

It is very common to record mild regurgitation by Doppler ultrasound across any of the cardiac valves. This may occur in the absence of any echocardiographic abnormality of the valve, or even in the absence of any audible murmur on physical examination. This finding suggests that Doppler ultrasound is very sensitive in detecting such abnormal flow patterns, which may be trivial and escape clinical detection on routine examination.

Continuous Murmurs

Murmurs that persist throughout the cardiac cycle are said to be continuous. Pseudocontinuous murmurs are frequently encountered in patients with multiple valvular abnormalities, whereby one valve causes a systolic murmur, and the other valve generates a diastolic murmur. Pseudocontinuous murmurs may also be encountered in patients with disease of a single valve that is stenotic as well as incompetent, such as combined aortic stenosis and regurgitation. Therefore, any of these combinations of valvular pathologic conditions may produce systolic as well as diastolic murmurs that superficially may seem continuous.

True continuous murmurs may occur in the rare adult patient who has persistent ductus arteriosus. In this context, the blood pressure in the aorta is always higher than the blood pressure in the pulmonary artery. Thus, a pressure gradient across the persistent ductus arteriosus persists throughout the cardiac cycle. This results in a continuous left-to-right shunt as well as a continuous murmur. A ruptured sinus of Valsalva into a right chamber is another example of a true continuous murmur. The aortic pressure is higher than the pressures in the right side of the heart throughout the cardiac cycle. The resulting left-to-right shunt typically causes a continuous murmur.

As noted earlier, combined two-dimensional echocardiography and Doppler ultrasound are very helpful in delineating the cardiac anatomy and identifying the site of the abnormal flow pattern causing the murmur.

21 Quantitative Applications of Doppler Ultrasonography

Knowledge of the velocity and direction of blood flow within the cardiac chambers and valves is an important step forward in the noninvasive evaluation of cardiovascular diseases. This information can be analyzed one step further in order to quantify hemodynamic abnormalities and thus provide a better understanding of the disease process being evaluated.

Mathematic Considerations

Going back to the analogy (in Chapter 8) of the water hose with a narrow nozzle opening, in order for the water to flow across this obstruction, the pressure within the hose should be higher than the pressure at the tip of the nozzle. The difference in pressure (pressure gradient) acts as the driving force that causes the water to flow across the obstruction. As was mentioned earlier, the velocity of water flow will be higher downstream to the nozzle as compared to the velocity within the hose itself (Figure 21.1). This increase in velocity has been shown to be proportionate to the pressure gradient. Hence, the higher the pressure gradient is, the greater the increment in the velocity distal to the obstruction is.

The Bernoulli Equation

The Bernoulli equation defines the mathematic relationship between the pressure gradient and velocity of flow. It in-

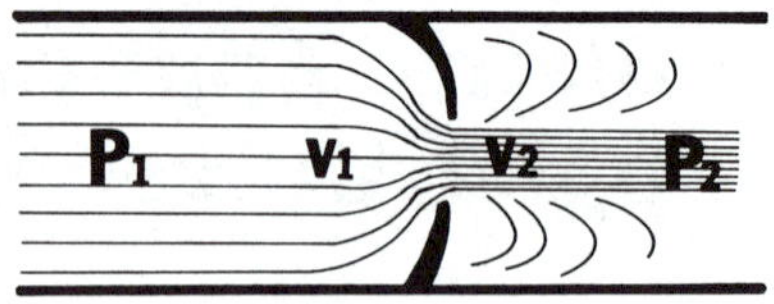

Figure 21.1
The difference in pressure and velocity of flow across an obstruction. P_1 and V_1 reflect the pressure and velocity upstream to the obstruction, respectively. P_2 and V_2 reflect the pressure and velocity downstream to the obstruction, respectively. A greater pressure gradient, whereby P_1 is greater than P_2, suggests more severe obstruction and will cause a proportionately higher value of V_2, whereby V_2 is greater than V_1.

cludes the effect of the viscosity of the fluid in resisting flow as well as the effect of inertial forces that also tend to resist change in the rate of flow. When applied to blood flow across a stenotic cardiac valve, this equation may be modified for simplicity. The inertial forces, as well as the effect of viscosity, may be neglected because these are of small magnitude. Therefore, the pressure gradient can be determined from the following equation:

$$\text{pressure gradient} = \tfrac{1}{2}\, d \times (V_2 - V_1) \qquad \text{(Equation 21.1)}$$

where d is the density of blood, and V_1 and V_2 are the velocities of blood flow proximal and distal to the stenosis in m/sec, respectively (Figure 21.1).

Usually, the velocity of blood upstream to the obstruction is minimal, compared to that downstream of flow, and may be deleted. By adjusting the units on both sides of this equation and substituting the numerical value of the density of blood, d, the modified Bernoulli equation can be simplified into:

$$\text{pressure gradient} = 4V^2 \qquad \text{(Equation 21.2)}$$

where V is the velocity distal to the obstruction in m/sec and 4 is a constant that allows the pressure gradient to be estimated in mm Hg.

Thus, the modified Bernoulli equation may be used in most clinical situations to estimate the pressure drop across a valvular or other obstruction, provided the velocity of flow is adequately measured by the Doppler shift. The basic principle to keep in mind is that blood flows from a high-pressure chamber to a low-pressure chamber throughout a certain interval in the cardiac cycle. For example, peak velocity of flow in early diastole from a patient with mitral stenosis, shown in Figure 8.5A, is 2 m/sec. By applying the modified Bernoulli equation, the estimated peak pressure gradient is equal to 4 × 2 × 2, which is 16 mm Hg. Moreover, peak systolic gradient from the patient with aortic stenosis and regurgitation, shown in Figure 8.11B, is equal to 4 × 3 × 3, which is 36 mm Hg.

Velocity Integral

Unfortunately, blood flow is pulsatile. At the beginning of left ventricular ejection, flow is minimal, and then it rapidly accelerates to a maximum value and rapidly decelerates to a minimum value at the end of ejection. This is accompanied by similar changes in the pressure gradient as well as the velocities as determined by the Doppler principle. Hence, estimation of the pressure gradient from a single velocity recording may not necessarily reflect the true severity of obstruction being evaluated. This may be simplified by the following analogy:

Consider a car moving at a constant velocity of 55 miles/hour on the highway. If one measures the velocity of this car at any particular point in time, this velocity will be an adequate representation since the rate of motion is constant. If this same car travels at the constant velocity of 55 miles/hour for 2 hours, then the total distance traveled is 110 miles.

$$\text{distance} = \text{velocity} \times \text{time} \qquad \text{(Equation 21.3)}$$

If this same car is moving down a busy street with many stop lights, its velocity will change frequently. In this situation, measurement of the velocity at any particular point in time is not representative of the overall rate of motion of the car. One way to resolve this problem is to determine the distance the car traveled and the time interval needed to go from one point to the other. By rearranging Equation 21.3:

$$\text{velocity} = \frac{\text{distance}}{\text{time}} \qquad \text{(Equation 21.4)}$$

Therefore, one may estimate the average velocity of the car, irrespective of how this velocity changed throughout the trip. Figure 21.2A shows velocity with respect to time for a car moving at constant speed. Since the distance traveled is the product of the velocity and time, one may realize that the shaded area represents the actual distance traveled. Figure 21.2B is another schematic illustration of variable velocities for different time intervals. The distance traveled in this

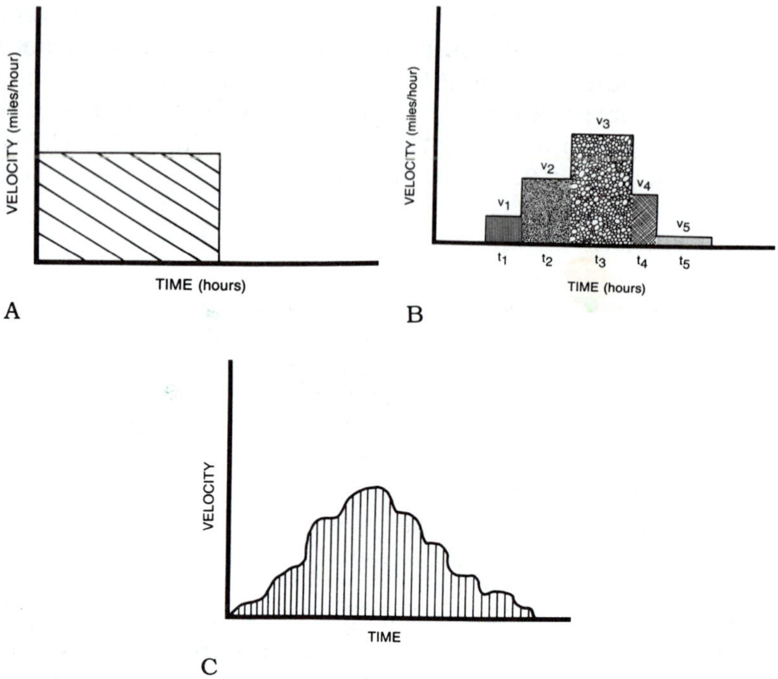

Figure 21.2
The method applied to estimate the mean velocity. In all of these examples, the mean velocity is estimated as the ratio of distance traveled to the time interval. A. At a constant velocity, the distance traveled is equal to the product of velocity and duration of travel. B. With a variable velocity, the distance traveled is equal to the sum of products of each velocity and the corresponding time interval. C. In this example with complex and variable velocity the distance traveled can be determined by planimetry of the area inscribed within the velocity-time diagram by using a planimeter, or more commonly, by computer analysis. See text for details. t = time; v = velocity.

situation is equal to the sum of the products of each particular velocity and the corresponding time interval. The shaded areas within this schematic illustration also represent the total distance traveled. Therefore, in a situation where the velocity is constantly variable, one may estimate the average or mean velocity by measuring the area inscribed within the velocity-time diagram and then dividing this value by the total time interval.

In mathematic terms, we are integrating the velocity with respect to time, and the area inscribed within this velocity-time diagram is referred to as the velocity integral.

$$\text{mean velocity} = \frac{\text{velocity integral}}{\text{duration of flow}} \quad \text{(Equation 21.5)}$$

In this example, the velocity integral is measured in miles since the velocity is represented in miles/hour and time is represented in hours. Doppler recordings of blood velocities are displayed in exactly the same fashion shown in this analogy; however, velocity is represented in m/sec or cm/sec and time is represented in seconds. The velocity integral will be represented in meters or in centimeters, respectively. One may actually measure the velocity integral of the Doppler recording using a planimeter (a small gadget used to measure areas with irregular borders) or a computer; the resultant number obtained is then divided by the total duration of flow to estimate the mean velocity (Figure 21.2C).

Mean Pressure Gradient

The mean velocity obtained in the manner described in the preceding section can be used in the modified Bernoulli equation to estimate the mean pressure gradient, which is a more physiologic parameter than estimation of the peak pressure gradient during the evaluation of obstructive valvular lesions. However, this method is only an approximate estimate of the true mean pressure gradient.

A more accurate estimate can be obtained by use of a computer that automatically measures the instantaneous velocity during short intervals throughout the duration of flow, and then applies the modified Bernoulli equation to determine the instantaneous pressure gradient during such short intervals. The average of all such instantaneous pressure gradients represents the mean pressure gradient during the duration of flow.

Flow-Velocity Interaction

The volume of a cylinder is equal to the product of the area of its base and the length of the cylinder. For the purpose of this discussion, the length will be referred to as the distance (Figure 21.3A).

$$\text{volume (cm}^3\text{)} = \text{area (cm}^2\text{)} \times \text{distance (cm)} \qquad \text{(Equation 21.6)}$$

Flow reflects the rate of change of volume with respect to time or the amount of volume output per unit of time.

$$\text{flow (cm}^3\text{/sec)} = \frac{\text{volume (cm}^3\text{)}}{\text{time (seconds)}} \qquad \text{(Equation 21.7)}$$

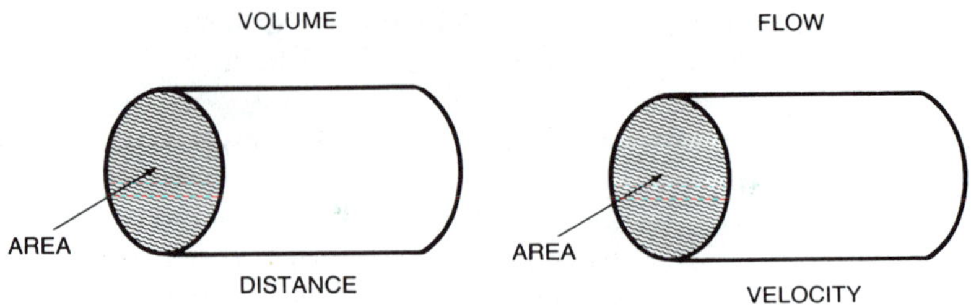

Figure 21.3
A. The volume of a cylinder is equal to the product of its cross-sectional area and its length (distance). B. Flow rate is equal to the product of the cross-sectional area and the velocity of the fluid passing through.

Combining Equations 21.6 and 21.7,

$$\text{flow} = \text{area} \times \frac{\text{distance}}{\text{time}} \qquad \text{(Equation 21.8)}$$

Since velocity has been shown to be equal to the ratio of distance to time (Equation 21.4), then

$$\text{flow (cm}^3\text{/sec)} = \text{area (cm}^2\text{)} \times \text{velocity (cm/sec)} \qquad \text{(Equation 21.9)}$$

Subsequently, in a steady-state situation, flow in a cylindrical vessel is equal to the product of the cross-sectional area of the vessel and the velocity of fluid passing through (Figure 21.3B).

The mathematic derivation of flow can be applied in cardiology to determine flow in the aortic root. To simplify matters, the aortic root is considered to behave like a rigid cylinder with a fixed cross-sectional area. However, since blood flow is pulsatile, the velocity of blood in systole is variable. For this reason, one has to use the mean velocity as determined in the previous section. There are certain errors introduced in this mathematic application. These will be discussed later.

A practical approach to quantitate flow is to determine the stroke volume (volume of blood ejected per beat [SV]) and the cardiac output (volume of blood ejected per minute [CO]). The stroke volume is usually reported as cm^3/beat. The duration of flow is just a fraction of the cardiac cycle. Therefore:

$$\text{SV (cm}^3\text{/beat)} = \text{A (cm}^2\text{)} \times \text{Vm (cm/sec)} \times \text{ET (sec/beat)} \qquad \text{(Equation 21.10)}$$

where A is the cross-sectional area, ET is the ejection time or duration of flow, and Vm is the mean velocity.

Since the mean velocity is equal to the ratio of the velocity integral (VI) to the duration of flow (Equation 21.5), then

$$SV = A \times VI \qquad \text{(Equation 21.11)}$$

and

$$CO = A \times VI \times HR \qquad \text{(Equation 21.12)}$$

where HR is the heart rate.

Usually the cardiac output is reported in liters/min rather than cm^3/min; therefore, the numerical value obtained from Equation 21.12 is divided by 1000 to adjust the units accordingly.

In the presence of atrial fibrillation, there may be significant beat-to-beat variation of the stroke volume. Therefore, one should estimate the average stroke volume from many cardiac cycles for a better estimation of the cardiac output.

The Gorlin Formula

The volume of flow across a stenotic valve depends on the severity of the obstruction (valve area) and the pressure gradient across the narrowed valve. This is mathematically represented in the Gorlin formula, which relates these parameters together:

$$A = \frac{CO}{K \times FT \times \sqrt{G}} \qquad \text{(Equation 21.13)}$$

where A is the cross-sectional area of the stenotic valve, CO is the cardiac output, FT is the flow time, G is the pressure gradient, and K is a constant that depends on the type of valve being examined, e.g., mitral or aortic.

Estimation of Cardiac Output: Clinical Applications

Following the guidelines discussed in the previous section, one may estimate the stroke volume and cardiac output. Several modifications have to be considered depending on the anatomic location from which the cardiac output is being measured.

Flow in the Ascending Aorta

The suprasternal location is the transducer position of choice to insonate the ascending aorta and record the velocity of systolic flow. Simultaneous two-dimensional imaging allows adequate measurement of the diameter of the ascending aorta to calculate its cross-sectional area, which is considered for purposes of simplicity to be circular:

$$\text{area of a circle} = \pi r^2 \qquad \text{(Equation 21.14)}$$

where r is the radius of the circle and is equal to one-half the diameter, D.

$$\text{area of a circle} = \frac{\pi D^2}{4} = \frac{3.14 D^2}{4} = 0.785\ D^2 \qquad \text{(Equation 21.15)}$$

Therefore, the volume of flow across the ascending aorta per beat is:

$$\text{stroke volume} = 0.785\ D^2 \times \text{velocity integral} \qquad \text{(Equation 21.16)}$$

The diameter of the ascending aorta may be measured from the parasternal views and aortic flow may be recorded from an apical location (Figure 21.4).

The drawbacks in estimating the cardiac output from the ascending aorta are:

1. The aorta is considered to be circular with fixed area throughout systole. It is known that this may not be true since the aortic wall is elastic and may distend slightly to

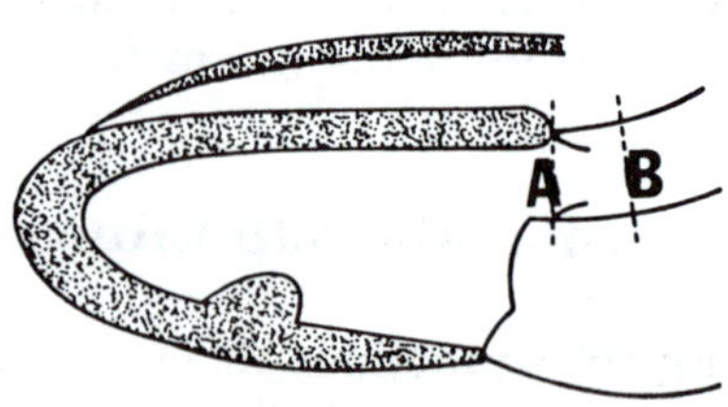

Figure 21.4
A parasternal long axis view, showing the method used to estimate the area of flow for purpose of estimation of stroke volume and cardiac output. Line A is at the aortic annulus. Line B is at the ascending aorta.

accommodate the volume of blood ejected by the ventricle in systole.

2. The volume of blood flow in the coronary arteries is not accounted for in measurements taken from the ascending aorta, as these arteries arise from the aortic root proximal to the usual anatomic site where ascending aortic flow is measured.

3. In low output states, the volume of flow is relatively diminished and the majority of blood flow may be centralized in the ascending aorta. Therefore, the true cross-sectional area of flow is significantly smaller than the cross-sectional area of the aorta, and the likelihood of overestimating stroke volume and cardiac output is increased.

Flow across the Aortic Annulus

This approach allows the measurement of flow without neglecting the volume of flow in the coronary arteries and seems to be more practical in these regards. The apical five-chamber or long axis view is used to measure the velocity of aortic flow, whereas the parasternal long axis view is used to determine the aortic annulus diameter (Figure 21.4).

Flow in the Pulmonary Artery

The diameter of the pulmonary artery can be easily determined in the pediatric age group. The parasternal short axis two-dimensional view may be used to determine pulmonary artery diameter and velocity of pulmonic flow. This approach may not be practical in the adult population because, in most instances, the anterior wall of the pulmonary artery is not adequately visualized.

Flow across the Mitral Valve

The area of the mitral valve annulus could be measured from the four-chamber or two-chamber apical views and is considered to be circular. Transmitral velocities of flow are recorded from the same apical view (Figure 21.5).

A successful attempt has been made to measure flow across the mitral valve leaflets. Using this technique, one can no longer consider the cross-sectional area of the mitral valve as circular or fixed throughout diastole. There is significant variation in this area when measured in early diastole and compared to the area during mid and late diastole. This issue is resolved in the following manner (Figure 21.6):

First, a short axis two-dimensional recording is obtained showing the tips of the mitral valve leaflets in full excursion

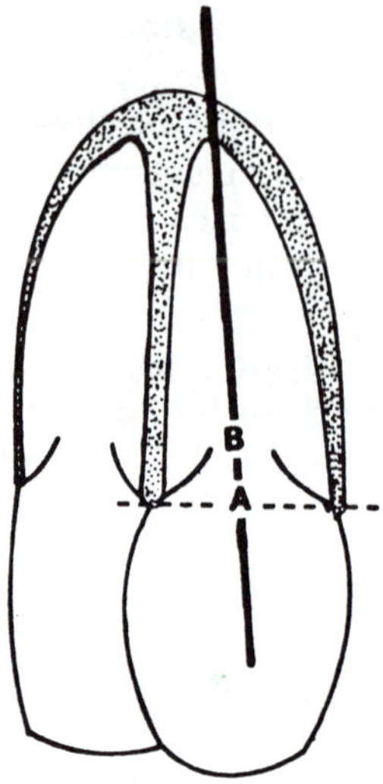

Figure 21.5
An apical four-chamber view, showing the method used to estimate the area of flow for purpose of estimation of the stroke volume and cardiac output. Line A is at the mitral annulus. B is at the tips of the mitral leaflets (see Figure 21.6).

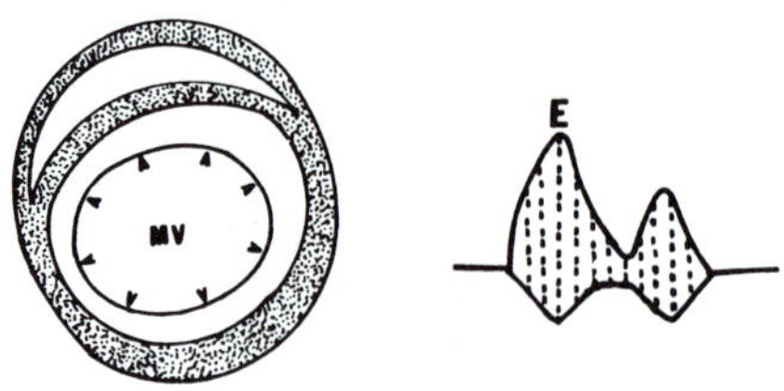

Figure 21.6
Estimation of mean diastolic mitral valve (MV) area: Maximal mitral valve area is measured from the short axis view in early diastole, at peak valve excursion (arrowheads). Mean valve excursion is determined by averaging the vertical distances measured between the anterior and posterior mitral leaflets from the M-mode echocardiogram. Mean valve area is estimated as the product of maximal area measured from the two-dimensional image and the ratio of mean valve excursion to peak valve excursion (at the E point) as determined from the M-mode recording.

in early diastole. The area inscribed within the leaflet opening is measured. Second, M-mode echocardiographic recording of the tip of the mitral valve leaflets is performed and the mean leaflet separation throughout the period of flow is determined. (This is done by dividing the duration of flow into equal time intervals and then measuring the vertical distance between the anterior and posterior leaflets at each interval and calculating the mean distance.) Third, the maximum valve area, as determined from the two-dimensional image, is multiplied by the ratio of mean leaflet separation to maximum separation as determined from the M-mode echocardiogram. The resulting value is considered to be an approximation of the average area of flow throughout diastole and is multiplied by the velocity integral. Similar to the estimation of cardiac output from the aortic root, estimation of cardiac output by the mitral valve method suffers from several drawbacks that could significantly affect the validity of this estimate. A detailed discussion of these issues is beyond the scope of this chapter. Suffice to mention that the method applied to estimate the mitral valve area and its variability throughout diastole is grossly inadequate. Moreover, because valve area and velocity of flow are constantly changing, the product of mean area and mean velocity does not truly reflect the volume of flow. In pure mathematic terms, the product of the means is not equal to the mean of the instantaneous products. Nevertheless, this method has been shown to reliably reflect the stroke volume in several clinical situations.

Evaluation of Valvular Stenosis

The severity of any valvular stenosis is usually assessed by evaluating the pressure gradient across the obstruction and determining the valve area. Using the modified Bernoulli equation, the pressure gradient can be estimated. Moreover, if one can determine the cardiac output, the valve area can also be predicted using the Gorlin formula. Rearranging Equation 21.12, the valve area can also be predicted noninvasively:

$$\text{area} = \frac{\text{cardiac output}}{\text{velocity integral} \times \text{heart rate}} \qquad \text{(Equation 21.17)}$$

However, the valve area predicted by the Gorlin formula is the anatomic valve area, and it is slightly larger than the effective area predicted from Equation 21.17. The leaflet edges of the stenosed valve cause certain physical distortions of flow so that the true area where flow exists (effective area) is slightly smaller than the true anatomic area of the stenotic valve.

In the absence of valvular regurgitation, the volume of flow across each cardiac valve should be equal. For example, the stroke volume across the mitral valve in diastole should be equal to the stroke volume across the aortic valve in systole. Thus, if aortic stenosis is present, in the absence of associ-

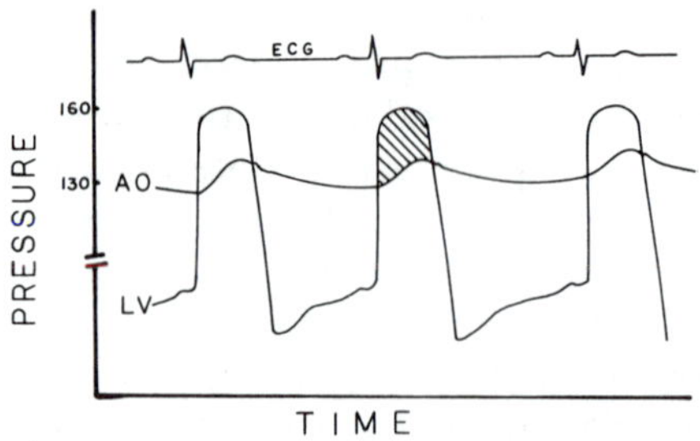

Figure 21.7
Simultaneous pressure recordings in the left ventricle (LV) and aorta (AO) in aortic stenosis. Due to the obstruction of flow at the aortic valve, left ventricular pressure generated in systole exceeds aortic pressure. The shaded area in between these two pressure tracings represents the pressure gradient in systole. Compare with Figure 1.7 whereby left ventricular and aortic pressures are identical in systole.

ated aortic regurgitation or mitral valve disease, one can estimate the cardiac output, by Doppler ultrasound, across the mitral valve and then apply the Gorlin formula noninvasively to predict the anatomic aortic valve area and the severity of the obstruction, e.g.,

$$\text{aortic valve area} = \frac{\text{mitral cardiac output}}{\text{aortic velocity integral} \times \text{heart rate}}$$

Stenosis of the Aortic Valve

Aortic valvular stenosis causes obstruction of flow in systole. The left ventricular pressure exceeds the pressure within the aorta (Figure 21.7). This pressure gradient varies throughout systole. There are two ways to measure the pressure gradient in the hemodynamic laboratory (Figure 21.8). The first way is to measure the difference between the highest pressure in the ventricle and the highest pressure in the aortic root. This is referred to as the peak-to-peak pressure gradient. This is a practical and easy method to determine the pressure gradient; however, it is not physiologic since these pressure measurements occur at different points in time during systole. The second more physiologic method is to determine the mean pressure gradient. This is done by measuring the area inscribed within the simultaneous left ventricular and aortic root pressure recordings and then dividing this value by the duration of flow. The third method employs Doppler ultrasound. As discussed earlier, Doppler examination in aortic stenosis will demonstrate a high velocity of flow. The highest velocity recorded by Doppler ultra-

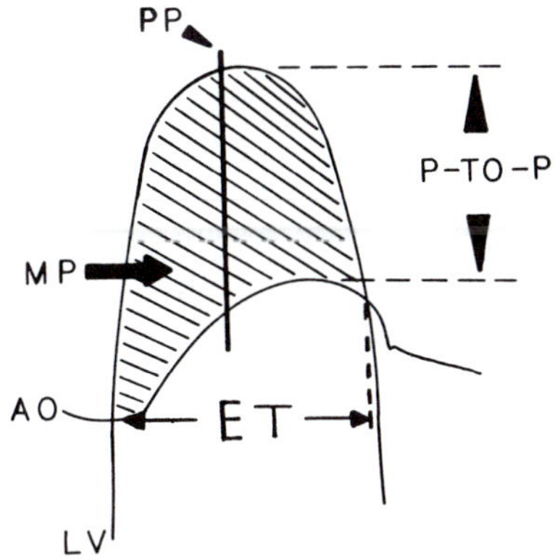

Figure 21.8
Simultaneous systolic pressure recordings in the left ventricle (LV) and aorta (AO) in aortic stenosis. The shaded area represents the pressure gradient in systole. Peak-to-peak (P-to-P) pressure gradient is the numerical difference between the highest pressure in the left ventricle and the highest pressure in the aorta. Note that these two pressure measurements do not necessarily occur at the same time interval. The peak pressure gradient (PP) represents the highest pressure difference achieved in systole. This value may be derived from the Doppler recordings across the stenotic aortic valve as the highest velocity achieved in systole. Mean pressure gradient (MP) is obtained by planimetry of the shaded area inscribed within these two pressure tracings, and by dividing this value by the duration of flow, i.e., ejection time (ET).

sound may be used in the modified Bernoulli equation to estimate the highest pressure gradient in systole, referred to as the peak pressure gradient. However, this pressure is not necessarily equal to the mean pressure gradient, or peak-to-peak gradient, obtained during cardiac catheterization. Therefore, one has to measure the velocity integral in order to determine the mean velocity and approximate the mean gradient. Another alternative is to divide the Doppler velocity recording into equal time intervals, determine the pressure that corresponds to each of these individual time intervals, and then obtain the average of these pressure determinations, as described earlier in this chapter. This will give a closer approximation of the true mean pressure gradient.

In the absence of associated aortic insufficiency or mitral valve disease, the cardiac output (CO) may be estimated using the mitral valve method described earlier. The duration of systolic flow can be measured directy from the Doppler tracing (from beginning to end of flow) and multiplied by the heart rate to determine the duration of systolic flow per minute (systolic ejection period [SEP]). Thus, the Gorlin formula

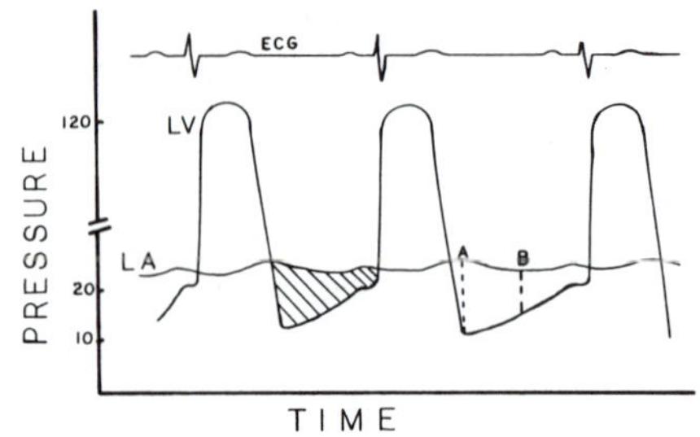

Figure 21.9
Simultaneous pressure recordings in the left ventricle (LV) and left atrium (LA) in mitral stenosis. Due to the obstruction of flow at the mitral valve, left atrial pressure is significantly greater than left ventricular pressure in diastole. The shaded area in between these two pressure tracings represents the pressure gradient in diastole. Compare with Figure 1.7 whereby left atrial pressure is only slightly greater than left ventricular pressure in diastole. A represents the point in time when the left atrial–left ventricular diastolic pressure gradient is highest in early systole. This corresponds to the peak velocity of flow obtained by Doppler ultrasound. B is the point in time where the left atrial–left ventricular pressure gradient is equal to one-half the pressure gradient at A. The time interval between A and B is referred to as the pressure half-time.

can be used to predict the anatomic aortic valve area using noninvasively determined parameters:

$$\text{aortic valve area (cm}^2\text{)} = \frac{\text{CO}}{44.5 \times \text{SEP} \times \sqrt{\text{gradient}}}$$

(Equation 21.18)

Then, combining Equations 21.2 and 21.18,

$$\text{aortic valve area (cm}^2\text{)} = \frac{\text{CO}}{89 \times \text{SEP} \times \text{mean velocity}}$$

(Equation 21.19)

The aortic valve area can be reasonably estimated from the continuity equation. In a steady state situation, it is expected that all systolic flow in the left ventricular outflow tract will be ejected across the stenotic aortic valve. In this approach, flow in the left ventricular outflow tract is estimated from measuring the velocity of flow in the outflow tract and its diameter obtained from an apical long axis 2-dimensional image by applying Equation 21.9. This estimate of flow in the left ventricular outflow tract is then applied in Equation 21.9, using the velocity of flow across the stenotic aortic valve, to solve for valve area.

$$\text{LVOT flow} = 3.14 \times (\text{LVOT R})^2 \times \text{LVOT V}$$

$$\text{AV flow} = \text{AV area} \times \text{AV V}$$

since flow in the outflow tract equals flow across the aortic valve;

$$\text{AV area} = \frac{3.14 \times (\text{LVOT R})^2 \times \text{LVOT V}}{\text{AV V}} \quad \text{(Equation 21.20)}$$

where LVOT flow, LVOT R, and LVOT V are the flow, radius, and velocity in the left ventricular outflow tract, respectively; and AV flow, AV area and AV V are the flow, area, and velocity across the aortic valve, respectively.

Stenosis of the Mitral Valve

The obstruction of flow in mitral stenosis occurs in diastole (Figure 21.9). The left atrial pressure exceeds left ventricular diastolic pressure, and this pressure gradient varies throughout diastole. In the presence of sinus rhythm, two peak velocities will be recorded, neither of which is an adequate reflection of the mean pressure gradient in diastole (Figure 8.5). One should follow the same procedure as that discussed for aortic stenosis in order to estimate the mean pressure gradient.

The Gorlin formula to estimate the anatomic mitral valve area is:

$$\text{mitral valve area} = \frac{\text{CO}}{38 \times \text{DFP} \times \sqrt{\text{G}}} \quad \text{(Equation 21.21)}$$

where CO is the cardiac output in cm^3/min, DFP is the diastolic filling period in sec/min, and G is the mean pressure gradient in diastole in mm Hg.

If the cardiac output is estimated by Doppler examination of the aortic valve or aortic root, then in the absence of associated mitral regurgitation or aortic valve disease, the noninvasive application of the Gorlin formula for the mitral valve yields:

$$\text{mitral valve area (cm}^2\text{)} = \frac{\text{CO}}{76 \times \text{DFP} \times \text{mean velocity}} \quad \text{(Equation 21.22)}$$

Another alternative method to estimate mitral valve area relies on the measurement of the pressure half-time (Figure

21.9). This is the time needed for the highest pressure gradient in early diastole to drop to one-half its initial value, which can be measured from the Doppler velocity recordings of mitral flow (see Appendix A).

$$\text{mitral valve area (cm}^2) = \frac{220}{\text{pressure half-time}}$$

(Equation 21.23)

This is an attractive approach because of its simplicity. The pressure half-time for a normal mitral valve is less than 60 milliseconds. A value greater than 120 milliseconds indicates definite stenosis. A pressure half-time value between 60 and 120 milliseconds is a gray zone, most commonly encountered in situations of minimal stenosis, or, as will be discussed later, possibly seen in mitral regurgitation.

A practical problem arises in patients with sinus tachycardia and short diastolic period. In this situation, peak velocity after the atrial kick occurs very close to the peak velocity in early diastole. This may not allow enough time for the initial pressure gradient to drop to one-half its value before the atrial kick causes the second increase in velocity (Appendix). Fortunately, this is not a problem in atrial fibrillation because there is no atrial kick. In fact, the pressure half-time is very helpful in this type of cardiac rhythm. The irregular rate causes significant beat-to-beat variation of flow and gradient, while pressure half-time is minimally affected.

Stenosis of the Tricuspid and Pulmonary Valve

The severity of tricuspid and pulmonary valve stenosis may be analyzed in a way similar to the analysis performed for mitral and aortic stenosis, respectively.

Estimation of Intracardiac Pressures

The clinical application of the modified Bernoulli equation to estimate pressure gradients may be useful in predicting the pressures within various cardiac chambers.

In aortic stenosis, the peak pressure gradient may be added to the aortic systolic pressure as measured by sphygmomanometry to predict peak left ventricular pressure in systole.

$$\begin{aligned}\text{left ventricular pressure} &= \text{aortic systolic pressure} \\ &\quad + \text{peak pressure gradient}\end{aligned}$$

(Equation 21.24)

In the presence of tricuspid regurgitation, peak right ventricular systolic pressure may be predicted by adding peak pressure gradient in systole (across the tricuspid valve) to the estimated right atrial pressure as determined by examination of the degree of jugular vein distension.

$$\text{right atrial pressure} = \frac{5\,(\text{cm } H_2O) + \text{JVP}\,(\text{cm } H_2O)}{1.36}$$

(Equation 21.25)

where JVP is the height of the column of blood seen within the jugular vein relative to the suprasternal notch with the head at 30-degree elevation.

The right-hand term of this equation is divided by 1.36 to convert the pressure measurement from cm H_20 to mm Hg. This approach is very practical in the estimation of the severity of pulmonary hypertension.

$$\text{right ventricular pressure} = \text{peak pressure gradient} + \text{right atrial pressure}$$

(Equation 21.26)

In patients with ventricular septal defect, right ventricular systolic pressure may be estimated. If left-to-right shunt is present, left ventricular pressure is greater than right ventricular pressure. In the absence of aortic stenosis, aortic systolic pressure, as measured by sphygmomanometry, may be substituted for peak left ventricular systolic pressure.

$$\text{right ventricular pressure} = \text{aortic systolic pressure} - \text{pressure gradient}$$

(Equation 21.27)

One cannot overemphasize the importance of obtaining good quality Doppler recordings of the highest velocities possible in order to estimate the intracardiac pressure just mentioned. Any error in determining these velocities may significantly affect the magnitude of the pressure gradient (since this is related to the square of the velocity); thus, the final pressure estimates may be inadequate.

Appendixes

Appendix A: Mitral Pressure Half-Time

The pressure half-time can be easily determined by use of computer applications software available with many commercial Doppler equipment (Figure A.1). The following is a step-by-step approach for manual determination of the pressure half-time and valve area from hard-copy Doppler recordings.

Velocity at Pressure Half-Time

The velocity of flow that corresponds to the pressure gradient at pressure half-time ($V_{1/2}$) is derived from the modified Bernoulli equation (Equation 21.2):

$$P = 4V^2 \qquad \text{(Equation A.1)}$$

where P is the peak gradient in early diastole and V is the peak velocity.

$$P_{1/2} = 4{V_{1/2}}^2 \qquad \text{(Equation A.2)}$$

where $P_{1/2}$ and $V_{1/2}$ are the pressure gradient and velocity at pressure half-time, respectively.

By definition:

$$P = 2P_{1/2} \text{ or } \frac{P}{2} = P_{1/2} \qquad \text{(Equation A.3)}$$

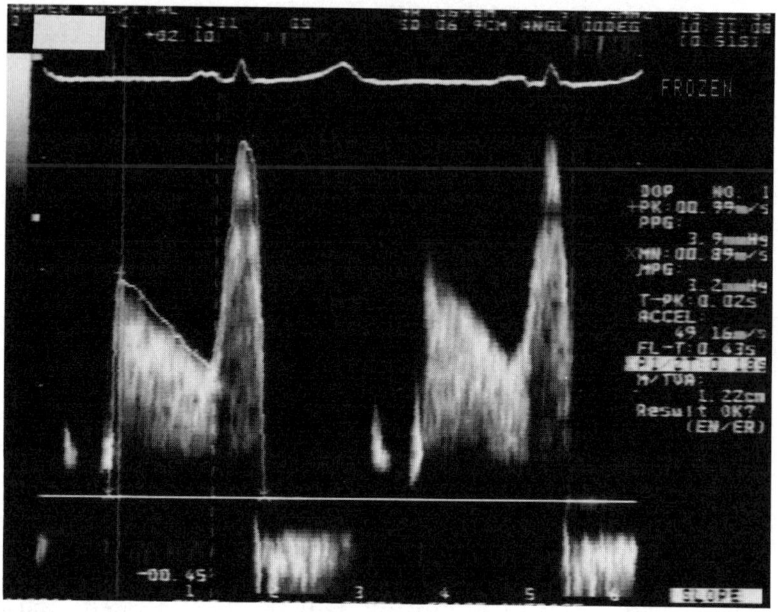

Figure A.1
Doppler recordings of transmitral flow in mitral stenosis. By use of a computer with a joystick or mouse, the spectral analysis signal is traced from beginning to end of flow, and peak velocity in early diastole is identified. The computer automatically performs the analysis and provides estimates of the peak and mean pressure gradients, pressure half-time, and valve area.

Combining Equations A.1, A.2, and A.3,

$$\frac{4V^2}{2} = 4V_{1/2}^{\ 2} \qquad \text{(Equation A.4)}$$

Solving Equation A.4 for $V_{1/2}$:

$$V_{1/2} = \frac{V}{\sqrt{2}} \text{ or } V_{1/2} = \frac{V}{1.4}$$

Hence, $V_{1/2}$ is equal to the ratio of V to 1.4, which is the square root of 2.

Pressure Half-Time

On the Doppler hard-copy recordings of transmitral flow, the peak velocity (V) is measured. This value is divided by 1.4 to determine $V_{1/2}$, which is then located on the spectral analysis recording. Vertical lines are drawn from V and $V_{1/2}$ to the baseline. The time interval between these two vertical lines is

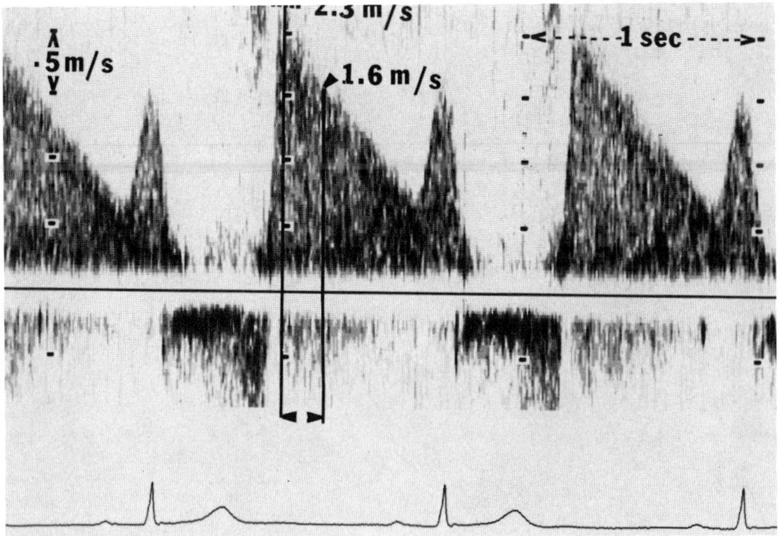

Figure A.2
Manual estimation of pressure half-time. See text for details.

the pressure half-time, and can be estimated by comparing this time interval to the time markings on the Doppler hard copy with a pair of calipers.

In Figure A.2, V is equal to 2.3 m/sec. When divided by 1.4, $V_{1/2}$ is equal to 1.6 m/sec. The distance between the two vertical lines drawn through V and $V_{1/2}$ is 0.19 seconds, or 190 milliseconds. By applying Equation 21.22, the estimated valve area is 1.1 cm^2.

It is important to note that the velocity is measured in m/sec and not cm/sec. Also, time is measured in milliseconds and not in seconds during the application of the pressure half-time.

Appendix B: Indications for Echocardiography and Cardiac Doppler Ultrasonography

General guidelines for the indications of echocardiography and cardiac Doppler ultrasonography follow. While these tests provide valuable information regarding the diagnosis and severity of cardiac pathology due to the economic costs involved, it is important to realize that the clinical situations in which these tests are indicated may be of limited value or not indicated for the proper diagnosis or management of patients with suspected cardiac disease. These guidelines may be modified when applied to specific individual circumstances and should be viewed as general recommendations.

Indications for Echocardiography

In general, an echocardiogram may be helpful to evaluate the following clinical symptoms when a cardiac cause is suspected:

- Cardiomegaly
- Chest pain
- Cyanosis
- Dizziness
- Dyspnea
- Edema
- Exercise intolerance
- Heart murmur
- Palpitations
- Shortness of breath
- Syncope

In general, an echocardiogram may be helpful for the diagnosis, determination of severity, or determination of associated cardiac abnormalities or complications of the following cardiac pathologies:

Abnormal electrocardiogram
Aortic aneurysm
Aortic dissection
Atrial fibrillation
Atrial flutter
Bacterial endocarditis
Cardiac contusion
Cardiac effects of cardiotoxic medications
Cardiac tamponade
Cardiac tumors
Cardiogenic shock
Chamber dilatation
Coarctation of aorta
Congenital heart disease
Congestive heart failure
Constrictive pericarditis
Coronary artery disease
Dilated cardiomyopathy
High-grade arrhythmia
Hypertrophic cardiomyopathy
Intracardiac thrombi
Left ventricular aneurysm
Left ventricular diastolic dysfunction
Left ventricular pseudoaneurysm
Myocardial infarction
Myocarditis
Penetrating cardiac injury
Pericardial cysts
Pericardial effusion
Pericardial tumors
Pericarditis
Peripheral embolization
Prosthetic cardiac valves
Pulmonary edema
Pulmonary embolism
Pulmonary hypertension
Restrictive cardiomyopathy
Rheumatic heart disease
Right ventricular infarction
Ruptured cardiac valve
Ruptured sinus of Valsalva
Stroke in a young patient
Systemic disease with suspected cardiac involvement

Systemic hypertension
Unexplained hypotension
Valvular heart disease
Ventricular tachycardia

Indications for Cardiac Doppler Ultrasonography

In general, a cardiac Doppler study is indicated for the diagnosis, determination of severity, determination of associated abnormalities or complications, or follow-up of the following cardiac pathologies:

Aortic dissection
Bacterial endocarditis
Cardiogenic shock
Chamber dilatation
Coarctation of aorta
Complicated myocardial infarction
Congenital heart disease
Constrictive pericarditis
Dilated cardiomyopathy
Heart murmur
Hypertrophic cardiomyopathy
Left ventricular diastolic dysfunction
Left ventricular pseudoaneurysm
Penetrating cardiac injury
Prosthetic cardiac valves
Pulmonary hypertension
Restrictive cardiomyopathy
Rheumatic heart disease
Right ventricular infarction
Ruptured cardiac valve
Ruptured sinus of Valsalva
Unexplained hypotension
Valvular heart disease

The symptoms or diseases listed above are not necessarily inclusive of all cardiac conditions in which an abnormal echocardiogram or cardiac Doppler study may be encountered. These lists serve as general reference only. There is considerable controversy in regard to the several indications for echocardiography or cardiac Doppler ultrasonography. Before ordering a test, one should ask the important question: Is this test going to confirm the diagnosis and aid in the management of the patient?

Index

Index

An italicized page number denotes a figure; the abbreviation t *denotes a table.*